Register Now ... s to Yo...

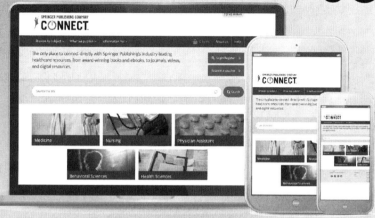

Your print purchase of *Review Manual for the Certified Healthcare Simulation Education™ (CHSE™) Exam, Second Edition,* **includes online access to the contents of your book**—increasing accessibility, portability, and searchability!

Access today at:

http://connect.springerpub.com/content/book/978-0-8261-3889-7
or scan the QR code at the right with your smartphone
and enter the access code below.

WTKFJ8LR

Scan here for quick access.

If you are experiencing problems accessing the digital component of this product, please contact our customer service department at cs@springerpub.com

The online access with your print purchase is available at the publisher's discretion and may be removed at any time without notice.

Publisher's Note: New and used products purchased from third-party sellers are not guaranteed for quality, authenticity, or access to any included digital components.

SPC

SPRINGER PUBLISHING COMPANY
View all our products at springerpub.com

Linda Wilson, PhD, RN, CPAN, CAPA, BC, CNE, CHSE-A, ANEF, FAAN, is an assistant dean for Special Projects, Simulation, and Continuing Nursing Education Accreditation and a clinical professor in the Division of Nursing at Drexel University, College of Nursing and Health Professions in Philadelphia, Pennsylvania. Dr. Wilson completed her BSN at Misericordia University in Dallas, Pennsylvania, and completed her MSN in critical care and trauma at Thomas Jefferson University in Philadelphia. She completed her PhD in nursing research at Rutgers, the State University of New Jersey in Newark. Dr. Wilson has also obtained a postgraduate Certificate in Epidemiology and Biostatistical Methods from Drexel University and a postgraduate Certificate in Pain Management from the University of California, San Francisco School of Medicine. She has dual certification in simulation: Certified Healthcare Simulation Educator™ (CHSE™) and Certified Healthcare Simulation Educator Advanced (CHSE-A), along with several additional certifications. She served as the president of the American Society of PeriAnesthesia Nurses (2002–2003) and has been serving as site appraiser for the American Nurses Credentialing Center Commission on Accreditation, American Nurses Association, from 2000 to the present. Dr. Wilson was the project director/primary investigator for SimTeam: The Joint Education of Health Professionals and Assistive Personnel Students in a Simulated Environment, a project funded by the Barra Foundation Inc. She was also the project director/primary investigator for Faculty Development: Integrating Technology into Nursing Education and Practice, a nearly $1.5 million, 5-year project funded by the Health Resources and Services Administration, Department of Health and Human Services. Dr. Wilson is also the coeditor of *Human Simulation for Nursing and Health Professions* and *Certified Nurse Educator (CNE) Review Manual, Third Edition,* published by Springer Publishing Company.

Ruth A. Wittmann-Price, PhD, RN, CNS, CNE, CHSE, ANEF, FAAN, is Dean of Health Sciences and professor of Nursing at Francis Marion University, in South Carolina. Dr. Wittmann-Price has been an obstetrical/women's health nurse for 40 years. She received her BSN degree from Felician College in Lodi, New Jersey (1981), and her master's in science as a perinatal CNS from Columbia University, New York, New York (1983). Dr. Wittmann-Price completed her PhD at Widener University, Chester, Pennsylvania (2006), and was awarded the Dean's Award for Excellence. She developed a midrange nursing theory, Emancipated Decision-Making in Women's Health Care. She was the coordinator for the nurse educator track in the DrNP program at Drexel University in Philadelphia (2007–2010) and the director of Nursing Research for Hahnemann University Hospital (2007–2010), overseeing all evidence-based practice projects for nursing. The Hahnemann University Hospital was awarded initial Magnet® status (American Nurses Credentialing Center) in December 2009. Dr. Wittmann-Price has taught all levels of nursing students over the past 20 years (AAS, BSN, MSN, DNP, PhD) and is a part of dissertation committees on decisional science. At Francis Marion University, she developed the simulation program, the MSN program, an interprofessional rural health initiative, a physician assistant program, the DNP program, and the speech-language pathology program. She has published over 20 articles and is coeditor and chapter contributor to 14 books, and is series editor of Nursing Test Success, a series of unfolding case studies, published by Springer Publishing Company. She has presented regionally, nationally, and internationally.

Review Manual for the Certified Healthcare Simulation Educator™ (CHSE™) Exam

Second Edition

Linda Wilson, PhD, RN, CPAN, CAPA, BC, CNE, CHSE-A, ANEF, FAAN

Ruth A. Wittmann-Price, PhD, RN, CNS, CNE, CHSE, ANEF, FAAN

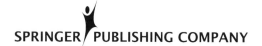

Copyright © 2019 Springer Publishing Company, LLC

All rights reserved.

No part of this publication may be reproduced, stored in a retrieval system, or transmitted in any form or by any means, electronic, mechanical, photocopying, recording, or otherwise, without the prior permission of Springer Publishing Company, LLC, or authorization through payment of the appropriate fees to the Copyright Clearance Center, Inc., 222 Rosewood Drive, Danvers, MA 01923, 978-750-8400, fax 978-646-8600, info@copyright.com or on the Web at www.copyright.com.

Springer Publishing Company, LLC
11 West 42nd Street
New York, NY 10036
www.springerpub.com

Acquisitions Editor: Margaret Zuccarini
Managing Editor: Cindy Yoo
Compositor: diacriTech

ISBN: 978-0-8261-3888-0
e-book ISBN: 978-0-8261-3889-7

18 19 20 21 22 / 5 4 3 2 1

The Certified Healthcare Simulation Educator™ (CHSE™) marks are trademarks of the Society for Simulation in Healthcare (SSH). This manual is an independent publication and is not endorsed, sponsored, or otherwise approved by the Society. SSH is not liable or responsible for any errors, omissions, or timeliness of the information or data available in this manual, any individual's negligence in connection with the manual, or any other liability resulting from the use or misuse of the manual.

The author and the publisher of this Work have made every effort to use sources believed to be reliable to provide information that is accurate and compatible with the standards generally accepted at the time of publication. The author and publisher shall not be liable for any special, consequential, or exemplary damages resulting, in whole or in part, from the readers' use of, or reliance on, the information contained in this book. The publisher has no responsibility for the persistence or accuracy of URLs for external or third-party Internet websites referred to in this publication and does not guarantee that any content on such websites is, or will remain, accurate or appropriate.

Library of Congress Cataloging-in-Publication Data
Names: Wilson, Linda, 1962- editor. | Wittmann-Price, Ruth A., editor.
Title: Review manual for the certified healthcare simulation educator™
 (CHSE™) exam / [edited by] Linda Wilson, Ruth A. Wittmann-Price.
Description: Second edition. | New York, NY : Springer Publishing Company,
 LLC, [2019] | Includes bibliographical references and index.
Identifiers: LCCN 2018028121 | ISBN 9780826138880 | ISBN 9780826138897
Subjects: | MESH: Patient Simulation | Health Occupations—education |
 Certification | Problems and Exercises
Classification: LCC RT51 | NLM W 18.2 | DDC 610.73—dc23 LC record available at
 https://lccn.loc.gov/2018028121

Contact us to receive discount rates on bulk purchases.
We can also customize our books to meet your needs.
For more information please contact: sales@springerpub.com

Publisher's Note: New and used products purchased from third-party sellers are not guaranteed for quality, authenticity, or access to any included digital components.

Printed in the United States of America.

Contents

Contributors   *vii*
Foreword   Gloria F. Donnelly, PhD, RN, FAAN, FCPP   *xi*
Preface   *xiii*
Acknowledgments   *xv*

SECTION I. INTRODUCTION

1. Overview of the Certification Examination, Advanced Certification, and Recertification   3
   Ruth A. Wittmann-Price and Brittny D. Chabalowski

2. The Certification Examination Test Plan   7
   Ruth A. Wittmann-Price

3. Test-Taking Strategies   13
   Dorie L. Weaver

SECTION II. DOMAIN I: PROFESSIONAL VALUES AND CAPABILITIES

4. Leadership in Simulation   27
   Ruth A. Wittmann-Price and Brittny D. Chabalowski

5. Special Learning Considerations in Simulation   35
   Ruth A. Wittmann-Price

6. Interprofessional Simulation   53
   Sharon Griswold, Kymberlee Montgomery, and Kate Morse

7. Ethical, Legal, and Regulatory Implications in Healthcare Simulation   67
   Bonnie A. Haupt and Colleen H. Meakim

SECTION III. DOMAIN II: HEALTHCARE AND SIMULATION KNOWLEDGE/PRINCIPLES

8. Human Patient Simulator Simulation   79
   Carol Okupniak

9. Moulage in Simulation   93
   John T. Cornele and Linda Wilson

10. Simulation Principles, Practice, and Methodologies for Standardized Patient Simulation   105
    Linda Wilson, H. Lynn Kane, and Samuel W. Price

11. Hybrid Simulation   125
    Anthony Errichetti

12. Part-Task Trainers   139
    Ruth A. Wittmann-Price and Deborah S. Arnold

13. Virtual Reality   147
    Rosemary Fliszar

SECTION IV. DOMAIN III: EDUCATIONAL PRINCIPLES APPLIED TO SIMULATION

14. Educational Theories, Learning Theories, and Special Concepts   165
    Ruth A. Wittmann-Price and Samuel W. Price

15. Implementing Simulation in the Curriculum   197
    Nina Multak

16. Planning Simulation Activities   209
    Karen K. Gittings

17. Debriefing   223
    Linda Wilson, John T. Cornele, and Ruth A. Wittmann-Price

18. Standardized Patient Debriefing and Feedback   237
    Anthony Errichetti

19. Evaluation of Simulation Activities   251
    Melanie Leigh Cason and Frances Wickham Lee

20. Fostering Professional Development in Healthcare Simulation   267
    Mark C. Crider and Mary Ellen Smith Glasgow

21. The Role of Research in Simulation   279
    Judy I. Murphy

SECTION V. DOMAIN IV: SIMULATION RESOURCES AND ENVIRONMENTS

22. Operations and Management of Environment, Personnel, and Nonpersonnel Resources   297
    Carolyn H. Scheese

23. Accreditation of Simulation Laboratories and Simulation Standards   323
    Anthony Battaglia, Fabien Pampaloni, and Beth A. Telesz

24. Practice Test   333
    Ruth A. Wittmann-Price, Linda Wilson, and Samuel W. Price

25. Answers and Rationales to End-of-Chapter Practice Questions   349

26. Answers and Rationales to Practice Test   397

Index   419

Contributors

Deborah S. Arnold, MSN, RN, CMSRN, CHSE Manager, Simulation and Interprofessional Education, Lehigh Valley Health Network, Allentown, Pennsylvania

Anthony Battaglia, MS, BSN, RN Corporate Counsel, Pocket Nurse, Monaca, Pennsylvania

Melanie Leigh Cason, MSN, RN, CNE Simulation Nurse Educator, Collaborative Partner Coordinator, Health Care Simulation South Carolina (HCSSC), Medical University of South Carolina, Charleston, South Carolina

Brittny D. Chabalowski, RN, MSN, CEN, CNE, CHSE Instructor, Program Director, Upper Division/2nd Degree Nursing Sequence Coordinator, Undergraduate Simulation, University of South Florida, Tampa, Florida

John T. Cornele, MSN, RN, CEN, EMT-P, CNE Director, Center for Interdisciplinary Clinical Simulation & Practice, Drexel University College of Nursing and Health Professions, Philadelphia, Pennsylvania

Mark C. Crider, PhD, MSN Assistant Professor and Chair of Undergraduate Programs, Duquesne University School of Nursing, Pittsburgh, Pennsylvania

Anthony Errichetti, PhD, CHSE Chief of Virtual Medicine, Director, MS in Medical/Health Care Simulation, New York Institute of Technology—College of Osteopathic Medicine, Old Westbury, New York

Rosemary Fliszar, PhD, RN, CNE Director, RN–BSN Program and Assistant Professor II, Rider University, Lawrenceville, New Jersey

Karen K. Gittings, DNP, RN, CNE, Alumnus CCRN Associate Dean Health Sciences, Francis Marion University, Florence, South Carolina

Mary Ellen Smith Glasgow, PhD, RN, CS, FAAN Dean and Professor, Duquesne University School of Nursing, Pittsburgh, Pennsylvania

Sharon Griswold, MD, MPH Associate Professor of Emergency Medicine, Director, Simulation Division, Department of Emergency Medicine; Director, Master's Degree in Medical/Healthcare Simulation, Drexel University College of Medicine, Philadelphia, Pennsylvania

Bonnie A. Haupt, DNP(c), MSN, RN, CNL, CHSE Clinical Nurse Leader, Veteran Affairs Connecticut Healthcare System; Acute Care Clinical Nurse Leader, Providence Veterans Administration Medical Center, Providence, Rhode Island

H. Lynn Kane, MSN, MBA, RN, CCRN Clinical Nurse Specialist, Thomas Jefferson University Hospital, Methodist Division, Philadelphia, Pennsylvania

Frances Wickham Lee, DBA, CHSE Professor, College of Health Professions, Director of Instructional Operations, Health Care Simulation of South Carolina (HCSSC), Medical University of South Carolina, Charleston, South Carolina

Colleen H. Meakim, MSN, RN, CHSE Director of Simulation and Learning Resources, Villanova University College of Nursing, Villanova, Pennsylvania

Kymberlee Montgomery, DrNP, WHNP-BC, CNE, FAANP, FAAN Nurse Faculty Leadership Fellow, Department Chair, Nurse Practitioner Program & Doctor of Nursing Practice Program, Associate Clinical Professor, Drexel University College of Nursing and Health Professions, Philadelphia, Pennsylvania

Kate Morse, PhD, CRNP-BC, CNE, CCRN Assistant Director of the Affiliate Program of the Center for Medical Simulation, Boston, Massachusetts

Nina Multak, PhD, MPAS, PA-C Associate Dean and Director of the University of Florida School of PA Studies, Gainesville, Florida

Judy I. Murphy, PhD, RN, CNE, CHSE Veteran Affairs Nursing Academic Partner Faculty and Simulation Coordinator, Providence Veterans Administration Medical Center and Rhode Island College, Providence, Rhode Island

Carol Okupniak, DNP, RN-BC Nursing Informatics Assistant Clinical Professor, Drexel University College of Nursing and Health Professions, Philadelphia, Pennsylvania

Fabien Pampaloni, BSN, RN International Business Affairs Specialist, Pocket Nurse, Monaca, Pennsylvania

Samuel W. Price, MFA Advisor, Drexel University College of Nursing and Health Professions, Philadelphia, Pennsylvania

Carolyn H. Scheese, MS, RN, CHSE Assistant Professor, Director, RN to BS in Nursing Program, College of Nursing, University of Utah, Salt Lake City, Utah

Beth A. Telesz, MSN, RN SimEMR Customer Service and Education Manager, Pocket Nurse, Monaca, Pennsylvania

Dorie L. Weaver, DNP, RN, CNE, FNP-BC Instructor of Nursing, Francis Marion University, Florence, South Carolina

Linda Wilson, PhD, RN, CPAN, CAPA, BC, CNE, CHSE-A, ANEF, FAAN Assistant Dean for Special Projects, Simulation and Continuing Nursing Education Accreditation; Clinical Professor Division of Nursing, Drexel University College of Nursing and Health Professions, Philadelphia, Pennsylvania

Ruth A. Wittmann-Price, PhD, RN, CNS, CNE, CHSE, ANEF, FAAN Dean of Health Sciences and Professor of Nursing, Francis Marion University, Florence, South Carolina

Foreword

The junior nursing student stood to speak at the dean's regular town hall meeting. "Is it possible to offer more simulation experiences to prepare us for clinical? I learn so much in our simulation sessions but more would be better, especially for labor and delivery and ER preparation. I must confess that I have purposely missed regular clinical days since learning that the required clinical makeup days are conducted in the simulation lab. What can be done?"

As dean of a college that has widely employed simulation as a teaching strategy since 2002, I was shocked at the student's observation, confession, and plea. However, after 15 years of integrating simulation into clinical curricula, my belief in its power to exquisitely promote clinical learning for nursing and health professions' students was reaffirmed by the student's request. An integrated program of clinical simulation not only propels student learning but also has significant impact on faculty, such as the contributors to this book:

- Faculty's imagination and enrichment occur as they design and refine simulation scenarios
- Faculty achieve more control of clinical learning processes because they are able to suspend practice, intervene, question, and give immediate feedback to students without fear of harming "real" patients
- Faculty assume control through the design of simulations for areas like labor and delivery and emergency departments—where there cannot be a guarantee of significant clinical experiences—or in designing disasters, which demand simulation
- Faculty exchange feedback on how best to critique and interact with students maneuvering through complex, clinical scenarios
- Faculty mine the rich data in archived clinical simulations to study patterns of student behavior and design scenarios that predict and prevent adverse events
- Faculty and students "reflect" as the scenario is suspended to discuss the rationale for action and to explore clinically inferential processes

For the past 15 years, the faculty contributors to this book have taken simulation learning to new levels with the development of interprofessional simulation scenarios that include students from undergraduate and graduate nursing, medicine, the physician assistant and behavioral health programs, and nurse anesthesia. They have acted as mentors to international faculty from Turkey, South Africa, Singapore, Puerto Rico, Costa Rica, Saudi Arabia, Guam, Jordan, Canada, Oman, Russia, Cameroon, and northern India, and to clinical faculty across the United States who attend Drexel University's Certificate in Simulation Program. They have provided guidance to many colleges and schools launching their own simulation labs and programs. The authors of this review manual have presented all of the essential elements of simulation from idea through evaluation. They have also presented the major content areas for the Certified Healthcare Simulation Educator™ (CHSE™) Exam.

In 1985, I completed my dissertation, *Language, Thought and Action in Children's Play*, during which I filmed and studied the play behavior of 48 preschoolers. The past 15 years of using simulation to promote clinical learning has intensified my conviction that play is one of the most important developmental processes facilitating human growth and learning. Simulation, as structured, purposive "play," enhances clinical learning resulting in thoughtful and safe patient care. As Alan W. Watts once said, *"This is the real secret of life: to be completely engaged with what you are doing in the here and now, and instead of calling it 'work,' realize that this is play."* (n.d., para. 7).

Gloria F. Donnelly, PhD, RN, FAAN, FCPP
Professor and Dean Emerita
College of Nursing and Health Professions
Drexel University
Philadelphia, Pennsylvania

Watts, A. W. (n.d.). The secret of life. Retrieved from https://genius.com/Alan-watts-the-secret-of-life-annotated

Preface

This book was created as part of an interprofessional, international project to assist healthcare simulation educators to become certified for the very important work that is being accomplished during every simulation experience around the world. Simulation is one of the teaching modalities needed to improve patient safety. Simulation effectively teaches healthcare providers interprofessional collaboration, communication, and cooperation like never before in the history of healthcare. Becoming certified in simulation is a wonderful step to promoting excellence in healthcare education, and we applaud your efforts.

This book is an invaluable resource in the certification process. The contributing authors have analyzed the certification test plan (Society for Simulation in Healthcare [SSH], 2018) to bring you all the important information that may be presented on the examination. The book is organized in a user-friendly format and the information is divided into short chapters. The authors are simulation and education experts who have added features to this text that will assist in critically analyzing the content.

The feature labeled *Teaching Tips* are provided for those educators who would like further explanation and exploration of topics, many of which provide practical hints to incorporate into simulation experiences. *Evidence-Based Simulation Practice* boxes assist you in focusing on the current simulation research and bring you state-of-the art evidence. *Case Studies* and *Practice Questions* at the end of each chapter promote critical thinking and situational decision-making.

Section I of this book includes Chapter 1, which covers the specifics of the examination and the activities needed to reach advanced certification, and recertification. Chapter 2 concentrates on the current 2018 certification test blueprint. Chapter 3 provides you with test-taking strategies, which are always beneficial for "the student in all of us."

Section II discusses Domain I of the certification examination blueprint (SSH, 2018): Professional values and capabilities in relation to teaching with simulation. Chapter 4 covers leadership in educational simulation. Chapter 5 includes special considerations about simulation experiences with learners and describes learning styles. Chapter 6 provides insight into simulation ethics, and Chapter 7 discusses the wonderful world of interprofessional simulation.

Section III addresses Domain II: Healthcare and Simulation Knowledge/Principles. This section reviews foundational knowledge about simulation and includes chapters on specific modalities and integrating simulation education into a professional healthcare curriculum.

Chapters 8 to 13 describe all the current modalities used in a simulation laboratory by experts that use them effectively on a consistent basis. Each modality is given a short chapter explanation that contains the knowledge and principles behind its use. This section addressed human patient simulation, moulage, standardized patients, hybrid simulation, part-task trainers, and the growing field of virtual reality.

Section IV focuses on Domain III of the certification examination blueprint: Educational Principles Applied to Simulation. In this section of the book the authors concentrate on the learner and delivering effective simulation by reviewing content on educational theory, curriculum development, debriefing and feedback techniques, planning simulation events, and evaluating learning outcomes.

Section V describes the information in Domain IV: Simulation Resources and Environments. Chapters 22 and 23 have content about simulation laboratory management including personnel and the standards of an accredited simulation environment. Chapter 24 is a simulated practice test, and the answers and rationales appear in Chapter 26. Chapter 25 contains the answers and rationales to the end-of-chapter tests. Good luck!

Our hope in developing and revising this review manual is that it will be another valuable tool to assist you in reaching your career goal of recognized excellence. We applaud your efforts as colleagues in the quest to educate the next generation of healthcare workers. We thank you for your efforts to recognize excellence in the simulation field and the very important role simulation plays in patient safety.

Linda Wilson
Ruth A. Wittmann-Price

Society for Simulation in Healthcare. (2018). *Certified Healthcare Simulation Educator Examination Blueprint, 2018 Version*. Retrieved from http://www.ssih.org/Portals/48/Certification/CHSE_Docs/CHSE_Examination_Blueprint.pdf

Acknowledgments

To H. Lynn Kane, Helen "Momma" Kane, Linda Webb, and Elizabeth Diaz, thank you for your amazing friendship and for being my family. To Lou Smith, Evan Babcock, and Steve Johnson, thank you for your friendship and support. To the Philadelphia Eagles, thank you for your inspiration.

—*Linda Wilson*

Thank you to all my colleagues and friends who so graciously contributed to this awesome project and, of course, thank you to Margaret Zuccarini, whose publishing assistance and support are invaluable.

—*Ruth A. Wittmann-Price*

Introduction

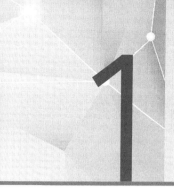

Overview of the Certification Examination, Advanced Certification, and Recertification

RUTH A. WITTMANN-PRICE AND
BRITTNY D. CHABALOWSKI

Do not go where the path may lead, go instead where there is no path and leave a trail.
—Ralph Waldo Emerson

[**LEARNING OUTCOMES**]

- Describe the benefits of certification.
- Review the requirements for initial certification.
- Review the recertification process.
- Describe the requirements for advanced certification.

Obtaining specialty certification is a well-recognized way to demonstrate expertise, both in clinical and academic settings. Healthcare educators have used simulation for many years for academic and clinical learning enhancement. Simulation can range from simple part-task trainers (PTTs) to high-fidelity simulated patient care experiences. The goal of complex patient-simulated experiences is to provide learners the opportunity to deliver care in high-risk, low-volume scenarios. These are situations that are seen infrequently in the clinical setting, but require swift and accurate intervention.

Unlike direct clinical instruction, simulation education requires a specialized skill set. Skilled healthcare simulation educators must be able to develop scenarios that are appropriate for the learners, administer the scenarios in a supportive atmosphere, and debrief the learners appropriately to complete an effective learning experience. It becomes clear that certification assists educators to understand the need for uniform simulation education and evaluation (Charles & Koehn, 2016).

Recognizing this need, the Society for Simulation in Healthcare (SSH) developed the basic certification examination and the advanced certification standards (SSH, 2016, 2018b). The benefits of these certifications go beyond the individual or the individual's organization. One of the goals is to identify, recognize, and pool the knowledge of best practices. This will serve to standardize the unique body of knowledge that belongs to healthcare simulation educators.

INITIAL CERTIFICATION

- Eligibility
  - Bachelor's degree or equivalent (any candidate who does not have a bachelor's degree may petition the committee for consideration of equivalency based on experience)
  - Minimum of 2 years' experience in healthcare simulation setting
  - Able to demonstrate that simulation experience is focused on learners in healthcare at any level
  - Continued use of simulation in healthcare education, research, or administration in the past 2 years (SSH, 2018b)
- Application
  - Can be completed online at www.ssih.org/certification/CHSE
  - Includes information about simulation experience, education, and employment
  - Narrative descriptions required include the following
    - Relevant simulation-based educational activity that demonstrates evidence of your capabilities as a simulation-based educator
    - Relevant activities that demonstrate your advocacy for simulation-based education (this would include your activities at your place of employment, activities at the local level, as well as in professional societies)
    - Scholarly activities relevant to simulation-based education (such as participation in research, abstract preparation, publications, posters, workshops, curriculum development, and course construction)
  - Contact information for at least three references so as to complete the Confidential Structured Report of Performance (CSRP) online
  - Application processing takes approximately 3 weeks (SSH, 2018b)
- Fees as of 2014
  - $395 for members of the SSH, the Association of Standardized Patient Educators (ASPEs), and the International Nursing Association for Clinical Simulation and Learning (INACSL)
  - $495 for all others (SSH, 2018b)
- Taking the test
  - Computer-based testing sites can be located on the ISO-Quality Testing, Inc. site: www.isoqualitytesting.com
  - Scheduled on a space-available basis
  - Must be taken within 90 days of application approval
  - Candidates are notified of results at the time of exam completion (SSH, 2018b)
- Certification
  - Valid for 3 years from the successful completion of the exam
  - The initials of certification may be used as a credential after the candidate's name (SSH, 2018b)

RECERTIFICATION/RENEWAL OF CERTIFICATION (SSH, 2018a)

- Retake the examination at or near the expiration date *or*
- Demonstrate ongoing professional development
  - Over the 3-year period, not just activity performed in a narrow time frame
  - In education- or simulation-focused activities
  - Including, but not limited to the following
    - Participation in continuing education (CE) activity such as attending conferences, webinars, or other education events
    - Publication of research, such as journal articles, chapters, books, or similar items
    - Presenting at educational events, such as conferences
- If the certification expires, candidates must reapply to take the exam and must meet the eligibility requirements in place at that time (SSH, 2018a)

> **SIMULATION TEACHING TIP 1.1**
>
> Charles and Koehn (2016) used peer study sessions for 7 weeks and all participants of the student sessions passed the Certified Nurse Educator (CNE) examination!

ADVANCED CERTIFICATION

- Eligibility
  - Possession of basic certification
  - Participation in healthcare simulation in an educational role
  - Focused simulation expertise with learners in undergraduate, graduate, allied health, or healthcare courses
  - Master's degree or equivalent experience (any candidate who does not have a master's degree may petition the committee for consideration of equivalency based on experience)
  - Five years of continued use of simulation in healthcare education, research, or administration
- Application
  - Submission of an extensive portfolio, including a media submission and reflective statements
  - Portfolio is peer reviewed and evaluated against the Advanced Standards and Elements (SSH, 2012, 2016).

SUMMARY

Deciding to take a certification examination will enhance your knowledge and ability as you achieve a personal and professional goal. Both the basic and advanced certifications promote facilitation of learning of future healthcare providers, and becoming certified will ultimately benefit patients receiving care. Congratulations on choosing to study and become a Certified Healthcare Simulation Educator.™ You will promote quality education that will benefit your students and all their patients.

REFERENCES

Charles, S., & Koehn, M. (2016). Using peer study to prepare for Certified Healthcare Simulation Educator certification. *Clinical Simulation in Nursing*, 12(6), 202–208. doi:10.1016/j.ecns.2016.02.009

Society for Simulation in Healthcare. (2012). *Certification standards and elements*. Washington, DC: Author. Retrieved from http://ssih.org/Portals/48/Certification/CHSE%20Standards.pdf

Society for Simulation in Healthcare. (2016). *SSH certified healthcare simulation educator-advanced handbook*. Washington, DC: Author. Retrieved from http://ssih.org/Portals/48/Certification/CHSE-A_Docs/CHSE-A%20Handbook.pdf

Society for Simulation in Healthcare. (2018a). *Certified healthcare simulation educator renewal & recertification materials*. Washington, DC: Author. Retrieved from http://ssih.org/Portals/48/Certification/CHSE_Docs/CHSE Recert Packet.pdf

Society for Simulation in Healthcare. (2018b). *SSH certified healthcare simulation educator handbook*. Washington, DC: Author. Retrieved from http://www.ssih.org/Portals/48/Certification/CHSE_Docs/CHSE%20Handbook.pdf

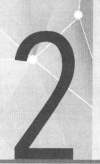

2

The Certification Examination Test Plan

RUTH A. WITTMANN-PRICE

> *We learn by example and by direct experience because there are real limits to the adequacy of verbal instruction.*
> —Malcolm Gladwell

[**LEARNING OUTCOMES**]

- Discuss the importance of certification in simulation for healthcare educators.
- Discuss the specifics of the test plan.
- Discuss case studies and practice questions as learning tools.

For many reasons, simulation in healthcare education is here to stay. Simulation experiences provide a wealth of benefits for learners of educational organizations. The Society for Simulation in Healthcare (SSH) has developed the preliminary and advanced certifications to recognize healthcare educators who are experts in this important and growing field of using simulation to teach all aspects of healthcare delivery to improve patient safety.

The test plan for the examination was developed in 2011 and revised in 2018 and can be found on the SSH website. There are four broad areas covered by the exam, which include professional values and capabilities; healthcare and simulation knowledge/principles; educational principles applied to simulation; and simulation resources and environments. The largest number of questions on the test (40%) concentrate on educational principles. The professional values and capabilities topics are 18% of the test, and simulation resources and environments are 14% of the test. Healthcare and simulation knowledge and principles comprises the last 28% of the test (SSH, 2018).

These four major test areas are further broken down into criteria that are less general and therefore easier to dissect and understand. Each of those areas is discussed. It is understood that not all healthcare educators who teach in simulation laboratories are expert in all four areas, but for the test, each educator needs a working knowledge of every area. For example, a healthcare educator working in a large simulation laboratory may not be responsible for the stocking, ordering, or maintenance of the laboratory, but will need to have an understanding of the resources needed and used for simulation education.

DOMAIN AREA I: PROFESSIONAL VALUES AND CAPABILITIES

The first area of the test is the display of professional values and capabilities (SSH, 2018). This area includes

- Demonstrating leadership
- Acting as a simulation advocate
- Displaying teamwork
- Understanding simulation roles
- Understanding regulatory compliance
- Participating in quality improvement and evidence-based practices

Professional values and capabilities comprise 18% of the test. So there will be 20 to 21 questions pertaining to this area. Section II of this book (Chapters 4 and 5) discusses these content areas in depth. Following is a quick synopsis of major content that falls under Domain I.

Leadership

Leadership in simulation is thoroughly addressed in Chapter 4.

Transformational leadership, first described by Burns (1978), is the current leadership theory discussed in organizations and education. Transformational leaders are described as exhibiting positive attributes, which include

- Vision for future development
- The ability to engage others in the vision
- Developing values surrounding the vision
- Moving people toward the vision
- Effecting positive change (Bass, 1985)

Transformational leadership is different from *transactional leadership*. Transactional leadership is equated with more authoritarian management that directs people without motivating them. Some of the attributes associated with transactional leadership are

- Hierarchical decisions
- Institution of a reward-and-punishment system
- Micromanaging from the top of the organization (Motacki & Burke, 2011)

Advocating for Simulation

It is generally understood that the use of simulation was developed for two major purposes: to improve healthcare safety and increase educational experiences for learners. Even with positive educational student learning outcomes (SLOs) contributing to simulation's success, there is still resistance for its use from some educators. Part of the controversy hinges on how much simulation is appropriate in a curriculum. The National Council of State Boards of Nursing (NCSBN; 2013) simulation study (Hayden, Smiley, Alexander, Kardong-Edgren, & Jeffries, 2010) demonstrated using a multisite project with 666 students that there was no significant difference in program outcomes among three groups using no simulation, 25% simulation, and 50% simulation for clinical learning experiences.

In addition, simulation experiences can be expanded to community activities for both the healthcare communities and the laity. Simulation can be an experience used in acute care, outpatient, and community settings. Disaster planning with simulation has made many groups aware of its educational ability. Whenever possible, all simulation educators should explain and demonstrate the positive learning experiences that can be attained through simulation.

DOMAIN AREA II: HEALTHCARE SIMULATION KNOWLEDGE AND PRINCIPLES

The second content area covered in the examination makes up 28% of the examination or approximately 32 or 33 questions (SSH, 2018). It is divided into 13 subcriteria. The chapters in this book address all 13 areas, and before the introduction to each chapter, the domain being addressed is stated. The second domain includes topics about simulation research, feedback and debriefing, realism, patient safety, and types of simulation activities.

DOMAIN AREA III: EDUCATIONAL PRINCIPLES APPLIED TO SIMULATION

Domain III is the largest part of the test and comprises approximately 46 questions (SSH, 2018). This section contains nine major criteria and many subcriteria. The content in this test section comprises questions regarding the actual use of simulation with learners. Questions contain education scenarios, and you have to choose the correct assessment, plan, intervention, or evaluation of the situation by the correct combination of educator and learner, learner and learner, learner and SP, or educator and SP. Expect application questions in which the knowledge from this area is applied to situations. Each of the criteria is also addressed in the upcoming, labeled chapters.

DOMAIN AREA IV: SIMULATION RESOURCES AND ENVIRONMENTS

Domain IV of the examination is made up of six criteria and comprises 14%—or 16 to 17 questions—of the examination (SSH, 2018). This content area is addressed in depth in Chapters 20 through 23. The criteria under this content area includes improving outcomes, planning and implementing operational changes in a simulation laboratory, using resources, and understanding risk reduction.

> **SIMULATION TEACHING TIP 2.1**
>
> Introducing simulation experiences in the first semester of healthcare education may increase the learners' comfort level with the methodology as it is repeated semester after semester.

> **EVIDENCE-BASED SIMULATION PRACTICE 2.1**
>
> Pisciottani, França da Rocha, da Costa, Figueiredo, and Magalhães (2017) studied the use of in situ cardiopulmonary resuscitation teaching to nursing students and compare groups using a researcher-made tool. Student *t*-test in-group comparison will be used to demonstrate the increased proficiency of students in the following criteria: ventilation with manual resuscitator, insertion of airway, monitoring and aiding defibrillation, and control of timing.

> **CASE STUDY 2.1**
>
> An expert clinician is hired as one of three educational coordinators for the simulation laboratory for undergraduate healthcare students. The person hired is an expert in the critical care units at the local acute care hospital. She is assisting in setting up a simulation experience for first-semester healthcare learners. During the experience, using a high-fidelity mannequin, the education coordinator uses the computer controls to cause the patient to "code," and then, in the debriefing, acknowledges that she thought the learners would know how to handle it better. How would you address this with the education coordinator using Benner's theory?

■ PRACTICE QUESTIONS

1. The most important element(s) of the simulation certification test for educators is (are):

   A. Professional values and capabilities
   B. Managing simulation resources
   C. Engaging in scholarship activity
   D. Education and assessment of learners

2. The healthcare simulation educator understands that acting as a role model at all times in the simulation laboratory is an expectation under the criteria of:

   A. Professional values and capabilities
   B. Managing simulation resources
   C. Engaging in scholarship activity
   D. Education and assessment of learners

3. The simulation educator is facilitating learning in the simulation laboratory for a group of healthcare students. The students are in a complex situation and have adjusted their plan of care according to the physical, psychological, and social needs of the patient. The simulation educator understands that the students are at which novice-to-expert level:

   A. Novice
   B. Advanced beginner
   C. Competent
   D. Proficient

4. The novice simulation educator needs additional understanding about the impact of simulation when he states:
   A. "Simulation should be used for difficult to find clinical learning experiences."
   B. "Students who use large percentages of simulation will not be able to perform as well in clinical practice."
   C. "Simulation can assist educators to teach professional values and standards."
   D. "Simulation should not be limited if it meets the students' learning outcomes."

5. The simulation educator is at a general faculty meeting and describes how simulation can be used as a recruitment tool for the university. The simulation educator is demonstrating which simulation certification examination criteria of professional values and capabilities:
   A. Mentorship
   B. Role modeling
   C. Leadership
   D. Advocating

6. One of the affective learning domains that simulation has been effectively used for is:
   A. Risk-management control
   B. Cultural humility
   C. Emotional adjustments
   D. Personality categorizing

7. A simulation educator rearranges the simulation space to depict a plane crash in order to teach triage. The simulation educator is guided by which simulation certification examination criteria:
   A. Professional values and capabilities
   B. Managing simulation resources
   C. Engaging in scholarship activity
   D. Education and assessment of learners

8. A simulation education team from an academic setting is presenting at a national conference. The educators are encouraging which simulation certification examination criteria by their work:
   A. Professional values and capabilities
   B. Managing simulation resources
   C. Engaging in scholarship activity
   D. Education and assessment of learners

9. The simulation educator has taught a group of students in the simulation laboratory for the past three semesters and has watched them develop their health assessment skills. The students now complete physical examinations from head to toe and understand that a finding in one patient may translate to the same healthcare issue in other patients they examine. The simulation educator understands that the students are at which novice-to-expert level in performing physical examination:

    A. Novice
    B. Advanced beginner
    C. Competent
    D. Proficient

10. The simulation educator presents a 5-year strategic plan for the simulation laboratory at a general faculty meeting. The simulation educator is demonstrating which simulation certification examination criteria of professional values and capabilities:

    A. Mentorship
    B. Role modeling
    C. Leadership
    D. Advocating

REFERENCES

Bass, B. M. (1985). *Leadership and performance beyond expectation*. New York, NY: Free Press.

Burns, J. M. (1978). *Leadership*. New York, NY: Harper & Row.

Gladwell, M. (2005). *Blink: The power of thinking without thinking*. Boston, MA: Little, Brown. Retrieved from https://www.goodreads.com/author/quotes/1439.Malcolm_Gladwell

Hayden, J. K., Smiley, R. A., Alexander, M., Kardong-Edgren, S., & Jeffries, P. R. (2010). The NCSBN National Simulation Study: A longitudinal, randomized, controlled study replacing clinical hours with simulation in prelicensure nursing education. *Journal of Nursing Regulation*, 5(2 Suppl.), S3–S40. doi:10.1016/S2155-8256(15)30062-4

Motacki, K., & Burke, K. (2011). *Nursing delegation and management of patient care*. St. Louis, MO: Mosby.

National Council of State Boards of Nursing. (2013). National simulation study. Retrieved from https://www.ncsbn.org/685.htm

Pisciottani, F., França da Rocha, D., da Costa, M. R., Figueiredo, A. E., & Magalhães, C. R. (2017). In situ simulation in cardiopulmonary resuscitation: Implications for permanent nursing education. *Journal of Nursing UFPE On Line*, 11(7), 2810–2815. doi:10.5205/reuol.9799-86079-1-RV.1106sup201722

Society for Simulation in Healthcare. (2018). *Certified Healthcare Simulation Educator Examination Blueprint, 2018 Version*. Retrieved from http://www.ssih.org/Portals/48/Certification/CHSE_Docs/CHSE_Examination_Blueprint.pdf

Wittmann-Price, R. A. (2012). *Fast facts for developing a nursing academic portfolio*. New York, NY: Springer Publishing.

3

Test-Taking Strategies

DORIE L. WEAVER

Education is not preparation for life; education is life itself.
—John Dewey

[LEARNING OUTCOMES]

- Identify the process to best prepare for the certification examination.
- Discuss tips for success to promote understanding of key concepts.
- Describe how to integrate standards from practice into information that is outlined in the examination blueprint.
- Discuss how to improve comprehension by eliminating anxiety related to test taking.

■ WHY BECOME CERTIFIED IN SIMULATION?

There is a significant need to prepare students to be competent to work within the current multifaceted, complex healthcare system. The advantage of simulation is that it allows learning to take place in a safe and controlled environment where there is no threat for patient harm (Turrentine et al., 2016). Clinical opportunities for students are random based on placement and increased practice restrictions by collaborating healthcare organizations.

A student told me that she was hired to work in an ICU immediately upon successful completion of the National Council Licensure Examination (NCLEX®).

The first day on the job, her patient coded. Although management of a patient in cardiac arrest was taught within the classroom through lecture as well as through discussion of a written case study, she was not given any opportunities to actually practice these essential skills in any type of setting. Any codes on the floor that did occur during clinical were dealt with by the licensed personnel.

Practicing in a simulation can better prepare the student for these types of situations and ultimately improve patient outcomes. Simulation promotes critical thinking and places students in scenarios that mimic situations they most likely will encounter in practice. The beneficial component of simulation is that it is carried out in a structured, controlled, and safe environment where mistakes can occur with no punitive damage to patients. The hands-on approach refines learning by helping to process knowledge for long-term retention.

It is common knowledge that there are students who can excel on written exams yet struggle within the clinical arena. In addition to skills training, simulation can enhance intraprofessional and interprofessional communication and collaboration. Because the lack of communication is one major source of error, simulation can indirectly reduce the number of preventable errors.

As educators and clinicians, it is our responsibility to provide simulations that develop individual and team skills as well as promote clinical reasoning to improve the competency of healthcare providers.

Educators and clinicians with years of experience in simulation can now validate their expertise and knowledge by certification. Obtaining a certification is an invaluable resource for future role models, mentors, and visionaries. Attainment demonstrates one's commitment to the nursing profession along with lifelong learning. In addition, it can provide the practitioner with a sense of both personal and professional accomplishment, competence, and credibility (Society for Simulation in Healthcare [SSH], 2018).

The following list outlines a few of the ways in which those who are certified can affect the healthcare environment:

- Support patient safety guidelines.
- Close the gap between theory and practice.
- Provide standardization of practice within healthcare.
- Impact patient outcomes and quality improvement.
- Develop evidence-based practice and research.

ARE YOU A QUALIFIED CANDIDATE TO TAKE THE EXAMINATION?

Ask yourself the following questions:

1. Have I participated in simulation within an educational role?
2. Was the simulation developed to focus on learners in undergraduate, graduate, allied health programs or healthcare practitioners?
3. Do I have a baccalaureate degree or an equivalent experience?
4. Have I used simulation in healthcare education, research, or administration continuously over the past 2 years?

The certification tests can be intimidating and anxiety provoking for many candidates. The more prepared one is, the better the chance for success.

HOW TO PREPARE FOR SUCCESS

- Set up a study schedule. Everyone studies differently, but it is best to set up a study calendar so you do not become overwhelmed. Make sure you have enough time to study before securing an examination date. Print the information that is available from the SSH Certified Healthcare Simulation Educator™ Handbook (2018) at www.ssih.org/chse/handbook. With knowledge of the test design and blueprint, the next step is to think about planning your effective study strategy.

- Use charts and diagrams to organize information so you can review at a glance. These visual aids also allow the learner to compare and contrast content. Images with key terms can enhance learning and memory.
- Practice answering questions on a routine basis. This will provide the learner with the ability to recognize gaps in knowledge. Schedule time to research the content that was incorrect on the practice exams.
- Look at the list of examination-preparation references, most of which are journal publications. It is to your advantage to read multiple articles related to the categories that carry the highest percentage of questions on the examination.
- Organize information that is related into groups. Focusing on one topic at a time will help you to remember information by comparing and contrasting content. Use the concept of the deep learning approach by critically examining new facts and making links between ideas. It is also helpful to relate new knowledge to previous knowledge. Adequate time management will allow you to understand content thoroughly and have confidence. If you are overworked and do not have enough time to study, there is a tendency to use the surface approach to learning, which is good for short-term memory only. This entails storing new facts as isolated information and may result in high anxiety (LeCun, Bengio, & Hinton, 2015).
- Organize a study group with your colleagues. Reviewing information while in a group may be worthwhile if all members of the group are committed and prepared for the study sessions. It is essential for the group to stay focused. Studying with representatives of various healthcare disciplines can be a valuable learning experience. Discussion and debate are critical for those who are auditory learners.
- Develop mnemonics or checklists. In order to promote patient safety and standardization of care, mnemonics and checklists have been developed as memory aids in specific situations. For example, mnemonics are used in Advanced Cardiac Life Support (ACLS) certification to recall algorithms. Healthcare professionals also use the SBAR mnemonic to promote optimal communication during patient handoff.

  S = Situation

  B = Background

  A = Assessment

  R = Recommendations

  There is a tremendous amount of information to remember, so you may want to develop your own mnemonics while you study.
- Healthcare professionals always care for others; now it is time to take care of yourself. Even though you feel that you deserve a sweet high-calorie dessert for all your hard work—think energy and brain power. Blueberries, strawberries, red beets, broccoli, tomatoes, pomegranate juice, vegetable juice, and nuts can enhance your brain power. Whole-grain foods, nuts, and legumes have a low glycemic index and release glucose into the bloodstream slowly, which

TABLE 3.1
Key Topics for Discussion in Your Review

The designing stage	Determine a needs assessment by deciding whether cognitive, behavioral, and technical issues will be incorporated into the scenario. Determine the participants—individual, team, systems. Define the goals for the activity. Develop measurable learning objectives. Write the scenario and integrate complications, distractions, and roles. Select the tool that will be used to evaluate the participants.
The planning stage	Organize the simulation team. Schedule the simulation laboratory with time allocated for setup, scenario, and reorganization of the environment. Determine whether the simulation will be videotaped. Reserve the capital equipment needed for the scenario. Schedule SPs if needed. Plan the scene setting. Determine the type of moulage needed. Make a list of supplies and drugs to be used in the scenario. Prepare written information for the simulation team.
The implementation stage	Provide an overview of the goals and objectives. Orient the participants to the environment and the equipment. Brief the participants about the scenario. Assess the participants related to the objectives. Determine how to respond to unforeseen issues during simulation, such as equipment failure, drugs or equipment missing, unprofessional behavior, and knowledge gaps.
The postsimulation stage	Debriefing can include evaluation by self, peers, or faculty. Provide time, and schedule the room to view the video (if indicated). Know the debriefing models. Understand the responsibility of the facilitator.

SPs, standardized (simulated) patients.

provides energy, for hours. Keep your body hydrated by drinking at least eight glasses of water daily (Table 3.1).

■ KNOW YOUR EQUIPMENT/TECHNOLOGY

- **Task trainers**—Used to practice procedures, such as wound care and intravenous (IV) insertion.
- **Human patient simulators**—Mannequin-based equipment in human form.
- **Virtual reality simulation**—Used to provide a computer-based simulation experience sometimes with the use of an avatar.

SIMULATION TEACHING TIP 3.1

When designing a simulation experience, think about activities to enhance different types of learning styles. Students can access the VARK website (http://vark-learn.com/the-vark-questionnaire/) to determine how they learn best (Fleming, 2001).

- **Standardized (simulated) patients (SPs)**—The use of actors to simulate patients in a standardized manner.
- **Hybrid simulation methodology**—A simulation that incorporates multiple types of simulation, with one being used to enhance the other. A task trainer can be used with an SP to provide a hybrid simulation experience.
- **Mixed simulation**—A simulation that incorporates multiple types of simulation, with each being a tool for educational purposes.

BECOME FAMILIAR WITH COMPUTERIZED TESTING

- Read directions for answering questions carefully. There is usually a tutorial for you to use to familiarize yourself with the process. Make sure you understand the directions that explain how to pause the test if you need to take a break.
- Pay attention to information such as how to change answers.
- Check the clock intermittently to ensure there is adequate time left to complete the exam. If you are unable to answer the question within 60 to 90 seconds, eliminate those answers you know are incorrect and guess using the remaining ones. Do not waste precious time. Keep in mind that there is no penalty for guessing. Bookmark the question and come back to it later if time allows.

INCORPORATE STRATEGIES TO EASE THE FEAR OF TEST ANXIETY

It is normal to have some test anxiety about taking a certification examination.
- Anxiety is a natural response to new challenges in our lives.
- Some anxiety will cause heightened awareness and may improve test taking, whereas anxiety that is uncontrolled will impede the ability to think critically.
- Everyone who takes tests experiences some anxiety; however, recognizing and controlling anxiety is an important factor in success.

Some strategies that can be used to ease test anxiety include the following:
1. Reduce anxiety related to time constraints.
   - Schedule the examination when your work schedule is less stressful.
   - Start a study group and plan to meet once a week for 2 hours.
     - Use a detailed test plan to divide assignments.
     - Each member of the study group can complete an assignment and share notes with the group.
     - Each member of the group can also share the sources of information.
2. Reduce anxiety related to having limited experience in taking tests.
   - Develop a checklist by writing a list of content that concerns you, and cross each item off when you have mastered it.
   - Practice the questions in the book and review the rationales, even if you answered the practice question correctly.

- Self-evaluation will assist you in refocusing on specific content.
- Practice will increase your proficiency. It also boosts your confidence level.

3. Reduce anxiety related to previous unfavorable testing experience.
   - Stop negative thoughts that begin with "what if." Read or repeat a positive message about being successful. Remember the mind is a powerful tool and can either serve as a motivator or an obstacle.

     You may reach a point when you have several consecutive difficult questions to answer in a row. Do not panic! Practice a calming technique such as deep breathing.
   - Use positive affirmations about your goal, such as "I can answer more questions correctly" or "I understand that information now."
   - Take time each day to exercise; practice yoga, or meditate. Avoid excessive caffeine intake while studying and before the exam. Caffeine can cause anxiety and can adversely affect one's ability to maintain focus. Avoid refined sugars and high-fat foods, which can drain one's energy decreasing concentration levels (Sefcik, Brice, & Prerost, 2013).

Practice these strategies on a regular basis so that reducing anxiety becomes easy to achieve. Engage in activities that you find relaxing on the evening prior to the examination, such as watching a movie or going out to dinner with friends. Do not attempt to open any books. If you do not know the material by this time, you will not learn it the evening prior to the exam. In addition, you will increase your anxiety level. Relaxation can help you to switch your focus from any external stressors. It is essential that you get an adequate amount of sleep the night prior to the exam.

USE STRATEGIES TO BE A SAVVY TEST TAKER

Read or Misread

Read each question carefully, and determine the key words that provide details for answering the question. Misreading the question can dramatically change the objective of the question. Know what the stem of the question is asking. This is extremely critical as it can help you more easily decide the correct option from a plausible distractor.

> **SIMULATION TEACHING TIP 3.2**
>
> If you begin to feel panicked because you just were given a few consecutive questions that were extremely difficult, say to yourself that these are experimental questions and will not count against you if you answered incorrectly. Always keep in mind that you devoted sufficient time to studying all the key concepts and that you entered the exam well prepared. Refuse to let the exam defeat you. Believe you have great potential to be successful.

Visualization

If a simulation is described and you are unsure of the answer, close your eyes. Picture the scenario in your mind prior to answering the question.

Changing Answers

The first answer that comes to mind is usually the correct answer. Do not second guess your "gut" feeling. If you are sure you need to change an answer—do it. However, if you usually change answers from correct to incorrect—do not do it.

Understand the Types of Questions Developed From Cognitive Levels of Learning

Bloom's taxonomy of learning is used to determine whether the candidate has mastered definitive skills or competencies. The easiest or lower level questions would be within the knowledge or comprehension category. These questions include recalling or demonstrating an understanding of concepts. Chances are that you will not be responsible for answering many of these types of questions because of their uncomplicated nature.

When you study—think application. Application questions expect the candidate to provide an intervention to the problem. There is usually a large percentage of these questions. In such questions it would be important to apply ideas, concepts, principles, or theories to solve a problem. Exhibit 3.1 demonstrates an application question.

Analysis questions will also be evident. These questions expect a logical response to the detailed cause and effect after examining information or reports. This provides an opportunity to break down the relationship between the parts and decide how the whole functions. Ask yourself why a solution worked or did not work. Your conclusion should always be supported by facts or results. Keep this in mind while you study for the certification exam. Exhibit 3.2 is an example of an analysis question.

Another category with high-level questions is synthesis (Exhibit 3.3). These types of questions are not used frequently in testing situations, but could be used in simulation because they require creating plans or constructing solutions to problems. All elements are combined into a unified whole to develop a tool or design a plan.

EXHIBIT 3.1

Example: During a simulation, the learners fail to recognize a negative response after a medication is administered. What action by the simulation facilitator would be most appropriate?

A. Decrease the other distractions in the environment.
B. Instruct the confederate to provide some information.
C. Continue the simulation as originally planned.
D. Stop the simulation.

The answer is C (Continue the simulation because this situation occurs in healthcare frequently).

It is important for the scenario to play out because it is a learning experience. The issue would be addressed and discussed during debriefing.

> **EXHIBIT 3.2**
>
> Example: A human simulation experience was designed as a formative assessment for learners who were midway through the nursing program. The learners stated that the experience was too difficult. Which information about the simulation experience should the educator examine first?
>
> A. Course grades of the learners involved in the simulation
> B. Training of the standardized (simulated) patients (SPs)
> C. Planning details of the encounter
> D. Feedback from the SPs
>
> The answer is D (Feedback from the SPs).
>
> Learners are usually very anxious about simulation, which may alter their evaluation of the experience. Verbal feedback from the SPs as well as the information from the checklists will provide accurate information.

> **EXHIBIT 3.3**
>
> Example: Data have determined that the patient wait time in the emergency department (ED) has increased by 20% within the last quarter. The patient visits and patient acuity have remained the same. Three extra full-time RNs and one clerk have been hired within the past 11 months. Six months ago, a boarding area was constructed to accommodate patients waiting for inpatient beds to open. The manager decides to design a simulation experience for the team to promote best practice. What should be the focus of the simulation?
>
> A. Perfecting skills
> B. Team building
> C. Effective communication
> D. Use of ancillary staff
>
> The answer is B (Team building).
>
> The data that were collected do not reflect the fact that the nursing staff has increased and the boarding area is operational. Staff must communicate effectively, perfect their skills, and use ancillary staff appropriately. These issues would all be encompassed in team building.

Evaluation will also be tested to provide the candidate with the opportunity to make value judgments based on effectiveness of a simulation design, scenario progression, patient outcomes, or equipment. Exhibit 3.4 provides an evaluation question.

Keep in mind that the simulation certification is available to all healthcare professionals who have met the eligibility requirements. Therefore, the global approach to reviewing information for this examination is critical. Positive patient outcomes rely on the multidisciplinary approach to quality care. Think about concepts in relation to the types of questions (application, analysis, synthesis, evaluation) that will be tested. Examine your own activities as an educator and in practice and relate them to the content in the questions.

EXHIBIT 3.4

Example: The RN-to-BSN (bachelor of science in nursing) nursing program has 375 learners at present. This is an increase of 20% in 1 year. Approximately 60% of the class attends online. After evaluating the program, determine what equipment/technology should be discussed during the upcoming budget meeting.

A. Nasogastric (NG) and tracheostomy care trainer
B. Harvey, the cardiopulmonary patient simulator
C. Wound care trainer
D. Virtual-reality simulation

The answer is D (Virtual-reality simulation).

Learners attending online classes continue to increase. This technology would be accessible to those attending the classes live as well as those attending online. If the learners are already RNs, they should have skills to care for patients with NG tubes and tracheostomies. Skills as well as heart and lung sounds are available in most virtual simulation programs.

CASE STUDY 3.1

A course chair requested that faculty teaching the course use a simulation the last week of the term. There were five sections of the course. The goal was to provide a safe environment for learners to use assessment techniques and fundamental nursing skills with the use of a high-fidelity mannequin. The educators were provided with a choice of four different scenarios, objectives, lists of equipment, and medications needed for each simulation. A self-evaluation tool was also available for learners to complete after the simulation.

After the completion of the term, the course chair received multiple emails from learners stating that their section never had an opportunity to experience a simulation. The two sections involved were taught by the same educator. How would you approach this issue if you were the course chair?

■ RECERTIFICATION

The credential gained by passing the certification examination is valid for a total of 3 years from the date it was awarded. In order to recertify, you must submit an application for renewal. There are two options to meet the recertification standards.

1. Retake the certification examination before the expiration date on the original certification.
2. Demonstrate ongoing continued professional development that focuses on education or simulation activities.

   Professional development includes

- Continued activity in simulation within the past 3 years
- Attendance at conferences, webinars, or other educational programs
- Presentations at educational conferences
- Publishing journals articles, book chapters, or books (SSH, 2018)

Simplify the recertification process.

- Keep a record of specific activities, their dates, and continuing education (CE) credits accrued.
- Keep the original hard copies of certificates of attendance in a folder. Scan the certificates into a folder to maintain an electronic copy. Additional copies are important because original copies can become lost or damaged.
- Submit an application for renewal and other specified information outlined by the SSH approximately 8 weeks before the due date.

PRACTICE QUESTIONS

1. Simulation educators understand that beside skills simulation can enhance the student's:
   A. Intrapersonnel and interpersonnel communication
   B. Cognitive test answering
   C. Test-taking skills
   D. Concept mapping

2. The novice simulation educator needs a better understanding of simulation principles when she states:
   A. "Simulation is safe space for learning."
   B. "Simulation can be less anxiety provoking."
   C. "Simulation is uncontrolled."
   D. "Simulation teaches safe patient care."

3. Which of the following is not considered a goal in the use of simulation?
   A. Provide standardization for evaluating a student's strengths and weaknesses
   B. Having participants reflect on their thoughts and feelings
   C. Widen the gap between theory and practice
   D. Discovery learning

4. Which of the following reasons to become simulation certified is not correct?
   A. Personal accomplishment and professional competence that can result in tangible and intangible benefits
   B. Ability to develop well-designed interdisciplinary scenarios for the purpose of enhancing collaboration and communication
   C. Publish about effective uses of simulation in nursing education
   D. It is mandated in order to conduct any simulation experience with nursing students

5. In which stage do the participants get oriented to the environment and obtain information on the scenario?
   A. Designing
   B. Planning
   C. Implementation
   D. Postsimulation

6. The simulation educator is in the process of completing a written scenario for a simulation experience and you have just identified the objectives. The simulation educator now needs to decide on the evaluation tool to be used to evaluate the participants. This describes which simulation stage?

    A. Designing
    B. Planning
    C. Implementation
    D. Postsimulation

7. The simulation educator is conducting a simulation using both a high-fidelity simulator as the patient and a standardized participant who is acting as a concerned and agitated family member. Which method of simulation is being used?

    A. Task trainer
    B. Human patient simulators
    C. Hybrid simulation
    D. Mixed simulation

8. A good test-taking strategy is to:

    A. Skim the references
    B. Just do a review course
    C. Do as many questions as possible
    D. Ask friends what was on the test

9. The simulation educator asks the following question on a test: "Identify the best type of simulation for developing interpersonal skills" and the answer is "standardized patients." This question is at what level of Bloom's taxonomy?

    A. Understanding
    B. Applying
    C. Comprehending
    D. Analyzing

10. The simulation educator understands that certification is a process that:

    A. Travels with nurses through their careers
    B. Can be revoked if wrong doing is noted in a career
    C. Is good for 3 years
    D. Tells others that you are proficient

REFERENCES

Fleming, N. (2001). VARK a guide to learning styles. Retrieved from http://www.vark-learn.com/english/page.asp?p=categories

Society for Simulation in Healthcare. (2018). *SSH certified healthcare simulation educator handbook.* Retrieved from http://www.ssih.org/Portals/48/Certification/CHSE_Docs/CHSE%20Handbook.pdf

Sefcik, D., Bice, G., & Prerost, F. (2013). *How to study for standardized tests.* Burlington, MA: Jones & Bartlett.

Turrentine, F. E., Rose, K. M., Hanks, J. B., Lorntz, B., Owen, J. A., Brashers, V. L., & Ramsdale, E. E. (2016). Interprofessional training enhances collaboration between nursing and medical students: A pilot study. *Nurse Education Today, 40,* 33–38. doi:10.1016/j.nedt.2016.01.024

Domain I: Professional Values and Capabilities

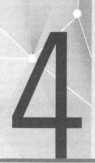

4 Leadership in Simulation

RUTH A. WITTMANN-PRICE AND
BRITTNY D. CHABALOWSKI

The task of the leader is to get people from where they are to where they have not been.

—Henry A. Kissinger

his chapter addresses Domain I: Professional Values and Capabilities (Society for Simulation in Healthcare [SSH], 2018).

[LEARNING OUTCOMES]

- Discuss the role of certification in simulation leadership.
- Discuss activities that contribute to leadership in simulation.
- Review resources available for faculty development in simulation instruction.

Simulation in healthcare requires experienced, confident, and well-trained educators. However, without any formal simulation education training available, experienced educators are responsible for passing along the bulk of this knowledge to novice educators through mentorship. Demonstration of leadership in the field includes development of future simulation educators.

In addition to building the unique body of simulation knowledge, educators are responsible for understanding and disseminating best practices. Leadership in the field of simulation education includes innovation and collaboration. Activities that demonstrate leadership include publication, presentation, and continued training. Sharing experiences in simulation and novel ideas builds the specialty and improves the delivery of simulation education on a large scale.

As a leader in the field of simulation education, being a champion of this pedagogy is a principal responsibility. The use of simulation as a teaching strategy can be intimidating for experienced educators because many did not use high-fidelity simulation in their own educational process. Being an enthusiastic mentor to novice simulation educators will have a monumental impact on the specialty of simulation education.

KNOWLEDGE ACQUISITION

Without a formal training program in place, how did we get to specialty certification? Some excellent ways to improve subject knowledge:

- Attend workshops.
- Work with an experienced individual or observing an experienced individual.
- Read about simulation.

More articles are appearing in reputable journals that instruct educators on how to set up and organize effective simulation scenarios (Sanner-Striehr, 2017).

FACULTY TRAINING

As stated in Chapter 2, the use of Patricia Benner's novice-to-expert theory (1982) has been proposed as a framework for faculty development in simulation education. Using those stages, the Bay Area Simulation Collaborative Model describes the steps for instructor training (Waxman & Telles, 2009):

- Novice
  - Technical training
  - May include training through simulator manufacturer
- Advanced beginner
  - Foundations of simulation methodology
  - May include written or online resources
- Competent
  - Begins observation with experienced simulation educator
  - Collaborates on scenario development
  - Practices facilitating simulation with feedback from experienced simulation educator
  - Leads debriefing sessions with feedback
  - Receives advanced technical training
  - Receives discipline-specific training
- Proficient
  - Facilitates simulations independently
  - Gains experience in simulation
  - Develops scenarios independently
- Expert
  - Acts as experienced simulation educator and mentor for novice simulation educators
  - Demonstrates innovation in simulation

FACULTY MENTORSHIP

In a fashion very similar to designing learning outcomes, mentorship for simulation educators begins with an assessment of learning style and current knowledge. There are a number of resources available, both in print and online, that are useful in the *advanced beginner* stage of training. When the educator moves into the *competent stage*, the mentor provides a comfortable learning environment for the educator.

Simulation should be a safe and supportive environment for the learners and the new educator. As with any new experience, learners can become frustrated if they feel they do not have the tools or support necessary to be successful. Some things to consider:

- Begin with observation of one or more experienced simulation educators.
- Start new simulation educators in their content area "comfort zone."
- Provide the new educator with a clear and concise template for the scenario.
- Allow new educators to engage at their own pace (initial interaction may be as minimal as controlling the technical aspect of a high-fidelity simulator).
- Model positive behaviors with the learners.
- Promote a supportive environment for the learners.
- Demonstrate effective debriefing techniques.

Once the new educator has reached the *proficient level* and is functioning independently, continue to serve as a resource for questions and support the development of innovation. As the new simulation educator designs and implements new scenarios, be sure to provide continuous guidance. As faculty grow into this role, there is a tendency to try to incorporate too much information into an experience. Emphasis on clear and concise learning outcomes is imperative. There should be between three and five objectives for each scenario. Having more than five objectives diminishes the experience for the learners and they may become easily overwhelmed.

While transitioning to independence as a new simulation educator, it is easy to fall back onto teaching methods that are more familiar. Experienced clinical faculty who transition to the role of simulation educators tend to interact with the learners during the scenario. This is the method that they might find the most comfortable and they may have difficulty allowing the learners to work independently without "real-time" guidance from the educator. As a mentor in simulation, it is important to continue to provide support to new educators. This includes the reassurance that the best learning experience develops by allowing the learners to work with minimal intervention from the educator.

That being said, one of the greatest challenges new simulation educators face when they begin to function independently is making modifications on the fly. What if the scenario does not go as planned? Anticipating and planning for the unexpected during simulation will improve the confidence of the new simulation educator.

Consider whether the learners:

- Do not perform the required behaviors to progress to the next phase of the simulation.
- Make an error that would cause great harm to the patient.
- "Kill" the patient.

As a mentor, it is important to discuss the "what ifs" with the new simulation educator. Although the goal is to provide all learners with a similar simulation experience, that is not always the case. Oftentimes, the learners' behaviors will drive the scenario down an unexpected path. After facilitating a scenario multiple times, the educator can begin to identify the most common errors. Those errors can be anticipated, and cues to refocus the learners can be developed.

There is evidence to suggest that unexpected death in simulation can negatively impact the learning experience. Some studies suggest that unless death is one of the learning objectives, the facilitator should not allow the simulator to "die" (Fraser et al., 2014), but simulation can be an effective method of teaching proper bereavement interactions with families (Colwell, 2017). Mentoring a new simulation educator should include the development of an escape plan for each scenario. These can include transfer to a higher level of care or intervention by a critical care team.

Mentorship for new simulation faculty is a continuous process. As a certified simulation educator, the expectation regarding leadership and mentorship extends to all levels of simulation. This includes continuing to ensure best practices and serving as a resource for educators, staff, and learners.

> **EVIDENCE-BASED SIMULATION PRACTICE 4.1**
>
> DeMaria et al. (2017) studied students' reactions when their simulated patient died during advanced cardiac life support training. Heart rates and salivary cortisol and dehydroepiandrosterone were collected during simulation on two groups of students. One group experienced a high-fidelity patient death and the other group did not. The physiological results indicated higher heart rates in the group who experienced the death.

RESOURCES FOR FACULTY DEVELOPMENT

As a leader in simulation, development of a formal training program may not be a feasible short-term goal. However, there are a number of training resources available for faculty development:

- SSH
  - Annual conference—International Meeting on Simulation in Healthcare (IMSH)
- CAE Healthcare
  - Annual conference—Human Patient Simulation Network (HPSN)
- National League for Nursing (NLN) Simulation Innovation Resource Center (SIRC)
  - Online training modules
  - Content continuously updated
  - Appropriate for novice-to-expert simulation educators
  - www.sirc.nln.org

- Drexel University's Certificate in Simulation
  - One-week-long training program
  - Offered throughout the year
  - On-site at Drexel University in Philadelphia, Pennsylvania
  - www.drexel.edu/cne/conferencesCourses/conferences/Certificate_in_Simulation
- *Simulation in Nursing Education: From Conceptualization to Evaluation*
  - Edited by Pamela Jefferies, PhD, RN, FAAN, ANEF
  - Published by the NLN, Washington, DC
- *Developing Successful Health Care Education Simulation Centers: The Consortium Model*
  - Written by Pamela Jeffries, PhD, RN, FAAN, ANEF, and Jim Battin, BS
  - Published by Springer Publishing Company, New York
- *Human Simulation for Nursing and Health Professions*
  - Edited by Linda Wilson, PhD, RN, CPAN, CAPA, BC, CNE, CHSE, CHSE-A, ANEF, FAAN, and Leland Rockstraw, PhD, RN
  - Published by Springer Publishing Company, New York

ADVOCATING FOR SIMULATION

Many healthcare training facilities have incorporated simulation into their programs on some level. However, advocating for simulation means increasing the use of simulation in a curriculum and cultivating new simulation educators. Acceptance of increasing simulation activities may initially be met with some resistance. Some anticipated challenges include the following:

- Time to prepare for simulation activities
- Lack of training
- Belief that it is not a useful teaching method
- Lack of space or equipment
- Complicated scheduling
- Lack of funding
- Lack of staffing
- Concerns about student engagement (Roh & Jang, 2017)

As a champion for simulation integration, acknowledging and addressing these challenges will be imperative. Some strategies include the following:

- Identify educators who are interested in being trained in simulation.
- Meet with content or course leaders to explore opportunities for simulation.
- Suggest simulation activities that do not require elaborate equipment or space (i.e., Second Life simulations or use of standardized [simulated] patients [SPs]).

- Review course or training objectives and identify ways to incorporate simulation to meet those objectives.
- Advocate for simulation as a tool to increase learner experience with diversity and high-risk, low-volume patient experiences.

SUMMARY

The responsibilities of being a certified educator in the discipline of simulation include continuous knowledge development and acquisition of the best practices of simulation. Furthermore, the dissemination of this knowledge serves to develop new simulation faculty and the field of simulation. Serving as a champion for simulation means

- Mentoring new faculty
- Promoting innovation in simulation
- Participating in building the specialty

CASE STUDY 4.1

A new simulation educator has been training with an experienced simulation educator and feels ready to start designing and implementing her own simulation scenarios. After reviewing the simulation design, the experienced educator finds there are 15 objectives for the 30-minute activity. What is the best approach to use to mentor the new educator?

PRACTICE QUESTIONS

1. An important quality needed in mentors to engage novice simulation educators is:

   A. Expert knowledge
   B. Enthusiasm
   C. Delegation skills
   D. Prioritization skills

2. A simulation educator who is requesting assistance of the manufacturer of the high-fidelity mannequin is probably on which level of expertise?

   A. Novice
   B. Advanced beginner
   C. Competent
   D. Proficient

3. A simulation educator's "comfort zone" includes:

   A. High-fidelity mannequin use
   B. Low-fidelity mannequin use
   C. Content that is familiar
   D. Environments that are familiar

4. Expert simulation educators understand that sometimes the best learning experiences for students include the following:

   A. Coaching through the scenario
   B. Minimal interventions
   C. Just-in-time instructions
   D. Clear prebriefing content review

5. A mentor for simulation educators should be in which stage of development?

   A. Advanced beginner
   B. Competent
   C. Proficient
   D. Expert

6. During a scenario a mannequin unintentionally "dies." The simulation educator can expert which type of student reaction?

   A. Physiological effects
   B. Emotional effects
   C. Cognitive effects
   D. Social effects

7. A good learning resource for novice simulation educators is:

   A. Observation
   B. Trial and error
   C. Reading how to books
   D. Training sessions by simulation organizations

8. One of the keys to developing simulation educator leaders is to determine:

   A. Who has seniority?
   B. Who is interested?
   C. Who is technically savvy?
   D. Who is the best didactic or clinical educator?

9. Student engagement in simulation is most influenced by:

   A. Time of day
   B. Attitudes of instructors
   C. Frequency of exposure
   D. Appropriate content

10. A simulation educator is collaborating on the development of a scenario. The simulation educator is most likely in which stage of development?

    A. Novice
    B. Advanced beginner
    C. Competent
    D. Proficient

REFERENCES

Benner, P. (1982). From novice to expert. *American Journal of Nursing, 82*(3), 402–407. doi:10.1097/00000446-198282030-00004

Colwell, P. (2017). Building confidence in neonatal bereavement: The use of simulation as an innovative educational approach. *Journal of Neonatal Nursing, 23*(2), 65–74. doi:10.1016/j.jnn.2016.07.005

DeMaria, S., Silverman, E. R., Lapidus, K. A. B., Williams, C. H., Spivack, J., Levine, A., & Goldberg, A. (2016). The impact of simulated patient death on medical students' stress response and learning of ACLS. *Medical Teacher, 38*(7), 730–737. doi:10.3109/0142159X.2016.1150986

Fraser, K., Huffman, J., Ma, I., Sobczak, M., McIlwrick, J., Wright, B., & McLaughlin, K. (2014). The emotional and cognitive impact of unexpected simulated patient death: A randomized controlled trial. *Chest, 145*(5), 958–963. doi:10.1378/chest.13-0987

Roh, Y. S., & Jang, K. I. (2017). Survey of factors influencing learner engagement with simulation debriefing among nursing students. *Nursing & Health Sciences, 19*(4), 485–491. doi:10.1111/nhs.12371

Sanner-Striehr, E. (2017). Using simulation to teach responses to lateral violence: Guidelines for nurse educators. *Nurse Educator, 42*(3), 133–137. doi:10.1097/NNE.0000000000000326

Society for Simulation in Healthcare. (2018). *Certified Healthcare Simulation Educator Examination Blueprint, 2018 Version.* Retrieved from http://www.ssih.org/Portals/48/Certification/CHSE_Docs/CHSE_Examination_Blueprint.pdf

Waxman, K. T., & Telles, C. L. (2009). The use of Benner's framework in high-fidelity simulation faculty development: The Bay Area Simulation Collaborative model. *Clinical Simulation in Nursing, 5*(6), e231–e235. doi:10.1016/j.ecns.2009.06.001

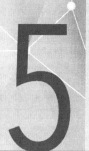

5. Special Learning Considerations in Simulation

RUTH A. WITTMANN-PRICE

> *It is time for parents to teach young people early on that in diversity there is beauty and there is strength.*
>
> —Maya Angelou

his chapter addresses Domain I: Professional Values and Capabilities (Society for Simulation in Healthcare [SSH], 2018).

[LEARNING OUTCOMES]

- Discuss the importance of recognizing diversity in learning styles, teaching styles, and generational differences.
- Develop simulation learning experiences for culturally diverse healthcare students.
- Discuss the enactment of the Americans With Disabilities Act (ADA; 2017) in the simulation laboratory.
- Describe diversity through a case study and practice questions.

Diversity can be defined as "the condition of having or being composed of different elements" (Merriam-Webster, n.d.). Diversity related to simulation experiences can include any or all of the following human attributes in any combination listed in Exhibit 5.1.

Simulation experiences used for learning and evaluation must consider the diversity inherent in all the participants of the experience. Personal characteristics and past experiences are "brought to the table" within any learning environment. The *realism* created within a simulation environment or scenario can easily trigger personal reactions that are guided by the participants' diversity. Simulation is a *social practice*. Dieckmann, Gaba, and Rall (2007) define it as a contextual event in space and time, conducted for one or more purposes, in which people interact in a goal-oriented fashion with each other, with technical artifacts (the simulator), and with the environment (including relevant devices). This chapter briefly outlines several elements of human diversity and relates them to the simulation environment. The outcome of understanding diversity and gaining tolerance for human differences can be reached through learning and reflection, which are hallmarks of simulation.

> **EXHIBIT 5.1**
>
> **Diversity Attributes**
>
> Diversity attributes can be exhibited by any of the humans or simulated humans, such as the patient (including family or community), learner, or educator. The attributes can include any of the following elements:
>
> - Demographic
>   - Age
>   - Gender
>   - Ethnicity
>   - Disabilities
> - Experiential
>   - Work–life experiences (e.g., adult learners)
> - Informational
>   - Educational background
>   - Learning–teaching styles
> - Fundamental
>   - Different beliefs and values
>   - Relationships with others

DIVERSITY IN LEARNING STYLES

All learners come to the simulation, skills laboratory, or the virtual environment with their own unique learning styles. A *learning style* refers to the ways and conditions under which learners most prefer to assimilate knowledge.

- The approach learners take to accomplish different tasks is also important.
- A learning style is an approach to learning that works for the individual learner.
- Learners may have more than one learning style.
- Educators must first assist learners in identifying their learning style(s) if they do not already know it, and then present information in a manner consistent with the students' learning styles (Lown & Hawkins, 2017).

The four most common learning styles are defined by the acronym VARK, as described by Fleming and Mills (1992).

- V = Visual
- A = Auditory
- R = Read/write
- K = Kinesthetic

Visual or Spatial Learners

- Learn best through what they *see*
- Pictures, diagrams, flow charts, timelines, maps, and demonstrations enhance their ability to learn

- A good learning assignment for a visual learner might involve concept mapping using computers and graphics
- May also be called *graphic* (G) learners
- Important to note that visual learners do not usually care to learn by viewing movies, videos, or PowerPoint presentations (Fleming, 2001)

Aural or Auditory Learners

- Prefer to learn through what is *heard or spoken*
- Learn best from lectures, tapes, tutorials, group discussions, speaking, web chats, emails, smart phone, and talking things through out loud
- By talking about a topic, these learners are able to process the given information (Fleming, 2001)

Reading or Writing Learners

- Prefer to have the information to be learned displayed as *written words*
- Prefer text-based input and output in all of its forms
- Many academics have a preference for this style of learning
- These learners are often fond of PowerPoint presentations, the Internet, lists, dictionaries, thesauri, quotations, or anything else featuring words (Fleming, 2001)

Kinesthetic or Active Learners

- Use their bodies and sense of touch to enhance learning while engaged in physical activity
- Like to think about issues while working out or exercising
- Like to participate, play games, role-play, act, and model experiences
- Appreciate demonstrations, simulations, videos, and movies of "real things," as well as case studies, practice sessions, and applications (Fleming, 2001)
- Felder and Solomon (1998) refer to these learners as *active learners*

Multimodal/Mixture (M) Learners

- Prefer to learn via two or more styles of learning or using a variety of modes
- Like information to be context specific or might choose a single mode to suit a certain occasion or situation
- Like to gather information from each mode and often have a deeper and broader understanding of topics (Fleming, 2001)

  In addition to the previous points, there are labels given to other learning styles by various authors, which include:

- Verbal (linguistic) learners
- Tactile learners

- Global learners
- Intuitive learners
- Sequential learners
- Reflective learners
- Analytical learners
- Accommodative learners

Table 5.1 displays the characteristics of these alternative types of learning styles identified by various learning specialists.

> **EVIDENCE-BASED SIMULATION PRACTICE 5.1**
>
> Lee, Lee, Lee, and Baem (2016) used high-fidelity simulation's effect on teaching nursing core competencies, problem solving, and academic self-efficacy using the four learning styles (VARK). The learning activities were more kinesthetic and the results demonstrated a significant improvement in the simulation-based nursing-core-competencies group compared to a group of students in classroom-based learning ($p = .008$).

TABLE 5.1 Various Diverse Learning Styles

Verbal (linguistic) learners (similar to auditory learning style)	• Get value from spoken words. • Enjoy talking through procedures. • Use recordings of content for repetition. • Frequently use mnemonics to retain information.
Tactile learners	• Learn by touching or manipulating objects. • Require movement. • Trace words and use letter tiles to learn to spell words (Scrabble).
Global learners	• Make decisions based on their emotions and intuition. • Are spontaneous and focus on creativity. • Do not consider tidiness important. • Enjoy learning. • Use humor, tell stories, and enjoy group work. • Like to participate in activities. • Tend to absorb material randomly. • Frequently do not see connections at first, but then suddenly "get it." • Are able to solve complex problems quickly or put things together in unique ways once they have grasped the big picture, but they may have difficulty explaining how they did it. • Lack good sequential thinking abilities (Felder & Solomon, 1998).
Intuitive learners	• Like to discover the possibilities in relationships. • Like solving problems using well-established methods. • Do not like complications or surprises. • Do not like repetition. • Work fast.

(continued)

TABLE 5.1

Various Diverse Learning Styles (*continued*)

	• Are innovative. • Do not like courses that involve memorization or routine calculations. • Easily become bored. • Are prone to careless mistakes on tests because they are impatient with details, such as checking math calculations (Felder & Solomon, 1998).
Reflective learners	• Prefer to think about new material by reflecting quietly. • Prefer to work alone, rather than with groups. • Do not like classes that cover large amounts of material quickly. • Do not like to be asked simply to read and memorize. • Like to stop periodically to review what they have read. • Find it helpful to write short summaries of readings or class notes in their own words to help them retain the material better (Felder & Solomon, 1998).
Analytical learners	• Base all of their decisions on logic. • Plan and organize well. • Focus on details and facts. • Like a tidy, well-organized environment. • Enjoy learning, take sequential steps, and follow "the rules."
Accommodative learners	• Like a combination of concrete experiences and active experimentation. • Complete tasks and are less concerned about the theories. • Are risk-takers. • Solve problems by trial and error. • Are concerned with abstract concepts and assimilate abstract conceptualizations with reflective observations.

Kolb's Learning Styles

Kolb describes *experiential learning* (Chapter 6) as a type of learning in which the student is actively engaged. Kolb also discusses learning styles in relation to experiential learning. Kolb's four learning styles are the following:

1. **Diverging:** This type of learner likes to work in groups and generate ideas. Students are fine with feedback and reflecting on activities learned. This learning style uses concrete experiences and reflective observation.

2. **Assimilating:** This type of learner prefers to read information, be presented with lectures, and then analyze topics. This learning style, according to Kolb, is generated by learners who prefer abstract conceptualization and reflective observation.

3. **Converging:** This type of learner likes to put ideas to practical application. This style of learning is generated from those who abstract, conceptualize, and actively experiment.

4. **Accommodating:** This type of learner enjoys hands-on work in teams to complete projects. This style of learning is derived from those people who use concrete experience and active experimentation (Kolb, 1984).

Generational Learners

In addition to learning styles, the era or context in which learners were born and reared will affect how they view receiving and retaining information. Just as homogeneous groups of healthcare learners are obsolete, having learners who all fall within one generation in higher educationis also not a reality in higher education. Characteristic learning attributes have been noted in different generational learners, but of course, as with any other categorization, individual differences and preferences may override any stereotypical attribute (Hart, 2017). Table 5.2 shows attributes of generational learners.

TABLE 5.2

Generational Learners

GENERATIONAL LABEL	LEARNER ATTRIBUTES	WHAT MAY FACILITATE LEARNING
Baby boomers (born between 1946 and 1964)	• Most healthcare educators fall into this category.	• Respond to competition due to large peer groups (80 million strong). • Are taught mainly by lecture. • May think technology is nice but not essential.
Generation X (born between 1965 and 1979)	• Challenge authority. • Are independent problem solvers. • Are multitaskers.	• Respond to self-learning modules. • Find demonstration is useful. • Are pragmatic and focus on the outcomes of learning. • Want real-world skills.
Generation Y **Millennials** **Nexters** **MTV generation** (born after 1975 or between 1981 and 1999) **This generation is:** • More culturally diverse • One third raised in single-parent homes • 81 million strong	• Need constant stimulation. • Respond to multimedia and instant information. • Are critical consumers. • Expect entertainment. • Are active, hands-on learners. • Prefer fast-paced experiences. • Seek instant gratification. • Respond to positive reinforcement. • Are resourceful. • Like the challenge of problem solving. • Prefer group activities. • May have poor reading and math skills. • Display poor work habits. • Are multitaskers. • Have no time for school. • Are visual learners due to computers.	• Use critical reading. • Use intertextuality—Reading multiple electronic sources to critically appraise the overlap for meaning. • Display self-preferentiality—Are better critiquing topics they are passionate about or can relate to in their own lives. • Consider different viewpoints or cultural interpretations. • Journal to foster reflection and critical thinking. • Like using technology. • Use concept mapping. • Respond to simulation of teamwork.

DIVERSITY IN TEACHING STYLES OF HEALTHCARE EDUCATORS

Jeffries (2007) emphasizes the importance of the teacher's role in simulation as well as the facilitator–learner relationship. The method by which the teacher designs the simulation experience and the educational practices used to organize and deliver the experience will affect the quality of the learning (Foronda, Baptiste, & Ockimey, 2017).

The teaching style used during the experience is another variable in its success. Teaching styles permeate the development and orchestration of the experience, and teaching styles have been classified by many different methods. Educators rarely ascribe to just one teaching style. Most educators use a variety of styles, even within a single learning session. This mixed approach can appeal to the variety of learning styles and improve learning outcomes. Reflecting on the type of style used encourages self-understanding the most and may serve to improve effectiveness.

> **EVIDENCE-BASED SIMULATION PRACTICE 5.2**
>
> Stirling (2017) studied how faculty ($N = 24$) use learning styles to assist students in learning information by using a cross-sectional study and found that faculty reported using a visual learning style approximately 33% of the time. This was compared to the learning style preferences of students, which were mainly kinesthetic and aural learning methods.

Individual teaching styles involve teaching behaviors and are noteworthy because behaviors have a direct effect on the simulation teaching–learning environment. The next section describes some of the ways teaching styles are categorized and what experts say are good teaching behaviors and personality traits for educators (Table 5.3).

TABLE 5.3

Helpful Teaching Strategies and Teacher Characteristics

TEACHING STRATEGIES	TEACHER CHARACTERISTICS
Uses repeat demonstrations	Knows learners
Role models good communication	Welcoming voice and demeanor
Is flexible about debriefing method	Dresses the part
Repeats instructions	Calm
Explains steps	Welcomes learners' questions
Does not rush	Experienced and current in practice
Discusses worst-case scenarios to alleviate fear	Willing to learn with and from students

(continued)

TABLE 5.3
Helpful Teaching Strategies and Teacher Characteristics (*continued*)

TEACHING STRATEGIES	TEACHER CHARACTERISTICS
Provides feedback to learners	Uses teachable moments and errors to learn
Maintains civil environment	Communicates well
Provides learners with opportunity to think through a situation	Enthusiastic and passionate
Role-plays thinking in action	Empathizes with learners' feelings

Grasha's Classification of Teaching Styles

Grasha's (1996) classification defines teaching styles as expert, formal authority, demonstrator, facilitator, and delegator. The characteristics of each teaching style are unique and are listed in Table 5.4.

Quirk's Classification of Teaching Styles

Another useful classification of teaching styles was devised by Quirk in 1994.

- **Assertive**—Communication is usually content specific and educator drives home information home.
- **Suggestive**—Educator uses experiences to describe a concept and then requests that the learners seek more information on the subject.

TABLE 5.4
Grasha's Teaching Styles

STYLE	CHARACTERISTICS
Expert	Uses vast knowledge base to inform learners. Challenges students to be well prepared. Can be intimidating to the learner.
Formal Authority	Educator is in control of the learners' knowledge acquisition. Educator is not concerned with student–teacher relationships. Focuses on the content to be delivered.
Demonstrator	Educator coaches, demonstrates, and encourages active learning.
Facilitator	Learner-centered, active learning strategies are encouraged. Accountability for learning is placed on the learner.
Delegator	Educator's role is that of a consultant. Learners are encouraged to direct the entire learning process.

Adapted from Grasha, A. (1996). *Teaching with style.* Pittsburgh, PA: Alliance.

- **Collaborative**—Educator uses skills to promote problem solving and a higher level of thinking in the learners.
- **Facilitative**—Educator challenges the learners to reflect and use affective learning, ask ethical questions, and demonstrate skill in interpersonal relationships and professional behavior.

Kelly's Teaching Effectiveness

Kelly (2008) also studied learners' perceptions of teaching effectiveness and found that there were three main important attributes for teaching effectiveness. The first of these, educator knowledge, was rated the most important and consists of four separate domains, as shown in Figure 5.1.

House, Chassie, and Spohn's Teaching Behaviors

House, Chassie, and Spohn (1999) provide examples of the following behaviors and their effect on learners:

- Making eye contact can encourage learner participation.
- Positive facial expressions that elicit a positive learner response, such as head nodding, can assist learners in feeling comfortable, whereas negative gestures, such as frowning, can discourage learners' class participation.
- Vocal tone is very important and can easily portray underlying feelings and encourage or discourage learner participation.

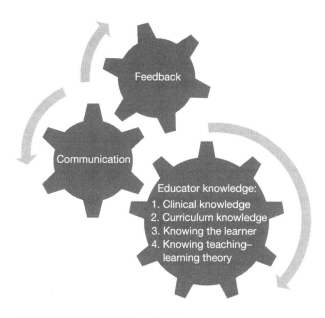

FIGURE 5.1 Kelly's attributes of teaching effectiveness.

Adapted from Kelly, C. (2008). Students' perceptions of effective clinical teaching revisited. *Nurse Education Today, 27*(8), 885–892.

Choo's Positive Characteristics for Educators

Choo (1996) researched teachers and identified characteristics that students rated positively.

- Values learning.
- Exhibits a caring relationship.
- Provides learner independence.
- Facilitates questioning.
- Tries different approaches.
- Accepts the differences among learners.

Hicks and Burkus

Hicks and Burkus (2011) describe attributes of "master teachers," which include the following:

- Clear communication
- Positive role modeling
- Professionalism demonstrated in lifelong learning and scholarship
- Reflective practice and making adjustments for improvement
- Use of philosophical, epistemological, and ontological influences in their practice of education

Story and Butts

Story and Butts (2010) discuss teaching delivery in the frame of the important four "Cs" shown in Figure 5.2.

The Myers-Briggs Type Indicator

The Myers-Briggs Type Indicator (MBTI) measures Jung's 16 personality types by classifying them into four bipolar dimensions; the educator's personality also affects instruction.

- Extroversion–introversion
- Sensing–intuition
- Thinking–feeling
- Judgment–perception (Schublova, 2017)

Silver, Hanson, and Strong

Silver, Hanson, and Strong (1996) developed a Teaching Style Inventory (TSI) based on Jung's theory of psychological types or personality types. It tests educators' propensity for one of four types.

- Sensing–thinking
- Sensing–feeling

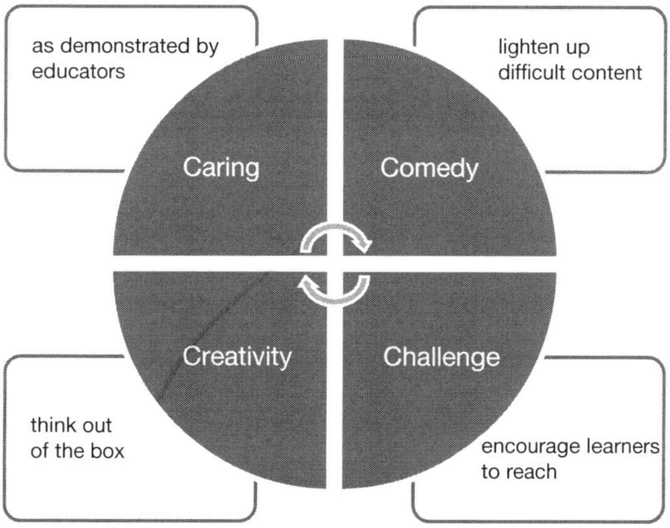

FIGURE 5.2 The four "Cs" of teaching methods.

Adapted from Story, L., & Butts, J. B. (2010). Compelling teaching with the four Cs: Caring, comedy, creativity, and challenging. *Journal of Nursing Education, 49*(5), 291–294. doi:10.3928/01484834-20100115-08

- Intuitive–thinking
- Intuitive–feeling

Knowing your teaching style and understanding your personality style and how those two personal aspects mix in the simulation or skills environment can be very enlightening. Reflecting on these attributes can assist healthcare educators to provide learners with excellent environments in which to facilitate their knowledge acquisition.

CULTURALLY DIVERSE LEARNERS

The culture of the individual encompasses an individual's values, attitudes, perceptions, interpersonal needs, roles, and cognitive styles. Cultural humility is needed by faculty to fully appreciate the experience of students (Clabby, 2017). It is important for simulation educators to recognize that cultural diversity can influence learning ability and needs and may influence how learning is perceived by individuals. Perceptions of individuals must be considered during any educational session.

Despite the growing diversity of the nation, the healthcare workforce continues to be underrepresented by minorities (Moreau, Sullivan-Bolyai, Ndiwane, & Jaffarian, 2017).

Moreover, culturally diverse learners face certain barriers that may impinge on their ability to achieve success in college. The most common of these barriers are:

- The lack of ethnically diverse faculty
- Finances

- Academic preparation
- Available role models
- Academic support
- Family support
- Peer support

Many times, needs of diverse or underrepresented students include the following (Alicea-Planas, 2017):

- Personal needs (lack of finances, time issues, family responsibilities and obligations, and difficulties related to language and communication)
- Academic needs (large or heavy workload)
- Language needs (difficulty reading and understanding assignments, a prejudice due to their accents, verbal communication barriers)
- Cultural needs (expectations related to assertiveness and cultural norms, lack of diverse role models, and difficulty with communication)

> **EVIDENCE-BASED SIMULATION PRACTICE 5.3**
>
> Bahreman and Swoboda (2017) used a simulation group method approach to successfully teach healthcare students culturally competent communication using scenarios with culturally diverse patients.

An important issue among culturally diverse learners is their level of knowledge of the English language, which, if inadequate, can be problematic. Barriers may also exist for the English-as-a-second-language (ESL) learner in progressing in healthcare programs, once accepted.

Hansen and Beaver (2012) discuss test development for ESL learners and provide the following tips:

- Use short simple sentences.
- Be direct when stating information.
- Use common vocabulary (K. King, Porr, & Gaudine, 2017).

EFFECT OF DIVERSITY ON SIMULATION SCENARIOS

Dieckmann, Lippert, Glavin, and Rall (2010) discuss simulation *lifesavers* (p. 219), that is, manipulations of a scenario when unexpected situations occur. Unexpected situations are listed in the following section as identified by Dieckmann et al. (2010) and are preempted many times by the diversity of the simulation learners. Causes for unexpected situations are the following:

- Comprehensiveness of the scenario is unclear to participants due to poor instructions or ambiguous clues during the scenario
- Inability to accept the scenario due to inexperience or distractibility of participants

- Unrealistic difficulty level of the scenario, which does not match the competency of the participants
- Participants in the scenario do not follow the procedural steps and produce unexpected actions
- Participants change the intended scenario to a familiar scenario that is also plausible

When unexpected occurrences take place during a scenario, debriefing (which will be discussed in depth in Chapter 15) may be affected. The lifesavers are the anticipated actions that may be needed during a scenario. Scenario lifesavers can be used to adapt to the situation or restore the scenario to its original form. These scenario-lifesaving actions are identified before the scenario and can come from "within" the scenario or simulation room itself by altering the patient or providing hints, or it can come from "outside" the scenario by using the director's voice to clarify, stop, or explain the scenario. Some lifesaving techniques are commonly used in many scenarios either to provide the participants with time or to emphasize missed clues, such as the patient asking learners to repeat information. Other lifesavers must be specific to the scenario, such as altering vital signs more drastically to gain the learners' attention.

LEARNER AND LEARNING DISABILITIES

Learning disabilities are the most common type of disability found on college campuses. Although increasing numbers of individuals with physical or affective disabilities are attending higher educational institutions and many disabilities are known and accommodated for before the learner enters college, other learners with learning disabilities begin college without their disability having been detected.

- In healthcare education, these disabilities are often noted when significant differences are noticed between a learner's classroom and simulation or clinical performance. Often, a learner may perform well in the simulation or clinical environment, but may be unable to demonstrate the same ability, skills, and competency in the classroom.
- Healthcare educators should always refer learners they suspect as having a learning disability to the appropriate counselors or office for accommodations for assistance (Joshi & Bouck, 2017).

Learners with documented disabilities are entitled to the same access to education as traditional learners. An office of academic services must be available to provide learners with *reasonable accommodations* and support services.

- Accommodations must be made for students with learning disabilities in accordance with the ADA.
- It is important for educators to be aware of learners with physical disabilities, such as learners with a documented or apparent physical limitation, substance abuse, chemical or alcohol impairments, and/or mental health problems (Rushton, 2017).

BELONGINGNESS

Learners who are marginalized are less likely to succeed; so simulation and virtual experiences must be inclusive, providing a valued role for each learner. Belongingness is conceptually related to motivation, and students who do not feel they belong may lose motivation to study and prepare for simulation (C. King, 2017).

> **EVIDENCE-BASED SIMULATION PRACTICE 5.4**
>
> de Jong, Favier, van der Vleuten, and Bok (2017) studied motivation in healthcare students and found that those who seek out information and had high self-determination were more likely to succeed.

SIMULATION LEARNING AS A SOCIAL PRACTICE

Goffman (1974) describes social meaning in terms of "frames" that are perceived by the individual about the reality that he or she is experiencing. Frames helps individuals understand what is happening at the moment and to make sense of the situation. Goffman breaks experiences down into two types of frames:

> **SIMULATION TEACHING TIP 5.1**
>
> Woods (2017) reminds us that simulation can evaluate the "human skills" which include social, cognitive, and personal skills.

1. **Primary frames:** Assist the individual to make sense out of the current situation.
2. **Modulation frames:** Bring in the individual's perception of the world and therefore will include individual differences (all diversity issues previously discussed). These frames must be addressed to ensure positive learning experiences (Dieckmann, Manswer, Wehner, & Rall, 2007).

SOCIALIZATION DURING SIMULATION

Walton, Chute, and Ball (2011) provide results of a grounded study with nursing learners that discusses socialization during simulation. Five phases of the process of "negotiating the role of the professional nurses" (p. 301) were identified and are as follows:

Phase I	Feeling like an imposter (includes anticipation, wanting further instructions, not knowing where to start, and anxiety)
Phase II	Trial and error (includes practice, replaying and reviewing, self-reflection, and mentoring)
Phase III	Taking the role seriously (includes having the scenario be realistic, dedication to learn, using nursing language, developing team leadership, analyzing, and better understanding of the situation)
Phase IV	Transference (includes gaining confidence, socializing into the healthcare role, feeling devastated after failing, then repracticing and rebuilding)
Phase V	Professionalism (includes growth in role as nurse and patient advocate, interprofessional collaboration, and career goal building)

The socialization aspects of simulation cannot be overlooked. Simulation is a powerful mechanism to provide learning environments in all three domains: cognitive, psychomotor, and affective.

CASE STUDY 5.1

A healthcare student tells the simulation educator that she needs time and a half to take tests, and she should have extra time to read and understand the patient history on the simulation scenario that is being used for evaluative purposes in a Capstone course. As the simulation educator, how would you respond, and what (if any) provisions would you make and under what circumstances?

PRACTICE QUESTIONS

1. The simulation educator observes a student crying after the death of a cardiac victim portrayed by a mannequin in the scenario. The simulation educator understands that this can happen because simulation is a:

    A. Social practice
    B. Learning experience
    C. Emotionally charged situation
    D. Unpredictable

2. Simulation learning activities lend themselves to a better understanding of human diversity because:

    A. There are faculty who can adjust scenarios
    B. Many laboratories have diverse mannequins
    C. It is a reflective learning environment
    D. There are standards that should be met

3. Student learning styles are important to understand so educational methodologies can reflect students' preferences. The simulation educator should be aware that a simulation scenario is most likely best suited for learners preferring which style?

    A. Visual
    B. Read/write
    C. Aural
    D. Kinesthetic

4. A simulation educator is facilitating learning about a procedure and one of the learners has difficulty following the steps. The learners may be displaying characteristics of which learning type?

    A. Tactile
    B. Intuitive
    C. Global
    D. Reflective

5. Many simulation educators are baby boomers or generation Xers and learners are millennials. One of the learning strategies that millennials respond positively to is:

    A. Modular learning
    B. Lecture before the scenario
    C. Independent problem solving
    D. Group activities

6. Grasha's teaching styles describe simulation educators who have different approaches. The best approach an educator can have with a group of learners in a simulation scenario is:

    A. Expert
    B. Formal
    C. Demonstrator
    D. Facilitator

7. A simulation educator provided students with a topic for the simulation for the following day and asks them to research the patient's care. According to Quirk, which teaching style is this?

    A. Assertive
    B. Suggestive
    C. Collaborative
    D. Facilitator

8. The novice simulation educator is reviewing her teaching effectiveness characteristic outlined by Kelly (2008) and needs further review when she states that _____ is included as a trait of an effective teacher.

    A. Feedback
    B. Communication
    C. Knowledge
    D. Sensitivity

9. Culturally diverse learners have social determinants that place them at risk. Among those determinants is:

    A. Lack of friends
    B. Family members who understand education
    C. Lack of diverse faculty
    D. Peer support

10. Lifesavers are sometimes needed in a scenario to promote positive learning and to:

    A. Decrease emotions
    B. Understand health and illness concepts
    C. Reach the learning outcomes
    D. Developed a care plan for the patient

REFERENCES

Alicea-Planas, J. (2017). Shifting our focus to support the educational journey of underrepresented students. *Journal of Nursing Education, 56*(3), 159–163. doi:10.3928/01484834-20170222-07

Americans With Disabilities Act (ADA). (2017). Information and technical assistance on the American with Disabilities Act. Retrieved from http://www.ada.gov

Bahreman, N. T., & Swoboda, S. M. (2017). Honoring diversity: Developing culturally competent communication skills through simulation. *Journal of Nursing Education, 55*(2), 105–108. doi:10.3928/01484834-20160114-09

Choo, L. A. (1996). Reflections: Learning at work. *Professional Nurse (Singapore), 23*(3), 8–11.

Clabby, J. F. (2017). Enter as an outsider: Teaching organizational humility. *International Journal of Psychiatry in Medicine, 52*(3), 219–227. doi: 10.1177/0091217417730285

de Jong, L. H., Favier, R. P., van der Vleuten, C. M. P., & Bok, H. G. J. (2017). Students' motivation toward feedback-seeking in the clinical workplace. *Medical Teacher, 39*(9), 954–958. doi:10.1080/0142159X.2017.1324948

Dieckmann, P., Gaba, D., & Rall, M. (2007). Deepening the theoretical foundations of simulation as social practice. *Simulation in Healthcare, 2*, 183–193. doi:10.1097/sih.0b013e3180f637f5

Dieckmann, P., Lippert, A., Glavin, R., & Rall, M. (2010). When things do not go as expected: Scenario life savers. *Simulation in Healthcare, 5*(4), 219–225. doi:10.1097/sih.0b013e3181e77f74

Dieckmann, P., Manswer, T., Wehner, T., & Rall, M. (2007). Reality and fiction cues in medical patient simulation: An interview study with anesthesiologists. *Journal of Cognitive Engineering Decision Making, 1*(2), 148–168. doi:10.1518/155534307x232820

Diversity. (n.d.). In Merriam-Webster's online dictionary (11th ed.). Retrieved from http://www.merriam_webster.com/dictionary/diversity

Felder, R. M., & Solomon, B. A. (1998). Learning styles and strategies. Retrieved from http://www4.ncsu.edu/unity/lockers/users/f/felder/public/ILSdir/styles.htm

Fleming, N. (2001). VARK: A guide to learning styles. Retrieved from http://www.vark-learn.com/english/page.asp?p=categories

Fleming, N., & Mills, C. (1992). Not another inventory, rather a catalyst for change. In D. Wulff & J. Nygist (Eds.), *To improve the academy: Resources for faculty, instructional, and organizational development* (Vol. 11, pp. 137–155). Stillwater, OK: New Forums.

Foronda, C. L., Baptiste, D., & Ockimey, J. (2017). As simple as Black and White: The presence of racial diversity in simulation product advertisements. *Clinical Simulation in Nursing, 13*(1), 24–27. doi: 10.1016/j.ecns.2016.10.007

Goffman, E. (1974). *Frame analysis: An essay on the organization of experience*. New York, NY: Harper & Row.

Grasha, A. (1996). *Teaching with style*. Pittsburgh, PA: Alliance.

Hansen, E., & Beaver, S. (2012). Faculty support for ESL nursing students: Action plan for success. *Nursing Education Perspectives, 33*(4), 246–250. doi:10.5480/1536-5026-33.4.246

Hart, S. (2017). Today's learners and educators: Bridging the generational gaps. *Teaching & Learning in Nursing, 12*(4), 253–257. doi:10.1016/j.teln.2017.05.003

Hicks, N. A., & Burkus, E. (2011). Knowledge development for master teachers. *Journal of Theory Construction and Testing, 15*(2), 32–35.

House, B. M., Chassie, M. B., & Spohn, B. B. (1999). Questioning: An essential ingredient in effective teaching. *Journal of Continuing Education in Nursing, 21*(5), 196–201.

Jeffries, P. (Ed.). (2007). *Simulation in nursing: From conceptualization to evaluation*. New York, NY: National League for Nursing.

Joshi, G., & Bouck, E. C. (2017). Examining postsecondary education predictors and participation for students with learning disabilities. *Journal of Learning Disabilities, 50*(1), 3–13. doi:10.1177/0022219415572894

Kelly, C. (2008). Students' perceptions of effective clinical teaching revisited. *Nurse Education Today, 27*(8), 885–892. doi:10.1016/j.nedt.2006.12.005

King, C. (2017). Promoting student belongingness: "WANTED"—The development, implementation and evaluation of a toolkit for nurses. *Australian Journal of Advanced Nursing, 34*(3), 48–53.

King, K., Porr, C., & Gaudine, A. (2017). Fostering academic success among English as an additional language nursing students using standardized patients. *Clinical Simulation in Nursing, 13*(10), 524–530. doi:10.1016/j.ecns.2017.06.001

Kolb, D. A. (1984). *Experiential learning: Experiences as the source of learning and development*. Englewood Cliffs, NJ: Prentice Hall.

Lee, J., Lee, Y. Lee, S, & Baem, J. (2016). Effects of high-fidelity patient simulation led clinical reasoning course: Focused on nursing core competencies, problem solving, and academic self-efficacy. *Japan Journal of Nursing Science, 13*(1), 20–28. doi:10.1111/jjns.12080

Lown, S. G., & Hawkins, L. A. (2017). Learning style as a predictor of first-time NCLEX-RN success: Implications for nurse educators. *Nurse Educator, 42*(4), 181–185. doi:10.1097/NNE.0000000000000344

Moreau, P., Sullivan-Bolvai, S., Ndiwane, A. N., & Jaffarian, C. A. (2017). Development and psychometric testing of a measure to evaluate faculty engagement with underrepresented minority nursing students. *Journal of Nursing Measurement, 25*(2), E108–E129. doi:10.1891/1061-3749.25.2.E108

Rushton, T. (2017). Understanding the experiences of occupational therapy students, with additional support requirements, while studying BSc (hons) in occupational therapy. *British Journal of Occupational Therapy, 80*, 2–3.

Schublova, M. (2017). Learning styles and personality types of freshman level pre-athletic training major students. *Internet Journal of Allied Health Sciences and Practice, 15*(4), 2–7.

Silver, H., Hanson, J. R., & Strong, R. W. (1996). *Teaching styles and strategies (Unity in Diversity Series, Manual No. 2)*. Alexandria, VA: Silver and Strong.

Society for Simulation in Healthcare. (2018). *Certified Healthcare Simulation Educator Examination Blueprint, 2018 Version*. Retrieved from http://www.ssih.org/Portals/48/Certification/CHSE_Docs/CHSE_Examination_Blueprint.pdf

Stirling, B. V. (2017). Results of a study assessing teaching methods of faculty after measuring student learning style preference. *Nurse Education Today, 55*, 107–111. doi:10.1016/j.nedt.2017.05.012

Story, L., & Butts, J. B. (2010). Compelling teaching with the four Cs: Caring, comedy, creativity, and challenging. *Journal of Nursing Education, 49*(5), 291–294. doi:10.3928/01484834-20100115-08

Quirk, M. E. (1994). *How to learn and teach in medical school: A learner-centered approach*. New York, NY: Charles C Thomas.

Walton, J., Chute, E., & Ball, L. (2011). Professional nurse: The pedagogy of simulation: A grounded study. *Journal of Professional Nursing, 27*, 299–310. doi:10.1016/j.profnurs.2011.04.005

Woods, T. (2017). Human factors: Role of cognitive and social skills in clinical practice. *Emergency Nurse, 24*(10), 18–19. doi:10.7748/en.24.10.18.s24

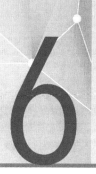

Interprofessional Simulation

SHARON GRISWOLD, KYMBERLEE MONTGOMERY, AND KATE MORSE

Alone we can do so little; together we can do so much.
—Helen Keller

his chapter addresses Domain I: Professional Values and Capabilities (Society for Simulation in Healthcare [SSH], 2018).

[LEARNING OUTCOMES]

- Discuss the history of interprofessional education (IPE) over the past century.
- Define IPE principles that foster a climate of patient/population care that is safe, timely, effective, and equitable.
  - Values and ethics (VE)
  - Roles and responsibilities (RR)
  - Interprofessional communication/Communication competency (IC/CC)
  - Teams and teamwork (TT)
- Discuss IC techniques in simulation-based education (SBE) to translate an improved team approach to daily patient care.
  - Application of closed-loop communication techniques in all professional interactions
  - Creation of a climate where providers apply a shared mental model
  - Support of learner understanding and respect of individual providers' roles and those of other professions to collaboratively address the healthcare needs of patients
- Discuss how IPE principles taught via SBE have begun to translate to patient care outcomes.

HISTORY OF IPE OR IE

The newly recognized and often-used acronym IPE has a variety of meanings and interpretations. The World Health Organization (WHO) defines *IPE* as a form of experiential learning whereby "students from two or more professions learn about, from, and with each other to enable effective collaboration and improve health outcomes" (WHO, 2010, p. 1). For many, learning through some type of active participation, experience, and reflection (experiential learning) provides a fresh lens in viewing the educational process (Kolb, 1984). To mimic real-life environments as the backdrop can be even more powerful. Thus, to practice together better, it is imperative that students have the opportunity to collaborate and learn together and from one another in a safe educational environment (Montgomery, Morse, Smith-Glasgow, Posmontier, & Follen, 2012).

BACKGROUND

The national recommendations to redesign the health education system to embrace the strengths of multidisciplinary skill sets are certainly not novel, nor did they develop out of a need to comply with the changes derived from healthcare reform. In fact, the origin of this challenge can be traced to the Flexner Report of 1910 (Flexner, 1910), and a call for healthcare educational transformations to include IPE initiatives has been a recurrent theme threaded through the following landmark reports of the Institute of Medicine (IOM) over the past half century (Table 6.1).

- *Educating for the Health Team* (IOM, 1972)
- *To Err Is Human: Building a Safer Health System* (Kohn, Corrigan, & Donaldson, 2000)
- *Crossing the Quality Chasm: A New Health System for the 21st Century* (IOM, 2001)

Unfortunately, although these reports provided the premise that IPE-based programs would decrease preventable medical errors through increased multidisciplinary team collaboration and communication and improved quality care delivery and patient safety outcomes, these challenges yielded slim results.

Years of escalating governmental spending, rising healthcare costs, numbers of uninsured and underinsured Americans, and fear of the individual's inability to afford basic healthcare spawned a unified consensus among governmental and private foundations to transform both the healthcare and health education system, strongly emphasizing the need for IPE in the United States (Montgomery, Morse, et al., 2012; Montgomery, Griswold-Theodorson, Morse, Montgomery, & Farabaugh, 2012). Rethinking the IPE's call-to-action initiatives was postulated in three well-respected and nationally recognized sentinel reports:

1. *The Future of Nursing: Leading Change, Advancing Health* (IOM, 2011)
2. "Framework for Action on Interprofessional Education and Collaborative Practice" (WHO, 2010)
3. "Health Professionals for a New Century: Transforming Education to Strengthen Health Systems in an Interdependent World" (Frenk et al., 2010)

TABLE 6.1

Historical Landmark Reports That Have Made Recommendations Regarding the Integration of Interprofessional Education (IPE) to the Healthcare Environment

LANDMARK REPORTS	IPE RECOMMENDATIONS
Flexner report (1910)	Suggests a full redesign of medical school education systems
Educating for the Health Team (IOM, 1972)	Challenges national healthcare educators and administrators to • Engage in IPE • Develop clinical settings to begin interprofessional innovation • Lobby governmental and professional support of IPE for healthcare delivery teams
To Err Is Human: Building a Safer Health System (Kohn, Corrigan, & Donaldson, 2000)	Encourages the reduction of preventable medical errors through • Provision of support to multidisciplinary teams of researchers, healthcare facilities, and organizations to determine the causes of medical errors • Development of new knowledge to assist in the creation of demonstration projects
Crossing the Quality Chasm: A New Health System for the 21st Century (IOM, 2001)	Provisions made to ensure licensing and accreditation organizations begin the evolution of our siloed educational processes through • Stressing evidence-based practice instruction • Providing opportunities for interprofessional training
Health Professions Education: Building a Bridge to Quality (Greiner & Knebel, 2003)	Reiterates the need for *all* healthcare professionals to be • Educated to deliver patient-centered care as members of an interprofessional team • Prepared to use evidence-based practice, quality-improvement approaches, and informatics
The Future of Nursing: Leading Change, Advancing Health (IOM, 2011)	Recommends that nurses need to be an integral part of the healthcare team by • Practicing to the full extent of their education and training • Intertwining advanced competencies within higher levels of training and education • Becoming equal partners in redesigning and improving healthcare • Participating in workforce planning and policymaking initiatives
Framework for Action on Interprofessional Education and Collaborative Practice (WHO, 2010)	Provides strategies to support global health workforce and • Identifies the necessity of IPE education and collaboration strategies to increase health profession workforce • Defines IPE as the future of health education and essential in the delivery of quality patient care

(continued)

TABLE 6.1

Historical Landmark Reports That Have Made Recommendations Regarding the Integration of Interprofessional Education (IPE) to the Healthcare Environment (*continued*)

LANDMARK REPORTS	IPE RECOMMENDATIONS
"Health Professions for a New Century: Transforming Education to Strengthen Health Systems in an Interdependent World" (Frenk et al., 2010)	Suggests that health education reform should • Promote interprofessional and transprofessional education that breaks down professional siloes • Encourage collaborative and nonhierarchical relationships in effective teams • Promote a new century of transformative professional education
Measuring the Impact of Interprofessional Education on Collaborative Practice and Patient Outcomes (IOM, 2015)	Examine the methods necessary to measure IPE impact on collaborative practice and heath and system outcomes. Develop a model template for the evaluation of IPE that is adaptable to a particular setting in which it is applied.

IOM, Institute of Medicine; IPE, interprofessional education; WHO, World Health Organization.

Many years after the initial IOM call to action for collaboration among healthcare professionals, six of the major national healthcare organizations convened an expert panel to produce documents containing the foundation of IPE (Montgomery, Morse, et al., 2012). *Team-Based Competencies: Building a Shared Foundation for Education and Clinical Practice* (The Josiah Macy Jr. Foundation, 2011) and *Core Competencies for Interprofessional Collaborative Practice* (American Association of Colleges of Nursing, 2011) define four measurable core competency domains and 38 subcompetencies for curriculum foundation for IPE and practice in all healthcare realms:

1. VE for interprofessional practice
2. RR
3. IC
4. TT

Since the development of these competencies, IPE has been gaining popularity and recognition across the country. Accreditation body endorsement, new IPE-specific faculty development and training program offerings, increased dissemination and promotion of the IPE competences, and the opening of the first National Center for Interprofessional Education and Practice are only a few of many indications that IPE is the future of healthcare education (Interprofessional Education Collaborative [IPEC], 2016).

In 2016, the IPEC Board, with an additional representation from nine new professions, reconvened to "reaffirm the original competencies, ground the competency model firmly under the singular domain of interprofessional collaboration, and broaden the competencies to better integrate population health approaches across the health and partner professions. This action will enhance collaboration for improving both individual care and population health outcomes" (IPEC, 2016, p. 3). This has resulted in the development of a Josiah Macy Jr. Foundation funded IPEC PORTAL Collection, a collection of peer-reviewed educational resources and materials supporting IPE instruction and the redesign of competencies that reflect the inclusion of population health competencies.

> **IPEC 2016 UPDATE**
>
> 1. Reaffirm the dissemination and impact of the 2011 core competencies.
> 2. Reorganize the competencies within the single domain of interprofessional collaboration instead of domains within IPE.
> 3. Attempt to achieve the Triple Aim (improve the patient experience of care, improve the health of populations, and reduce the per capita cost of healthcare) by expanding the interprofessional competencies with a population health focus.

GENERAL IPE COMPETENCIES

The aforementioned competencies for IPE in health professions were developed by the IPEC, an expert panel that included the American Association of Colleges of Nursing, the American Association of Colleges of Osteopathic Medicine, the American Association of Colleges of Pharmacy, the American Dental Education Association, the Association of American Medical Colleges, and the Association of Schools of Public Health. The overarching goal of this collaboration was to develop individual-level core interprofessional competencies. Originally developed with an authentic patient-practice focus, these definitions are also foundational to IPE in simulated environments. IPEC defined *interprofessional competencies* in healthcare as "integrated enactment of knowledge, skills and values/attitudes that define working together across the professions, with other healthcare workers, and with patients, along with families and communities as appropriate to improve health outcomes in specific care contexts" (The Josiah Macy Jr. Foundation, 2011, p. 1).

The collaborative identified that core IPE competencies were needed in order to coordinate and direct the curricular revisions needed in health professions, including pedagogy and assessment strategies to promote success, to lay the foundation for a teaching curriculum in IPE that was connected to the development of student lifelong learning, to foster discussion regarding the divide between authentic patient care demands and IPE core competencies, to identify opportunities to integrate IPE content with current accreditation expectations, to provide a framework of common IPE competencies that would eventually link to a common set of accreditation standards, to provide licensing and credentialing bodies with potential testing content, and to promote the conduct of evaluation and research in this area to support outcomes (IPEC Expert Panel, 2011).

The competencies are based on a single, unifying concept, interprofessionality, which was originally defined as part of the work by Health Canada (D'Amour &

Oandasan, 2005). It refers not merely to practicing in the same room or on the same team, but to a deliberate practice of professionals to reflect and develop an integrated practice model focused on addressing the needs at the level of patient/family or population. The key elements include constant knowledge sharing between professionals and an emphasis on active patient participation. This is a paradigm shift from traditional care teams and educational models in most health professions. Thus, the development of core IPE competencies to describe the unique attributes of IPE practice was needed. The intent of the publication and competencies was to remain general in nature to provide for individual profession and institutional flexibility. In 2016, as part of the competencies revisions, the four domains listed earlier (VE, RR, IC, TT) now reside under the single domain of interprofessional collaboration (Figure 6.1).

Exhibit 6.1 demonstrates IPE core competencies from the IPEC (Dieckmann, Molin Friis, Lippert, & Østergaard, 2009).

Each of the four core competencies or domains is further delineated into specific IPE competencies that are outlined here.

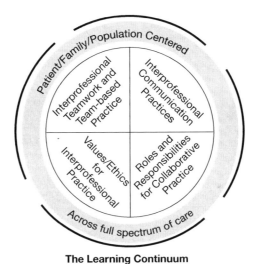

Figure 6.1 Interprofessional collaborative practice core competency domains.

Source: Reprinted under creative commons permission from the 2016 IPEC©.

EXHIBIT 6.1

Core Competencies for Interprofessional Collaborative Practice From the IPEC

1. VE. Work with individuals of other professions to maintain a climate of mutual respect and shared values.
2. RR. Use the knowledge of one's own role and those of other professions to appropriately assess and address the healthcare needs of the patients and to promote and advance the health of populations.

> **EXHIBIT 6.1 (continued)**
>
> 3. CC. Communicate with patients, families, communities, and professionals in health and other fields in a responsive and responsible manner that supports a team approach to the promotion and maintenance of health and the prevention treatment of disease.
> 4. TT. Apply relationship-building values and the principles of team dynamics to perform effectively in different team roles to plan, deliver, and evaluate patient/population-centered care and population health programs and programs that are safe, timely, effective, and equitable.

IC/CC, interprofessional communication; RR, roles and responsibilities; TT, teams and teamwork; VE, values and ethics.

Detailed VE Competencies

This domain moves beyond the individual's professional ethics and focuses on the development of interprofessional ethics.

- VE 1. Place the interests of patients and populations at the center of the IPE healthcare delivery and population health programs and policies, with the goal of promoting health and health equity across the life span.
- VE 2. Respect the dignity and privacy of patients while maintaining confidentiality in the delivery of team-based care.
- VE 3. Embrace the cultural diversity and individual differences that characterize patients, populations, and the health team.
- VE 4. Respect the unique cultures, values, roles/responsibilities, and expertise of other health professions and the impact these factors can have on health outcomes.
- VE 5. Work in cooperation with those who receive care, those who provide care, and those who contribute to or support the delivery of prevention and health services and programs.
- VE 6. Develop a trusting relationship with patients, families, and other team members.
- VE 7. Demonstrate high standards of ethical conduct and quality of care in one's contribution to team-based care.
- VE 8. Manage ethical dilemmas specific to interprofessional patient/population-centered care situations.
- VE 9. Act with honesty and integrity in relationships with patients, families, communities, and other team members.
- VE 10. Maintain competence in one's own profession appropriate to scope of practice.

Detailed RR Competencies

The interaction between understanding your own and others' RR within an interprofessional team while providing patient-centered or population-focused care are delineated in the RR-specific competencies. Each profession's RR is delineated within a legal scope of practice that may be significantly influenced by practice environment, region, or location. However, within the appropriate scope of practice, RR may vary depending on the particular situation. The specific RR subcompetencies are:

- RR 1. Communicate one's RR clearly to patients, families, community members, and other professions.
- RR 2. Recognize one's limitations in skills, knowledge, and abilities.
- RR 3. Engage diverse professionals who complement one's own professional expertise, as well as associated resources, to develop strategies to meet specific patient health and healthcare needs of patients and populations.
- RR 4. Explain the RR of other care providers and how the team works together to provide care, promote health, and prevent disease.
- RR 5. Use the full scope of knowledge, skills, and abilities of professionals from health and other fields to provide care that is timely, safe, effective, and equitable.
- RR 6. Communicate with team members to clarify each member's responsibility in executing components of a treatment plan or public health intervention.
- RR 7. Forge interdependent relationships with other professions within and outside the health system to improve care and advance learning.
- RR 8. Engage in continuous professional and interprofessional development to enhance team performance and collaboration.
- RR 9. Use unique and complementary abilities of all members of the team to optimize health and patient care.
- RR 10. Describe how professionals in health and other fields can collaborate and integrate clinical care and public health interventions to optimize population health.

Detailed IC Competencies

These subcompetencies expound on the critical nature of effective verbal, written, and health literacy communication to promote interprofessional collaboration. This includes using a shared language that is known to all team members. The following is a list of positive communication techniques (Cochrane, Baker, & Meudell, 1998):

- CC 1. Choose effective communication tools and techniques, including information systems and communication technologies, to facilitate discussions and interactions that enhance team function.
- CC 2. Communicate information with patients, families, community members, and health team members in a form that is understandable, avoiding discipline-specific terminology when possible.
- CC 3. Express one's knowledge and opinions to team members involved in patient care and population health improvement with confidence, clarity, and respect, working to ensure common understanding of information and treatment and care decisions, and population health programs and policies.
- CC 4. Listen actively, and encourage ideas and opinions of other team members.
- CC 5. Give timely, sensitive, instructive feedback to others about their performance on the team, responding respectfully as a team member to feedback from others.

- CC 6. Use respectful language appropriate for a given difficult situation, crucial conversation, or interprofessional conflict.
- CC 7. Recognize how one's own uniqueness (experience level, expertise, culture, power and hierarchy within the health team) contributes to effective communication, conflict resolution, and positive interprofessional relationships.
- CC 8. Communicate the importance of teamwork in patient-centered care and population health programs and policies.

Detailed TT Competencies

The last subcompetencies address the concepts of effective team members and team behaviors that may influence, positively or negatively, the team's overall effectiveness.

- TT 1. Describe the process of team development and the roles and practices of effective teams.
- TT 2. Develop consensus on the ethical principles to guide all aspects of teamwork.
- TT 3. Engage health and other professionals in shared patient-centered and population-focused problem-solving.
- TT 4. Integrate the knowledge and experience of health and other professions to inform health and care decisions, while respecting patient and community values and priorities/preferences for care.
- TT 5. Apply leadership practices that support collaborative practice and team effectiveness.
- TT 6. Engage self and others to manage constructively disagreements about values, roles, goals, and actions that arise among

> **SIMULATION TEACHING TIP 6.1**
>
> *Pearls and Pitfalls Implementing Interprofessional SBE*
>
> **Pearls**
>
> Medical errors can often be traced back to common root causes: lack of team communication or provider knowledge or organizational transfer of knowledge to a relevant clinical encounter (Agency for Healthcare Research and Quality [AHRQ], 2003).
>
> One of the greatest changes in the healthcare communication culture may be advanced by bringing multidisciplinary healthcare professionals together to practice improved situational awareness, a shared mental model, or "huddle" as defined by TeamSTEPPS (AHRQ, 2012). The TeamSTEPPS curriculum is jointly developed by the Department of Defense and the AHRQ in the United States to improve institutional collaboration and communication relating to patient safety. The cultural implications of any team member speaking up when concerned and open sharing of situational monitoring of the STEP (*s*tatus of the patient, *t*eam status, *e*nvironment, and *p*rogress toward the goal) are best practiced in the simulation environment. The TeamSTEPPS educational materials are readily available in the public domain: teamstepps.ahrq.gov.
>
> **Pitfalls**
>
> The enormity of bringing healthcare providers together to practice without risk to patients and to improve patient care is systematically challenging. The practical issues of scheduling and time commitment may be some of the most significant barriers to successful implementation. Successful implementation requires a committed interprofessional team of educators.

health and other professionals and with patients, families, and community members.
- TT 7. Share accountability with other professions, patients, and communities for outcomes relevant to prevention and healthcare.
- TT 8. Reflect on individual and team performance for individual as well as team performance improvement.
- TT 9. Use process-improvement strategies to increase the effectiveness of interprofessional teamwork and team-based services, programs, and policies.
- TT 10. Use available evidence to inform effective teamwork and team-based practices.
- TT 11. Perform effectively on teams and in different team roles in a variety of settings.

> **EVIDENCE-BASED SIMULATION PRACTICE 6.1**
>
> Teamwork training, including IPE principles conducted using simulation and debriefing, has begun to translate to improved patient care process outcomes (Marr et al., 2012; Riley et al., 2011; Starmer et al., 2014). Although it is extremely difficult to understand the specific methodology used in each of these studies to definitively understand what, when, and how IPE principles practiced outside of the patient care environment lead to patient care improvements, the following studies are promising. In 2010, Capella et al. (2010) studied trauma team performance after simulation-based TeamSTEPPS Training. In this study, the time to CT, time to tracheal intubation, and appropriateness of time to the operating room were all significantly improved after training. Additional studies (Marr et al., 2012; Steinemann et al., 2011) have been able to demonstrate similar patient care process outcomes after multidisciplinary providers practiced high-stress clinical situations in a simulated environment.
>
> Riley et al. (2011) demonstrated that a simulation-based intervention in addition to interprofessional team training resulted in a statistically significant 37% improvement in perinatal morbidity scores. The authors used the Weighted Adverse Outcome Score measure of perinatal morbidity and a culture-of-safety survey (safety attitudes questionnaire) before and after intervention to compare three hospital groups. The first group served as a control, and the second hospital received the U.S. AHRQ-supported curriculum, the TeamSTEPPS didactic training program. The third hospital received both the TeamSTEPPS program and a series of in situ simulation training exercises. The authors found that a comprehensive interprofessional team training program using in situ simulation in addition to interprofessional educational team training in nontechnical skills improved perinatal safety in the hospital setting. They also reinforced the idea that didactic instruction alone without simulation was not effective in improving perinatal outcomes.
>
> In 2013, Theilen et al. (2013) published a prospective cohort study of all deteriorating inpatients of a tertiary pediatric hospital requiring admission to pediatric intensive care unit the year before and after the introduction of pediatric

> **EVIDENCE-BASED SIMULATION PRACTICE 6.1 (*continued*)**
>
> rapid-response medical emergency team (pMET) and concurrent team training. The article suggests improvements in patient outcomes were specifically related to the in situ simulation training. Lessons learned by ward staff during regular training that brought physicians and nurses together for weekly, in situ team training led to significantly improved recognition and management of deteriorating inpatients with evolving critical illness. A follow-up study published in 2017 (Theilen, Fraser, Jones, Leonard, & Simpson, 2017) demonstrated a sustained improvement in the hospital response to critically deteriorating inpatients, significantly improved patient outcomes, and substantial cost savings after exposure to an IPE simulation education curriculum.
>
> It is imperative to understand the methodology of these recent studies to determine how IPE and other simulation-based interventions have contributed to each study's success and limitations to improve patient care via simulation.

> **CASE STUDY 6.1**
>
> A Certified Healthcare Simulation Educator™ (CHSE™) is arranging an interprofessional simulation experience with multiple disciplines in a teaching hospital laboratory. All the healthcare professionals are licensed and needed for the simulation experience of a prolapsed cord on a laboring patient. It is imperative that nursing, medicine, the obstetrical operating-room team, respiratory, and neonatology disciplines respond. The simulation experience is scheduled three separate times, and all three times, one of the participants cancels due to "being busy in the labor-and-delivery suites." What pitfall is the CHSE falling into and how can this be overcome?

■ PRACTICE QUESTIONS

1. Which of the following is the overarching domain identified for interprofessional education (IPE)?

    A. Interprofessional collaboration
    B. Team communication
    C. Interprofessional teamwork
    D. Scope of practice

2. The simulation educator overhears a participant of the interprofessional education (IPE) experience raising her voice loudly and stating an order to someone in a different discipline without addressing this person by name. The simulation educator would best handle this situation initially by:

    A. Exploring the action observed in the debriefing following the case
    B. Ignoring the behavior and focusing on the medical management of the case
    C. Reporting the participant to her supervisor for remediation
    D. Stopping the scenario, removing the participant, and restarting the scenario

3. The most common cause of error in authentic patient care is which of the following?

    A. Lack of knowledge
    B. Inadequate resources
    C. Lack of communication
    D. Lack of leadership

4. Experiential learning includes components of:

    A. Laboratory experimentation
    B. Surface memory acquisition
    C. Active participation
    D. Didactic education

5. The goal of all the Institute of Medicine (IOM) reports is:

    A. Better patient care
    B. Reduction of healthcare retirements
    C. Increasing technology knowledge
    D. Decreasing healthcare errors

6. The essence of interprofessional education (IPE) is:

    A. Cooperation
    B. Knowing scopes of practice for each role
    C. Collaboration
    D. Meeting accreditation standards

7. The Interprofessional Education Collaboration (IPC) program places mutual respect in which core competency?

    A. Values and ethics
    B. Roles and responsibilities
    C. Communication
    D. Teamwork

8. The Interprofessional Education Collaboration (IPC) program places relationship-building into which core competency?

    A. Values and ethics
    B. Roles and responsibilities
    C. Communication
    D. Teamwork

9. The Interprofessional Education Collaboration (IPC) program places expressing one's knowledge and opinion into which core competency?

    A. Values and ethics
    B. Roles and responsibilities
    C. Communication
    D. Teamwork

10. The Interprofessional Education Collaboration (IPC) program places integrating knowledge into which core competency?
   A. Values and ethics
   B. Roles and responsibilities
   C. Communication
   D. Teamwork

REFERENCES

Agency for Healthcare Research and Quality. (2003). *AHRQ's patient safety initiative: Building foundations, reducing risk* (Chapter 2). Retrieved from http://www.ahrq.gov/research/findings/final-reports/pscongrpt/psini2.html

Agency for Healthcare Research and Quality. (2012). TeamSTEPPS: National implemenation. Retrieved from http://teamstepps.ahrq.gov

American Association of Colleges of Nursing. Team-Based Competencies Building a Shared Foundation for Education and Clinical Practice. (2011). Health Resources Service Administration. Retrieved from http://www.aacn.nche.edu/leading-initiatives/IPECProceedings.pdf

Capella, J., Smith, S., Philp, A., Putnam, T., Gilbert, C., Fry, W., & Remine, S. (2010). Teamwork training improves the clinical care of trauma patients. *Journal of Surgical Education, 67*(6), 439–443. doi:10.1016/j.jsurg.2010.06.006

Cochrane, H. J., Baker, G. A., & Meudell, P. R. (1998). Simulating a memory impairment: Can amnesics implicitly outperform simulators? *British Journal of Clinical Psychology, 37*(Pt 1), 31–48. doi:10.1111/j.2044-8260.1998.tb01277.x

D'Amour, D., & Oandasan, I. (2005). Interprofessionality as the field of interprofessional practice and interprofessional education: An emerging concept. *Journal of Interprofesssional Care, 19*(Suppl. 1), 8–20. doi:10.1080/13561820500081604

Dieckmann, P., Molin Friis, S., Lippert, A., & Østergaard, D. (2009). The art and science of debriefing in simulation: Ideal and practice. *Medical Teacher, 31*(7), e287–e294.

Flexner, A. (1910). *Medical education in the United States and Canada: A report to the Carnegie Foundation for the Advancement of Teaching*. New York, NY: The Carnegie Foundation for the Advancement of Teaching.

Frenk, J., Chen, L., Bhutta, Z. A., Cohen, J., Crisp, N., Evans, T., ... Zurayk, H. (2010). Health professionals for a new century: Transforming education to strengthen health systems in an interdependent world. *Lancet, 376*(9756), 1923–1958. doi:10.1016/s0140-6736(10)61854-5

Greiner, A. C., & Knebel, E. (Eds.). (2003). Health professions education: A bridge to quality. Washington, DC: Institute of Medicine of the National Academies.

Institute of Medicine. (1972). *Educating for the health team*. Washington, DC: Institute of Medicine of the National Academies.

Institute of Medicine. (1999). To err is human: Building a safer health system. Retrieved from https://www.iom.edu

Institute of Medicine of the National Academies. (2001). *Crossing the quality chasm: A new health system for the 21st century*. Retrieved from http://iom.edu/Reports/2001/Crossing-the-Quality-Chasm-A-New-Health-System-for-the-21st-Century.aspx

Institute of Medicine. (2011). The future of nursing: Leading change, advancing health. Washington, DC: National Academies Press.

Institute of Medicine. (2015). *Measuring the impact of interprofessional education on collaborative practice and patient outcomes*. Washington, DC: National Academies Press.

Interprofessional Education Collaborative Expert Panel. (2011). *Core competencies for interprofessional collaborative practice: Report of an expert panel*. Washington, DC: Interprofessional Education Collaborative.

Interprofessional Education Collaborative Expert Panel. (2016). *Core competencies for interprofessional collaborative practice*. Update. Washington, DC: Interprofessional Education Collaborative.

Kohn, L. T., Corrigan, J. M., & Donaldson, M. S. (Eds.). (2000). *To err is human: Building a safer health system*. Washington, DC: National Academies Press.

Kolb, D. A. (1984). *Experiential learning: Experience as the source of learning and development* (Vol. 1). Englewood Cliffs, NJ: Prentice Hall.

Marr, M., Hemmert, K., Nguyen, A. H., Combs, R., Annamalai, A., Miller, G., … Cohen, S. M. (2012). Team play in surgical education: A simulation-based study. *Journal of Surgical Education, 69*(1), 63–69. doi:10.1016/j.jsurg.2011.07.002

Montgomery, K., Griswold-Theodorson, S., Morse, K., Montgomery, O., & Farabaugh, D. (2012). Transdisciplinary simulation: Learning and practicing together. *Nursing Clinics of North America, 47*(4), 493–502. doi:10.1016/j.cnur.2012.07.009

Montgomery, K., Morse, C., Smith-Glasgow, M. E., Posmontier, B., & Follen, M. (2012). Promoting quality and safety in women's health through the use of transdisciplinary clinical simulation educational modules: Methodology and a pilot trial. *Gender Medicine, 9*(Suppl. 1), S48–S54. doi:10.1016/j.genm.2011.11.001

Riley, W., Davis, S., Miller, K., Hansen, H., Sainfort, F., & Sweet, R. (2011). Didactic and simulation nontechnical skills team training to improve perinatal patient outcomes in a community hospital. *Joint Commission Journal on Quality and Patient Safety, 37*(8), 357–364. doi:10.1016/s1553-7250(11)37046-8

Society for Simulation in Healthcare. (2018). *Certified Healthcare Simulation Educator Examination Blueprint, 2018 Version*. Retrieved from http://www.ssih.org/Portals/48/Certification/CHSE_Docs/CHSE_Examination_Blueprint.pdf

Starmer, A. J., Spector, N. D., Srivastava, R., West, D. C., Rosenbluth, G., Allen, A. D., … Landrigan, C. P. (2014). Changes in medical errors after implementation of a handoff program. *New England Journal of Medicine, 371*(19), 1803–1812. doi:10.1056/NEJMsa1405556

Steinemann, S., Berg, B., Skinner, A., DiTulio, A., Anzelon, K., Terada, K., … Speck, C. (2011). In situ, multidisciplinary, simulation-based teamwork training improves early trauma care. *Journal of Surgical Education, 68*(6), 472–477. doi:10.1016/j.jsurg.2011.05.009

Theilen, U., Fraser, L., Jones, P., Leonard, P., & Simpson, D. (2017). Regular in-situ simulation training of paediatric medical emergency team leads to sustained improvements in hospital response to deteriorating patients, improved outcomes in intensive care and financial savings. *Resuscitation, 115*, 61–67. doi:10.1016/j.resuscitation.2017.03.031

Theilen, U., Leonard, P., Jones, P., Ardill, R., Weitz, J., Agrawal, D., & Simpson, D. (2013). Regular in situ simulation training of paediatric Medical Emergency Team improves hospital response to deteriorating patients. *Resuscitation, 84*(2), 218–222. doi:10.1016/j.resuscitation.2012.06.027

World Health Organization. (2010). *Framework for action on interprofessional education & collaborative practice*. Geneva, Switzerland: Author. Retrieved from http://apps.who.int/iris/bitstream/handle/10665/70185/?sequence=1

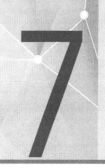

Ethical, Legal, and Regulatory Implications in Healthcare Simulation

BONNIE A. HAUPT AND COLLEEN H. MEAKIM

Excellence calls for character . . . integrity . . . fairness . . . honesty . . . a determination to do what's right. High ethical standards, across the board.

—Price Pritchett

his chapter addresses Domain I: Professional Values and Capabilities (Society for Simulation in Healthcare [SSH], 2018).

[LEARNING OUTCOMES]

- Discuss the regulatory requirements and issues that affect simulation practice.
- Outline the ethical and legal implications associated with healthcare simulation.
- Review the case studies and practice questions as they relate to legal, ethical, and regulatory issues that may arise during simulation scenarios.

Simulation use in healthcare education was developed to improve patient safety, enhance professional performance, reduce errors, and improve overall patient outcomes. Calhoun, Boone, Miller, and Pian-Smith (2013) believe that simulation permits consequences of errors from real-life events to be studied and recreated without causing patient harm. Simulation education must not only focus on creating a safe learning environment to protect patients from harm but it should also protect learners. Establishing trust in the learner–educator relationship is crucial to implementing successful simulation experiences. This chapter explores the importance of ethical, legal, and regulatory implications in healthcare simulation education, including the role of simulation in the development of the learner's personal professional integrity.

HISTORY

What thoughts come to mind when you hear the word "Tuskegee"? Do you think of the famous Tuskegee airmen, the African Americans who were trained to maintain and fly combat planes (Tuskegee Airmen, 2013)? Or do you think of the U.S. Public Health Service syphilis study at the Tuskegee Institute from 1932 to 1972 (Centers for Disease Control and Prevention, 2012)? The researchers involved in the study caused distress and pain for African Americans and their families by withholding treatment to those who had the disease. Are you familiar with the name Henrietta Lacks? In 1951, Ms. Lacks' cells were used without her permission or knowledge. The cells were used by the scientific community to develop cloning, gene mapping, and other historical research (Skloot, 2010). Ethical dilemmas created in the scientific community have led to changes in research involving human subjects to prevent ethical and moral harm. A code of ethics was developed by the American Educational Research Association (AERA) in 2011. This code governs the ethical standards and principles for researchers working in education (AERA, 2017). Hundreds of books and articles have been published to guide educators in educational ethics.

> **EVIDENCE-BASED SIMULATION PRACTICE 7.1**
>
> Reeves et al. (2017) developed a successful interprofessional simulation experience with medical, nursing, and physician assistant students using structured communication techniques to improve patient safety in the clinical area.

CREATING A SAFE ENVIRONMENT

The Agency for Healthcare Research and Quality (AHRQ) recognizes simulation as an educational tool used to enhance skills and allow healthcare providers to test new clinical procedures in a safe learning environment (AHRQ, 2016). According to Truog and Meyer (2013), for simulation to be credible, it must be developed on a strong foundation of safety and trust. Globally, simulation centers are developing standards and guidelines to create a safe environment focusing on creating protection of learners' ethical, legal, and regulatory rights. A review of simulation centers within universities and healthcare institutions found specific guidelines, including:

- Codes of conduct and confidentiality guidelines
- Learner evaluation processes
- Use of recording- and photo-use consent forms in release contracts

Codes of Conduct and Confidential Guidelines

Codes of conduct and confidential guidelines developed by simulation centers stress the importance of abiding by the Health Insurance Portability and Accountability Act of 1996 (HIPAA) regulations during simulation scenarios. Simulation experiences are to be considered as real-life events. Learners are expected

- To act in a professional manner
- To be prepared to participate
- Not to discuss the information outside of the simulation center

Sharing of information could impede the confidentiality of participants or affect other participants' learning opportunities. The International Nursing Association for Clinical Simulation and Learning (INACSL) Standards of Best Practice: Simulation^{SM} Professional Integrity (INACSL Standards Committee, 2016b) address the need for and the details associated with professional integrity, which needs to be maintained by everyone who is involved in simulation-based experiences.

> **SIMULATION TEACHING TIP 7.1**
>
> Many simulation centers ask learners to sign a contract letter prior to courses, agreeing to the confidentiality of the simulation experience, thereby creating an ethical environment for all learners.

Learner Evaluations

How learners are evaluated has received a great deal of interest from simulation educations and learners alike. Formative evaluation occurs during the learning activity or program with a goal of achieving specific objectives (INACSL Standards Committee, 2016a). The purpose of formative evaluation is to promote self-assessment along with constructive feedback for individual and/or group improvement (INACSL Standards Committee, 2016c; Jeffries & McNelis, 2010).

Summative evaluation takes place at the end of a learning period or other defined time frame, or can be used for a competency determination (INACSL Standards Committee, 2016c). Summative evaluations are used to award a grade, or degree, or to certify competency, using a standardized criterion (INACSL Standards Committee, 2016c; Jeffries & McNelis, 2010). When evaluating learners, they must be informed as to whether they are participating in a formative or summative simulation experience. When developing scenarios, healthcare simulation educators should determine the goals/purpose of the simulation and match them with the appropriate evaluation type. The INACSL Standards of Best Practice: Simulation^{SM} Participant Evaluation (INACSL Standards Committee, 2016a) outlines the details associated with participant evaluation for formative, summative, and high-stakes evaluation.

Recording and Photo Use

Wang (2011) believes learners can be guided by healthcare simulation educators during debriefing in reviewing learner objectives and performances. Recording of simulation experiences for debriefing purposes is widely used in healthcare simulation education. Cantrell (2008) highlights that video recording use during scenarios captures learner performance, which can be viewed with learners after the experience. Video recording may provide a moment of clarity for the learner during a debriefing session. Recording can recall precise interactions during the simulation to focus on what went well and what needs improvement, to allow for critical reflection. Recording consents and releases should emphasize the following:

- How long the material(s) will be stored
- Purpose of the recording
- That participants have no right to compensation

Simulation centers are also challenged with issues regarding religious objections to being recorded, and, in some instances, standardized (simulated) patients (SPs) who are members of the Screen Actors Guild who decline being recorded or photographed.

> **SIMULATION TEACHING TIP 7.2**
>
> Having a policy "up front" about expectations regarding video recording and picture taking will allow learners, standardized patients, and healthcare simulation educators to decide whether they can meet the learning outcomes or expectations of the experience if recorded debriefing is not done.

PROFESSIONAL DEVELOPMENT THROUGH SIMULATION

Part of the simulation process includes the development of the individual learner's understanding of the chosen profession's value system. Therefore, initially, learners and the healthcare simulation educator must come to a common understanding of what the group's professional value system entails. In the broadest sense, professionalism includes requirements for practitioners to be honest and responsible, which ultimately can lead to a sense of professional integrity (Wiseman, Haynes, & Solicitor, 2013).

However, both learners and educators share responsibility for the learning activities associated with simulation. Both must participate in preparation for simulation, as well as identifying knowledge gaps and strategizing to address these gaps. If these activities are integrated throughout the curriculum and constructed based on the profession's code of conduct, this process can lead to an enhanced moral reasoning process (Gillespie, 2005; Wiseman et al., 2013). If learners can develop their own personal and social responsibility within the simulated clinical environment, they should be more able to reflect and analyze situations to assist in clinical decision making (Wiseman et al., 2013). A complicating factor associated with the development and defining of norms for ethical behavior is the globalization of cultures. As the world becomes more global, clearly identified norms of professionalism become more difficult because of differences in cultural values and practices (Logar, Le, Harrison, & Glass, 2015).

Educators play a key role in the process of developing learners' moral and ethical reasoning processes. There are varieties of ways that moral and ethical situations can be woven into simulation activities, including simulations with overriding issues that have these components embedded in them. Scenarios focusing on specifically complex healthcare issues can include the following:

- Informed consent
- Patient confidentiality
- End-of-life care

- Care of vulnerable populations
- Genetic and reproductive issues
- "Do not resuscitate" or "allow natural death" orders

Such simulations can generate critical thinking, enhance communication, and allow for consideration of complex ethical issues from various participants. Participation in a mock ethics committee, in which learners assume various roles as committee or family members, is another example of an activity that can teach participants about communication-related issues for both medical personnel and families (Gisondi, Smith-Coggins, Harter, Soltysik, & Yarnold, 2004; Gropelli, 2010; Rostain & Parrott, 1986). In addition, microethical situations (those involving decisions that are more routine and everyday and include things such as poor infection control practices, unsafe or borderline medication administration practices, and/or breeches in confidentiality [Krautscheid, 2017]) can be embedded in a variety of simulation scenarios. Discussion of these issues as part of other simulation scenarios can strengthen overall ethical decision making.

SUMMARY

Simulation experiences were created to improve patient safety, enhance professional performance, reduce errors, and improve overall patient outcomes. However, it is extremely important to remember that protection of human rights applies to the learners as well. When developing simulation experiences, not only should there be an emphasis on objectives, methods, and outcomes, but healthcare simulation educators must also consider the importance of ethical, legal, and regulatory concerns when developing these experiences.

CASE STUDY 7.1

Review the following case study and answer questions 1 and 2.

The healthcare simulation team is excited to have received funding and equipment to develop a simulation training center. The group has worked tirelessly on developing and coordinating the first simulation scenario that will be piloted this fall with undergraduate students. The scenario objectives, methods, and outcomes focusing on a failure-to-rescue case will be presented. The simulation environment consists of high-fidelity mannequins and learners will be recorded during each session. The team has decided not to inform learners of the recording or that the findings of the scenario will be shared with administrators and could potentially cause learners to be removed from the program.

1. Reflect on what major ethical, legal, and regulatory implications the simulation training center team has overlooked in their planning phases for the simulation experience.
2. The simulation team wants to try a new product during a simulation scenario. Would the team need to obtain learner consent to participate?

PRACTICE QUESTIONS

1. Participation in ethical simulation experiences is important for healthcare professionals because they can assist participants to:
   A. Develop moral reasoning and recognize professional values.
   B. Learn to work out healthcare problems in a neutral way.
   C. Focus on the negative aspects of the healthcare professions.
   D. Rationalize behavior when making moral decisions.

2. A student is participating in a summative simulation activity and has failed in an area that has been identified as a "critical element." It is clearly stated in the testing guidelines that if a student misses a "critical element," the student must fail the exam. The evaluator is rationalizing that the student's omission is an oversight, and therefore the student should not be failed. What is the best action for the simulation leader/manager?
   A. Leave it alone as the faculty are the experts.
   B. Call in an administrator to lead the discussion about the situation.
   C. Inform the evaluator that his or her behavior will be reported to administration.
   D. Lead a discussion of the situation, identifying the policy and ramifications if the omission is ignored.

3. You are completing a summative testing session with students in an educational program. The testing session is about to start, but one of the faculty evaluators is not present because of traffic issues. She has phoned in and will be at least 60 minutes late. The Simulation Center leader/manager's best decision is to:
   A. Have the students wait until the faculty evaluator can arrive.
   B. Step in as a substitute evaluator until the faculty member arrives.
   C. Call in a substitute faculty evaluator with similar content expertise and testing training.
   D. Inform the students that they will have to return and be tested on a different day.

4. A student is participating in a simulation scenario and must give a medication. The correct calculation to give the patient should have been 0.5 mL of the medication and the student drew up and administered 0.6 mL. During debriefing, the student's response is that it was not a big deal because it was only 0.1 more milliliters than the desired dose of the medication. The facilitator's best response should be
   A. Well, it was not a critical medication, but next time please be more cautious.
   B. Any medication error is ethically important and should be considered serious.
   C. All medications should be given using the five rights of medication administration.
   D. If this were real life, this would be considered inappropriate and an event report would need to be completed as soon as possible.

5. A group of educators is creating an end-of-life scenario. In addition to creating the details about the patient and family, what other considerations related to designing the simulation are critical to make the scenario appropriate for the participants?

   A. Standards of care and culture of the region should be considered.
   B. Family-centered care is an essential element of the simulation design.
   C. The scenario must be based on a real-life situation.
   D. The scenario must include all healthcare disciplines.

6. A student is in the hall discussing the last simulation scenario with her peers. She states that the standardized patient had HIV and was being told for the first time about the disease. The healthcare simulation educator overhears the conversation. The appropriate action by the healthcare simulation educator would be to:

   A. Ask the students to take the conversation into a private room.
   B. Call the student who was discussing the patient later and explain that her conversation breeched confidentiality.
   C. Stop the conversation and explain that it breeches confidentiality.
   D. Explain to the students that if it were a real patient this would be a Health Insurance Portability and Accountability Act (HIPAA) violation.

7. A healthcare student states that he has had a bad day and does not want to participate in the simulation scenario that is scheduled. The healthcare simulation educator should:

   A. Remind him of the code of conduct to act professionally at all times.
   B. Excuse him for the day.
   C. Have him observe the scenario.
   D. Tell him he can make it up by writing a response to a case study.

8. The healthcare simulation educator wants to determine the intravenous administration competency level of junior healthcare students and then develop a module for remediation for identified weaknesses. This is an example of:

   A. Summative evaluation
   B. Ongoing assessment
   C. Competency-based simulation
   D. Formative evaluation

9. Graduates from a healthcare educational program see an advertisement for the educational organization on a billboard with their pictures in it from a simulation experience. The students did not give consent for the pictures to be used as external advertisements. This is an example of:

   A. Free trade
   B. Extended use of educational material
   C. Lack of consent
   D. Academic freedom

10. An example of a microethical situation embedded in a simulation scenario would be:

   A. Administering the wrong medication to a patient that causes an allergic reaction
   B. Forgetting to wash hands before touching a patient
   C. Forgetting to identify the patient
   D. Leaving a Foley in all night that was supposed to come out the evening before

■ REFERENCES

Agency for Healthcare Research and Quality. (2016). *Healthcare simulation dictionary*. Retrieved from https://www.ahrq.gov/sites/default/files/publications/files/sim-dictionary.pdf

American Educational Research Association. (2017). *Research ethics*. Retrieved from http://www.aera.net

Calhoun, A. W., Boone, M. C., Miller, K. H., & Pian-Smith, M. C. (2013). Using simulation to address hierarchy issues during medical crises. *Simulation in Healthcare, 8*(1), 13–19. doi:10.1097/SIH.0b013e318280b202

Cantrell, M. A. (2008). The importance of debriefing in clinical simulations. *Clinical Simulation in Nursing, 4*(2), e19–e23. doi:10.1016/j.ecns.2008.06.006

Centers for Disease Control and Prevention. (2012). *U.S. public health service syphilis study at Tuskegee*. Retrieved from http://www.cdc.gov/tuskegee

Gillespie, M. (2005). Student–teacher connection: A place of possibility. *Journal of Advanced Nursing, 52*(2), 211–219. doi:10.1111/j.1365-2648.2005.03581.x

Gisondi, M., Smith-Coggins, R., Harter, P. M., Soltysik, R. C., & Yarnold, P. R. (2004). Assessment of resident professionalism using high-fidelity simulation of ethical dilemmas. *Academic Emergency Medicine, 11*(9), 931–937. doi:10.1197/j.aem.2004.04.005

Gropelli, T. M. (2010). Using active simulation to enhance learning of nursing ethics. *Journal of Continuing Education in Nursing, 41*(3), 104–105. doi:10.3928/00220124-20100224-09

INACSL Standards Committee (2016a). INACSL standards of best practice: Simulation[SM] participant evaluation. *Clinical Simulation in Nursing, 12*(S), S26–S29. doi:10.1016/j.ecns.2016.09.009

INACSL Standards Committee (2016b). INACSL standards of best practice: Simulation[SM] professional integrity. *Clinical Simulation in Nursing, 12*(S), S30–S33. doi:10.1016/j.ecns.2016.09.010

INACSL Standards Committee (2016c). INACSL standards of best practice: Simulation[SM] Simulation glossary. *Clinical Simulation in Nursing, 12*(S), S39–S47. doi:10.1016/j.ecns.2016.09.012

Jeffries, J. R., & McNelis, A. M. (2010). Evaluation. In W. M. Nehring & F. R. Lashley (Eds.), *High-fidelity patient simulation in nursing education* (pp. 405–424). Sudbury, MA: Jones & Barlett.

Krautscheid, L. C. (2017). Embedding microethical dilemmas in high-fidelity simulation scenarios: Preparing nursing students for ethical practice. *Journal of Nursing Education, 56*(1), 55–58. doi:10.3928/01484834-20161219-11

Logar, T., Le, P., Harrison, J. D., & Glass, M. (2015). Teaching corner: "First do no harm": Teaching global health ethics to medical trainees through experiential learning. *Bioethical Inquiry, 12*, 69–78. doi:10.1007/s11673-014-9603-7

Reeves, S. A., Denault, D., Huntington, J. T., Orgrinc, G., Southard, D., & Vebell, R. (2017). Learning to overcome hierarchical pressures to achieve safer patient care: An interprofessional simulation for nursing, medical, and physician assistant students. *Nurse Educator, 42*(5S), S27–S31. doi:10.1097/NNE.0000000000000427

Rostain, A. L., & Parrott, M. C. (1986). Ethics committee simulations for teaching medical ethics. *Journal of Medical Education, 61*(3), 178–181.

Skloot, R. (2010). *The immortal life of Henrietta Lacks*. New York, NY: Broadway Paperbacks, Random House.

Society for Simulation in Healthcare. (2018). *Certified Healthcare Simulation Educator Examination Blueprint, 2018 Version*. Retrieved from http://www.ssih.org/Portals/48/Certification/CHSE_Docs/CHSE_Examination_Blueprint.pdf

Truog, R. D., & Meyer, E. C. (2013). Deception and death in medical simulation. *Simulation in Healthcare, 8*(1), 1–3. doi:10.1097/SIH.0b013e3182869fc2

Tuskegee Airmen Inc. (2013). Tuskegee airmen history. Retrieved from http://tuskegeeairmen.org/explore-tai/a-brief-history/

Wang, E. E. (2011). Simulation and adult learning. *Disease a Month, 57*(11), 664–678. doi:10.1016/j.disamonth.2011.08.017

Wiseman, A., Haynes, C., & Solicitor, S. H. (2013). Implementing professional integrity and simulation-based learning in health and social care: An ethical and legal maze or a professional requirement for high-quality simulated practice learning? *Clinical Simulation in Nursing, 9*(10), e437–e443. doi:10.1016/j.ecns.2012.12.004

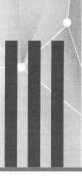

Domain II: Healthcare and Simulation Knowledge/Principles

Human Patient Simulator Simulation

CAROL OKUPNIAK

Simulation is fiction—your decisions are real.

—*John Cornele*

his chapter addresses Domain II: Healthcare and Simulation Knowledge/Principles (Society for Simulation in Healthcare, 2018).

[LEARNING OUTCOMES]

- Discuss the principles of human simulator simulation learning in healthcare education.
- Describe the variety of methodologies for the use of human simulator simulation.
- Describe the principles of interprofessional teamwork.

When considering the incorporation of human simulator simulations for the education of healthcare professionals, it is important to understand the principles, practice, and methodologies necessary for a successful simulation experience. Included in this understanding is knowledge of the relationship between the learner and the environment and how healthcare decisions will be assessed and evaluated. When using human simulators as an educational tool, the designer of the simulation scenario incorporates learning methodologies into the process of planning, implementation, and evaluation of the learning that takes place with human simulator simulation experiences. Among the outcomes measured during simulation scenarios are participation, attitude, knowledge, and skills (Issenberg, McGaghie, Petrusa, Gordon, & Scalese, 2005).

SIMULATION PRINCIPLES

Simulation-Based Learning

Simulation-based learning (SBL) is a process that occurs in a safe and carefully controlled setting that enhances skill acquisition and training using a simulated environment as the platform for learning (Lateef, 2010). Many healthcare institutions and academic settings are using SBL to educate and evaluate healthcare professionals and those in educational programs to become future healthcare professionals. Simulation is a technique that replicates real-life experiences with scenarios that immerse the learner in an environment that attempts to closely duplicate the clinical environment (Lateef, 2010). In addition to task and technical skills, SBL can also be used to identify problem-solving and decision-making skills. Team education, communication, and interpersonal skills are evaluated during SBL. To use simulation effectively, sound teaching–learning principles are needed. Without sound principles and planning, adverse consequences can easily occur during a simulation experience. For example, Lateef (2010) has identified common problems detected during simulation scenarios involving teams:

- Group does not understand that each team member has a unique role
- Lack of clear role definition resulting in role confusion
- No plan in place to use when mistakes or errors occur
- No method to measure individual or team performance

The success of using simulator scenarios to educate healthcare professionals should be measured in relationship to the improvement in clinical competence and the potential or actual impact on patient safety and outcomes.

Deliberate Practice

Using human simulator experiences gives the learner an opportunity to practice and acquire clinical skills without practicing on live human patients (McGaghie, Issenberg, Petrusa, & Scalese, 2010). A core principle of human simulator education is the concept of *deliberate practice* (*DP*). *DP* is defined as a learner's endeavor to practice for the purpose of improving a task or skill beyond the current level of proficiency (Gonzalez & Kardong-Edgren, 2017).

Using the concept of DP, simulation can improve the effectiveness of the learning experience. An integral component of DP is *critical reflection*. A student must recognize a deficit in knowledge in an effort to seek learning opportunities to narrow this gap in knowledge. With the assistance of a healthcare simulation educator, the learner becomes actively engaged in practicing and improving a task, skill, or decision-making process. When a learner engages in DP, feedback from the healthcare simulation educator is necessary to communicate improvement and identify areas that continue to need refinement (Ericsson, 2008).

Team Training

Many events in a healthcare environment require a cohesive team to accomplish their tasks (Andreatta, Bullough, & Marzano, 2010). Like a real clinical environment, human simulator scenarios most often include a small group of participants rather than just an individual learner. Knowing how to incorporate principles of team education and crisis resource management (CRM) into a scenario involving more than one learner will build this competency. The first step in team education in simulation is to articulate the specific competencies targeted toward acquiring team-building skills (Salas, Rosen, & King, 2009). Once these competencies are recognized, a level of measurement can be calculated to guide the debriefing process.

> **EVIDENCE-BASED SIMULATION PRACTICE 8.1**
>
> Badowski and Oosterhouse (2017) completed a quasi-experimental pretest/posttest design, a simulation-based, peer-coached, deliberate practice clinical substitution was implemented to compare nursing students' knowledge, skills, and attitudes for promoting safety. The results demonstrated improved knowledge and skill acquisition in the intervention and control groups. There was a trend toward improved team communication attitudes and skill performance.

Team-learning principals can be applied with a team of students from the same discipline or an interprofessional group using human simulator education. The Agency for Healthcare Research and Quality (AHRQ) developed a framework for building teams: Team Strategies and Tools to Enhance Performance and Patient Safety, or TeamSTEPPS (AHRQ, 2017). This process of team training is designed for healthcare professionals to improve patient safety and achieve better patient outcomes. Simulation aids in the acquisition of team skills by allowing the learner to practice in a simulated, safe environment. Using TeamSTEPPS in simulation is one way to aid in the design, measurement of objectives, and evaluation of team training (Table 8.1).

> **SIMULATION TEACHING TIP 8.1**
>
> If at all possible, when assigning learners to teams, make every team diverse. Diversity in race, gender, as well as role should be considered for every interprofessional team in order to teach cultural awareness and sensitivity as well as group collaboration.

Within TeamSTEPPS training is a principle known as *CUS*, which stands for

- "I am **c**oncerned!
- I am **u**ncomfortable!
- This is a **s**afety issue!" (AHRQ, 2017)

The purpose of CUS is to empower individuals to speak up if they are concerned about an actual or potential breach in safety. Included in the CUS course of action is a two-challenge rule (AHRQ, 2017). Under this rule, if individuals feel that their concern has not been recognized, they should:

- Verbalize this concern at least twice. If, after the second exchange, the team member concludes that the response is not acceptable, the team member is expected to take a different, more assertive course.

- This alternate course may include following the chain of command to ensure a safe environment.

TABLE 8.1
Components of Team Training in Human Simulator Simulations

Leadership	Delegates tasks to other team members, plans, organizes, and motivates other team members
Peer observation	Uses a shared understanding of group dynamics and team roles; is able to recognize errors and openly communicate ideas and suggestions for correction
Flexibility	Able to adapt or change as the scenario unfolds or the group dynamics change
Group membership	Recognizes that the work of the team is paramount and individual goals are secondary
Balance	The workload of all team members should be balanced and match the knowledge and skills of each individual
Trust	An atmosphere of mutual trust should exist in which individuals are able to share knowledge and speak about errors in judgment and action and accept constructive feedback
Communication	All members of the team are able to openly communicate, confirm that their message was heard and understood, and clarify the message if necessary

The use of the CUS rule can be employed during a simulation scenario and measured as part of the evaluation criteria.

Crisis Resource Management

Another method of assessing teams is through a process of CRM. When CRM began in the aviation industry, it was originally called *crew resource management*. CRM has been incorporated throughout healthcare education (Lucas & Edwards, 2017). A team is identified as two or more individuals with specific roles and tasks who make decisions by interacting and coordinating with one another (Baker, Gustafson, & Beaubien, 2010). The key principles of CRM are:

- Having a clear leader and well-defined roles
- Knowing your environment and resources
- Having a plan and sharing and adapting the plan as needed
- Requesting help early
- Distributing the work and supporting all members of the team
- Prioritizing and delegating tasks to others (Joshi, 2013)

Using the principles of CRM within a simulation scenario will help the team perform in a coordinated and efficient manner in the care of the simulated patient.

Closed-Loop Communication

When communicating to members of the team during simulator simulations, it is imperative that each individual's message is heard and understood. *Closed-loop communication* is a method of communication in which there is a sender and receiver of a specific message. The receiver of the message confirms the message that was communicated by the sender, thereby ensuring that the message was received and understood (Paramalingam et al., 2017).

EXHIBIT 8.1

Closed-Loop Communication

- A sender delivers a message to a receiver.
- The receiver of the message acknowledges that the message was received and ascribes meaning to the message.
- The sender communicates with the receiver to ensure that the expected meaning was conferred through the message.
- If the sender does not feel that the message was interpreted as intended, the conversation continues until the loop is closed.

ISBAR Communication

The acronym ISBAR stands for introduction, situation, background, assessment, and recommendation. ISBAR communication is an organized, structured method of two-way communication in a healthcare setting. The person conferring the information provides:

- I = Introduction, or who is providing the report and his or her role
- S = A short, but relevant summary of the current situation
- B = The patient's background relevant to the information exchange
- A = Important assessment findings
- R = A recommendation for action on the part of the receiver of the information

In many simulator simulations, it is expected that the participants communicate with each other, other disciplines, and those outside of the simulated environment using ISBAR communication (Marmor & Li, 2017).

SIMULATION METHODOLOGY

Experiential Learning

A methodology is the theoretical analysis of the body of methods and principles associated with a body of knowledge. Kolb's model of experiential learning is often applied to simulation learning (Kolb & Fry, 1975). Kolb's model places the learner into one of four learning styles. These styles are converger, diverger, assimilator, and accommodator (Wain, 2017).

- Convergers are best at problem solving and making decisions.
- Divergers are more creative and able to form new ideas.
- Assimilators apply inductive reasoning to a situation.
- Accommodators are those who are actively engaged and able to adapt quickly when the situation changes.

Each of these learning styles can be an asset during a simulation scenario (D'Amore, James, & Mitchell, 2012).

Contrasted with traditional, didactic learning, experiential learning requires the learner to solve real-world problems by discovering his or her own solutions based on his or her unique knowledge and understanding (Canhoto & Murphy, 2016). Inherent within the concept of experiential learning is how experience contributes to the process of learning. For learning to occur it is imperative that there is active participation with reflection on decisions made. In simulation, experiences are artificially constructed with the purpose of eliciting defined outcomes. Learning takes place through the simulation experience, during the debriefing process, and when participants conceptualize events and become involved in decision making (Koivisto, Miemi, Multisilta, & Eriksson, 2017).

Because the learners are living the experience during simulation, they are able to increase their engagement. Due to the reality of the setting, the learner is more engaged and interacts more fully in the activity. The goal of experiential learning is to gain new knowledge and understanding of key concepts or principles. During experiential learning, learners are asked to perform within a defined role in an activity that has context and meaning for the learners.

Adult Learning

Simulation is a technique that uses a guided experience to replicate the real world in a manner that is thoroughly interactive. Adult learners practice the concepts of andragogy (teaching of adults) in the simulation environment. Knowles (1950) developed the concept of andragogy. Adult learners are self-directed and independent and consider that they are responsible for their own learning. Adult learners also have experience and previously learned knowledge that can be used as a resource for future learning (Sanchez, 2017). Ensuring a proper environment for learning is another principle of adult learning. This is also the basis of using simulation to educate healthcare professionals.

Because simulation allows adults to practice skills and behaviors in a team environment, it has the ability to motivate adults to learn (Sarikoc, Ozcan, & Elcin, 2017). Adult learners expect their performance is confidential after a simulation is concluded. This is especially challenging when both the simulation and the debriefing are group experiences. The simulation educator, while providing a safe, rich learning environment, must maintain respect and support for the adult learner during simulation and maintain the confidentiality of all involved. In addition, the participants of the simulation must also respect the need to maintain confidentiality of the actions during the simulation scenario and debriefing to protect the privacy of all participants.

There are additional concepts related to adult learners not originally considered by Knowles (1950). Not all adults learn in the same way. Learning is situation specific, and there are many factors that affect the adult learner. One important factor of adult learning is how a person's culture affects learning and professional growth (Bleich, 2017). It is also assumed that adults experience information overload and are not capable of additional learning. It has been found that adults who perceive themselves as overloaded will continue to learn if they consider the activity an important and meaningful part of their development (Clapper, 2010). In addition to using simulation pedagogy to teach tasks, it can also be used to develop interpersonal relationships such as caring, compassion, empathy, comfort, and communication (Eggenberger, Krumwiede, & Young, 2015). The challenge for educators using simulation is to convey the importance and value of the experience for the adult learner.

Situational Awareness

Situational awareness is a method of continuous assessment of the environment. A construct of situational awareness in team activities is to inform all members about the individual's perception of the situation and environment so that everyone has the same understanding (Green et al., 2017).

This shared cognizance helps each team member to see the larger picture during a simulation scenario rather than concentrating only on an individual task. When situational awareness is employed during a scenario, all team members are kept informed and updated on the plan of care and all new developments in patient status. Having knowledge of available resources within the simulated environment will reduce the uncertainty of the learner and allows the learner to concentrate on making appropriate decisions (Tanoubi et al., 2016).

Perfect Practice

A novel approach to simulation learning is a methodology termed *perfect practice* or *do-overs*. This process allows the learner to complete a human simulator simulation, discover new knowledge from the debriefing session, and return to the simulated environment to repeat the same simulation with the new insight gained from the debriefing. Ishoy, Epps, and Packard (2010) found increased learner satisfaction and improved self-confidence when learners are permitted to repeat the simulation and are given the opportunity to provide feedback on their repeat performance. Repeated practice using simulation gives the healthcare simulation educator the opportunity to assess the student's skills to observe improvement while the student becomes more confident (Khunger & Kathuria, 2016).

■ HIGH-FIDELITY SIMULATION

The concept of simulation is not new in medical education. However, the use of high-fidelity simulators used in healthcare provider education has been a relatively new phenomenon. *Fidelity* is the measure to which the simulator or the simulation match the real environment the scenario is attempting to simulate (Maran & Glavin, 2003). Due to significant advancements in simulator technology, it is now possible to create a simulated environment using many high-fidelity strategies to construct a setting very close to the real world. Today's high-fidelity mannequins are capable of a multitude of physiologic functions. In addition to mannequin fidelity, there is also physical, functional, psychological, and task fidelity, which add to the realism for the learner. The higher the fidelity of the simulation, the more human and physical resources and time are needed when preparing and executing the simulator scenario (Alinier, 2011).

Current high-fidelity mannequins are available in models representing different stages of the life span from fetal and neonatal through adult. High-fidelity mannequins can be used for specific tasks, such as central-line placement, or whole-body mannequins can be used to respond with complex, multisystem, physiologic adaptation to the learner's actions or inactions. Advancement in the science of designing high-fidelity human simulators continues as technology improves. What is available today may seem primitive in only a few years as improvements in computerization, robotics, and materials science improve our ability to create a more realistic human simulator.

Functional Fidelity

Functional fidelity is the degree of accuracy in the operation of the simulated system. When operating a computerized, high-fidelity mannequin, the physiologic manifestations should be as close as possible to how a real person would respond. Responses to medication administration, oxygen delivery, and other treatments should be manifested in the mannequin as in a real human. An important consideration is the training of the simulator operator. Adequate training is imperative to be able to present a mannequin with high-function fidelity to the learner. As the simulation progresses, participants initially perceive the mannequin as a technically based nonhuman. The reality of the scenario improves and the responses become more meaningful as the participants interact with other people and objects within the environment (Kelly, Berragan, Husebo, & Orr, 2016).

Task Fidelity

Task fidelity is the measure of how authentic the simulated task is to the real task. It is important to match the task to the knowledge of the learner. During simulation, learners should not be expected to perform a task for which they have not been educated or that is outside of their scope of practice. Using complex simulators to educate a novice in basic skills is not necessary and may not be appropriate (Maran & Glavin, 2003). When using a simulator to learn a skill, the task fidelity should be very close to what the learner will experience within a real setting to avoid transferring negative motor skills and to promote transferring positive motor skills (Maran & Glavin, 2003).

Physical Fidelity

Physical fidelity refers to the environment where the simulation takes place. This includes the visual, auditory, kinesthetic or tactile, and spatial surroundings. When able, the setting should resemble the real clinical structures as closely as possible. Equipment and furnishings within the setting should be fully functioning. Attention to detail is an important part of physical fidelity. Some simulation centers take every aspect of the physical environment into consideration when preparing for a simulation scenario. Changing the room temperature, changing time on the clocks, and adding authentic odors are some examples of increasing the physical fidelity of a simulation scenario.

Psychological Fidelity

Psychological fidelity is the degree to which the learner perceives the scenario as real. This aspect of simulation fidelity is not always easy to secure. Simulations ask the learner to forget temporarily that the scenario is not real and engage in the activity, believing in its authenticity. It can take great effort to plan the physical, functional, and task fidelity, but it is up to the learner to consider the psychological fidelity of the scenario.

CASE STUDY 8.1

John is the healthcare simulation educator and he is running an interprofessional high-fidelity simulation experience that involves learners of medicine, nursing, respiratory therapy, and unlicensed assistive personnel (UAP). The scenario involves a patient with sepsis whose respiratory and circulatory status is declining to the point of circulatory collapse, and a "code" is initiated. During the code, the medical learner shouts orders to the other members and the nursing learners who are having difficulty finding the equipment in the "code cart" where it should be. The respiratory therapist is asking for guidance as to what he should be doing for the team effort. The UAP is recording the times of events. If you were the Certified Healthcare Simulation Educator™, how would you handle this situation? What aspects of team collaboration need to be emphasized? How would you prepare the next interprofessional team for the simulation experience?

■ PRACTICE QUESTIONS

1. The healthcare simulation educator identifies which common problem during a team-based scenario in which a student does not adequately check a patient's carotid pulse before beginning cardiopulmonary resuscitation (CPR) and another student begins to assist the first student with CPR?

   A. The group does not understand that each team member has a unique role.
   B. There was a lack of clear role definition resulting in confusion.
   C. There was no plan in place to use when errors occur.
   D. There is no method to use to measure individual or team performance.

2. Which student is participating in deliberate practice? The student who is:

   A. Thinking about his mistakes and trying again
   B. Doing a task over and over again without a break in between
   C. Reading up on the task that he is about to perform
   D. Discussing the task with the healthcare simulation educator

3. The student understands the goal of crises resource management when she states:

    A. "I should keep trying to figure out the correct patient intervention."
    B. "The team members need to provide each other with direction and I will do the intervention."
    C. "I should request help as soon as possible when a serious situation occurs."
    D. "I should flex my role during a serious situation and do what is needed."

4. The healthcare simulation educator realizes a student needs additional team training when he states:

    A. "When I become uneasy about an intervention being done, I will say something."
    B. "My only role is to remain at the bedside and calm the patient and family members."
    C. "Patient safety includes both physical and psychological safety."
    D. "Understanding CUS provides me with more autonomy as a practitioner."

5. During a simulation scenario, the team leader provides orders to another member who requests clarification of the medication dosage. This is an example of:

    A. ISBAR communication
    B. Reflective practice communication
    C. TeamSTEPPs communication
    D. Closed-loop communication

6. The student demonstrates the proper method of using ISBAR communication in a simulation scenario when he states:

    A. "I know you can give me an order to help."
    B. "The current vital signs are 99-92-24-86/40."
    C. "The past health history of this patient includes all of the following . . ."
    D. "The referrals made so far for this patient's discharge are . . ."

7. Having a high-fidelity mannequin that can close its eyes during a simulator simulation is an example of what kind of fidelity?

    A. Physical fidelity
    B. Functional fidelity
    C. Task fidelity
    D. Psychological fidelity

8. What type of experiential learner would a student be if, during a simulation scenario, he decides to try a new innovative intervention because the patient's condition is worsening using traditional methods?

    A. Convergent
    B. Divergent
    C. Assimilator
    D. Accommodator

9. The healthcare simulation educator allows a learner to repeat a procedure as many times as she would like. Studies demonstrate that "perfect practice" assists students to:

   A. Memorize procedures.
   B. Provide efficient patient care.
   C. Increase self-confidence.
   D. Decrease healthcare errors.

10. During a simulation scenario, a member of the team who has been actively engaged in the care of the patient quickly recognizes a change in the patient's condition, calls for rapid response, delegates tasks to the other team members, and administers prescribed medications before the patient's condition deteriorates. Which of Kolb's learning styles is this learner demonstrating?

    A. Converger
    B. Diverger
    C. Assimilator
    D. Accommodator

REFERENCES

Agency for Healthcare Research and Quality. (2017). TeamSTEPPS®: National implementation. Retrieved from http://teamstepps.ahrq.gov/about-2cl_3.htm

Alinier, G. (2011). Developing high-fidelity health care simulation scenarios: A guide for educators and professionals. *Simulation Gaming, 42*(9), 9–26. doi:10.1177/1046878109355683

Andreatta, P. B., Bullough, A. S., & Marzano, D. (2010). Simulation and team training. *Clinical Obstetrics and Gynecology, 53*(3), 532–544. doi:10.1097/GRF.0b13e3181ec1a48

Badowski, D. M., & Oosterhouse, K. J. (2017). Impact of a simulated clinical day with peer coaching and deliberate practice: Promoting a culture of safety. *Nursing Education Perspectives, 38*(2), 93–95. doi:10.1097/01.NEP.0000000000000108

Baker, D. P., Gustafson, S., & Beaubien, J. M. (2010). *Medical teamwork and patient safety: The evidence-based relation.* Rockville, MD: Agency for Healthcare Research and Quality. Retrieved from https://www.ahrq.gov/research/findings/final-reports/medteam/references.html

Bleich, M. (2017). Reducing stereotyping when developing leaders. *Journal of Continuing Education in Nursing, 48*(11), 492–493. doi:10.3928/00220124-20171017-04

Canhoto, A. I., & Murphy, J. (2016). Learning from simulation design to develop better experiential learning initiatives: An integrative approach. *Journal of Marketing Education, 38*(2), 98–106. doi:10.1177/0273475316643746

Clapper, T. C. (2010). Beyond Knowles: What those conducting simulation need to know about adult learning theory. *Clinical Simulation in Nursing, 6*(1), e7–e14. doi:10.1016/j.ecns.2009.07.003

D'Amore, A., James, S., & Mitchell, E. K. L. (2012). Learning styles of first-year undergraduate nursing and midwifery students: A cross-sectional survey utilizing the Kolb learning style inventory. *Nurse Education Today, 32*(5), 506–515. doi:10.1016/j.nedt2011.08.001

Eggenberger, S. K., Krumwiede, N. K., & Young, P. K. (2015). Using simulation pedagogy in the formation of family-focused generalist nurses. *Journal of Nursing Education, 54*(10), 588–593. doi:10.3928/01484834-20150916-08

Ericsson, K. A. (2008). Deliberate practice and acquisition of expert performance: A general overview. *Society for Academic Emergency Medicine*, *15*(11), 988–994. doi:10.11/j.1553-2712.2008.00227.x

Gaba, D. M. (2004). The future vision of simulation in health care. *Quality and Safety in Health Care*, *13*, i2–i10. doi:10.1136/qshc.2004.009878

Gonzalez, L., & Kardong-Edgren, S. (2017). Deliberate practice for mastery learning in nursing. *Clinical Simulation in Nursing*, *13*(1), 10–14. doi:10.1016/j.ecns.2016.10.005

Green, B., Parry, D., Oeppen, R. S., Plint, S., Dale, T., & Brennan, P. A. (2017). Situational awareness—What it means for clinicians, its recognition and importance in patient safety. *Oral Diseases*, *23*(6), 721–725. doi:10.1111/odi.12547

Ishoy, B., Epps, C. D., & Packard, A. (2010). "Do-overs" and double debriefing: A pilot study evaluating a different design for student simulation experiences. *Clinical Simulation in Nursing*, *6*(3), e117. doi:10.1016/j.ecns.2010.03.041

Issenberg, S. B., McGaghie, W. C., Petrusa, E. R., Gordon, D. L., & Scalese, R. J. (2005). Features and uses of high-fidelity medical simulations that lead to effective learning: A BEME systematic review. *Medical Teacher*, *27*(1), 10–28. doi:10.1080/01421590500046.924

Joshi, N. (2013). Crisis resource management. *Academic life in emergency medicine*. Retrieved from http://academiclifeinem.com/crisis-resource-management

Kelly, M. A., Berragan, E., Husebo, S. E., & Orr, F. (2016). Simulation in nursing education—International perspectives and contemporary scope of practice. *Journal of Nursing Scholarship*, *48*(3), 312–321. doi:10.1111/jnu.12208

Khunger, N., & Kathuria, S. (2016). Mastering surgical skills through simulation-based learning: Practice makes one perfect. *Journal of Cutaneous and Aesthetic Surgery*, *9*(1), 27–31. doi:10.4103/0974-2077.178540

Knowles, M. S. (1950). *Informal adult education: A guide for administrators, leaders, and teachers*. New York, NY: Association Press.

Koivisto, J. M., Niemi, H., Multisilta, J., & Eriksson, E. (2017). Nursing students' experiential learning process using an online 3D simulation game. *Education Information Technology*, *22*, 383–398. doi:10.1007/s10639-015-9453-x

Kolb, D. A., & Fry, R. (1975). Toward an applied theory of experiential learning. In C. Cooper (Ed.), *Theories of Group Process*. London, UK: John Wiley.

Lateef, F. (2010). Simulation-based learning: Just like the real thing. *Journal of Emergencies, Trauma, and Shock*, *3*(4), 348–352. doi:10.4103/0974-2700.70743

Lucas, A. & Edwards, M. (2017). Development of crisis resource management skills: A literature review. *Clinical Simulation in Nursing*, *13*(8), 347–358. doi:10.1016/j.ecns.2017.04.006

Maran, N. J., & Glavin, R. J. (2003). Low- to high-fidelity simulation—A continuum of medical education? *Medical Education*, *37*, 22–28. doi:10.1046/j.1365-2923.37.s1.9.x

Marmor, G. O. & Li, M. Y. (2017). Improving emergency department medical clinical handover: Barriers at the bedside. *Emergency Medicine Australasia*, *29*(3), 297–302. doi:10.1111/1742-6723.12768

McGaghie, W. C., Issenberg, S. B., Petrusa, E. R., & Scalese, R. J. (2010). A critical review of simulation-based medical education research: 2003–2009. *Medical Education*, *44*, 50–63. doi:10.1111/j.1365-2923.2009.03547.x

Paramalingam, V., Swift, S., Smith, O., Williams, M., Greco, P., Every, H., . . . Baker, A. (2017). Improving quality and safety in the ICU through the introduction of a procedural checklist and pause. *Canadian Journal of Critical Care Nursing*, *28(2)*, 64.

Salas, E., Rosen, M. A., & King, H. B. (2009). Integrating teamwork into the "DNA" of graduate medical education: Principles for simulation-based training. *Journal of Graduate Medical Education*, *1*(2), 243–244. doi:10.4300/JGME-D-09-00074.1

Sanchez, L. M. (2017). The Power of 3: Using adult learning principles to facilitate patient education. *Nursing*, *47*(2), 17–19. doi:10.1097/01.NURSE.0000511819.18774.85

Sarikoc, G., Ozcan, C. T., & Elcin, M. (2017). The impact of using standardized patients in psychiatric cases on the levels of motivation and perceived learning of the nursing students. *Nurse Education Today, 51*, 15–22. doi:10.1016/j.nedt.2017.01.001

Society for Simulation in Healthcare. (2018). *Certified Healthcare Simulation Educator Examination Blueprint, 2018 Version.* Retrieved from http://www.ssih.org/Portals/48/Certification/CHSE_Docs/CHSE_Examination_Blueprint.pdf

Tanoubi, I., Belanger, M. E., Georgescu, M., Perron, R., Germain, J. F., Robitalle, A., & Drolet, P. (2016). Identification tags and learners' situational awareness during high-fidelity simulation. *International Journal of Medical Education, 7*, 93–94. doi:10.5116/ijme.56ed.1060

Wain, A. (2017). Learning through reflection. *British Journal of Midwifery, 25*(10), 662–666. doi:10.12968/bjom.2017.25.10.662

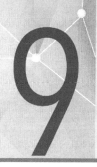

Moulage in Simulation

JOHN T. CORNELE AND LINDA WILSON

Start by doing what's necessary; then do what's possible; and suddenly you are doing the impossible

—Francis of Assisi

his chapter addresses Domain II: Healthcare and Simulation Knowledge/Principles (Society for Simulation in Healthcare, 2018).

[LEARNING OUTCOMES]

- Discuss the value of realism and the use of moulage in simulation.
- Describe the established methods of creating simulated injuries and medical conditions.
- Discuss the sources of moulage materials and possibilities of adding moulage to simulation sessions.

Moulage is a French term that means casting or molding; today, it is the art of applying mock injuries for the purpose of training healthcare personnel. The formal practice dates back to the 18th century, when wax figures and castings of body parts were used for this purpose (Riva, Conti, Solinas, & Loy, 2010). The concept of using models in education can also be seen in early Greek culture. Thus, the use of simulated injuries and illnesses, or moulage, to educate healthcare practitioners is not new, but its utilization in modern education is expanding.

This chapter provides an overview of moulage and its use in casualty and illness simulation. The chapter discusses makeup as well as an indication of the educational basis for its choice as a tool for use in simulation. Several broad areas are addressed, covering ideas involving the use of moulage in specific situations, with human patient simulators (HPS) or mannequins and with standardized patients (SPs), setting the stage by adding props and standardized participants (confederates), and some of the specific techniques as well as the process of clean up.

The more advanced concept of making your own moulage supplies and materials are also addressed. The chapter outline includes

- Educational basis for moulage
- Basic moulage supplies
- Actors and makeup—moulage for SPs
- Mannequins and makeup—moulage for HPS
- Special effects basics—creating props and setting the stage
- Striking the set—clean up and resetting the scenario

The use of moulage in a simulation scenario is limited only by the scenario developer's imagination and expertise. Care must be taken, however, to keep this imagination from running wild as excessive or inappropriate moulage or makeup can detract from the simulation or provide incorrect cues to the learners.

EDUCATIONAL BASIS FOR THE USE OF MOULAGE IN SIMULATION

Although there is a paucity of actual research on the use of moulage and makeup in educational simulation, anecdotal reports are plentiful. It seems logical that when speaking of simulation as an experiential learning tool, anything that enhances the reality of the learning environment is supportive of the learner's experience. The appropriate level of authenticity and realism can contribute to the degree of the engagement of the learner in the simulation and that in turn can enhance the learning (Stokes-Parish, 2017). Moulage, then, is one more tool that the educator can use to enhance the reality of the learning environment (Figure 9.1).

> **SIMULATION TEACHING TIP 9.1**
>
> In a study of critical care simulations for undergraduate nursing learners, Mould, White, and Gallagher (2011) were able to show that high-fidelity simulations increased both the confidence and competency of the learners. Although Mould et al. do not specifically mention moulage or makeup, the concept of increased realism is explored and found to be beneficial.

Caution should be exercised though, as improperly done moulage can detract from the experience. The choice to use or not use moulage should be driven by the objectives of the simulation and not solely by the expertise of the moulage artist. Makeup and props used for their own sake or to surprise or deliberately confuse or trick the learner will not support the learning outcomes and may send the learners down a false path by providing incorrect cues or information. This is not to say that moulage cannot be used as a distractor to add a higher level of difficulty to a scenario, but just that caution should be used. In fact, the use of varying complexities of moulage can quite nicely adjust the presentation to create several

> **SIMULATION TEACHING TIP 9.2**
>
> A word of caution: This is quite a captivating component of simulation and the more that you find yourself involved with moulage, the more tricks you will collect and the larger your makeup kit will grow until you find yourself pushing it around on a cart.

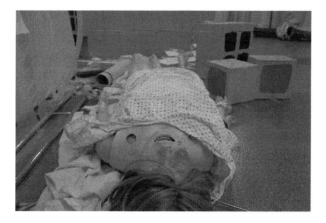

FIGURE 9.1 The Drexel University simulation lab.

Courtesy of Drexel University College of Nursing of Health Professions.

different versions of the same scenario, altering the amount and consistency of wound drainage, for example, leading the learners in one case to deal with an uncomplicated postoperative wound and in another with a grossly infected one. One must remember to match the need and type of moulage with the learning outcomes for the scenario.

■ BASIC MOULAGE SUPPLIES

Assembling a good, basic moulage kit does not have to be time-consuming or expensive. It is best to start small and keep the kit consistent with the state of one's moulage skills. In the beginning, you may only be focusing on one or two items or appliances, such as

- A few application sponges
- A color wheel of makeup
- Some glycerin and water
- A premolded commercial wound

In the beginning, some sweat, vomit, blood, and a wound or two may be all you need.

Table 9.1 contains a short list of some equipment you might need. As experience increases, the materials used to create injuries and illnesses become more varied. Advanced materials may include

> **SIMULATION TEACHING TIP 9.3**
>
> An easy recipe for sweat or diaphoresis is to mix approximately one-third glycerine and two-thirds water by volume in a bottle with a spray attachment. This allows easy application on either SP actors or mannequins. The more glycerine used, the more the solution will bead on the skin. Some experimentation may be needed to get a mixture that works just the way that you want it to. As a caution, the glycerine does tend to build up and get gooey and sticky if not cleaned thoroughly at the end of the day. Soap and water are usually all that is necessary for cleanup. As always, care should be taken around the eyes when working with actors.

TABLE 9.1
Suggested Basic Supplies for a Moulage Kit

SUPPLIES	POSSIBLE SOURCES
Makeup (a bruise wheel and burn wheel) Sponges (application) Sponges (stipple) Cotton-tipped applicators (lots) Makeup brushes (inexpensive to start) Liquid latex Spirit gum Cold cream Glycerin Petroleum jelly Tongue depressors (lots) Stage blood, both thick and thin Cleanup products Baby wipes Tissues	Halloween stores, theatrical supply stores, online stores, makeup counters, drug stores, etc.

- Liquid latex—exercise caution with regard to allergies.
- Silicone—both as premade purchased wounds as well as silicone adhesive used to assist in application.
- Gelefects and molding wax

■ PREPARING SUBSTANCES

When trying a new product, be sure to review its properties and characteristics before using it in an actual simulation. Working with a platinum silicone rubber compound is quite different when compared with a liquid latex preparation with regard to setting time and compatibility with plastics. Whatever you choose to work with, time should be set aside well in advance of the event to allow for familiarization with the product and the techniques needed to produce a realistic result. Substances that need time to dry or set may change your preparation timeline; moulage of the mannequins may need to be started hours or even days ahead of the simulation event. If using actors, in addition to the need for more time for application, new materials require a reassessment of sensitivities and allergies. The time to find out that the blood does not "run" correctly or that the pus is the wrong color or that the adhesive you chose makes the actor itch and breakout in a rash is not when students are in the scenario. Gauging the effect of moulage in a scenario is part of the testing process that should be done with any new or revised scenario.

■ MOULAGE FOR SPs

Using moulage with an SP can produce a greatly enhanced learning experience for the learner. The combination of the natural conversational interaction with a person as a patient, coupled with properly applied makeup or an appliance, can produce a very realistic environment. As Garg (2009) noted in a study of second-year medical students, simulation education improved the learner's ability to correctly recognize skin lesions as well as retain the clinical skill longer. The quality of the makeup used can have an impact on this process; the better the makeup or appliance (prosthetic), generally, the better the result.

MAKEUP

Although it is generally true that makeup used in simulations does not need to be expensive, a modest increase in investment can have a positive impact. A higher quality of theatrical-grade makeup from manufacturers, such as Ben Nye or Mehron to name but two, will produce more consistent results and be easier to work with. Frequently, companies, such as these, will package makeup in wheels or stacks that have colors grouped for specific purposes; bruise or burn wheels, for example. This makes the challenge of choosing the correct colors for the desired illness or injury easier. Makeup that is designed and tested to be used on people also can have a lower risk of allergic or sensitivity reactions. Quite a few of the commercial products are manufactured with this in mind, but it is always prudent to check using small amounts and allowing time for any reaction. Good-quality makeup can also be obtained from the obvious sources of makeup counters and drugstores; however, at times, the color selection for illness and injury can be a bit sparse. Although there are many good-quality sources of makeup available, determining what works best requires trial and error, and in the end, choices are frequently made by personal preference. The application of moulage on a live person will produce more satisfactory results mostly due to the fact that makeup blends better on the skin of the actor, and this process allows for more natural coloration and appearance. Materials that are designed for use on the skin work best in that environment. SPs are favorable to work with for several reasons.

> **SIMULATION TEACHING TIP 9.4**
>
> As you are learning moulage techniques, remember to take pictures of your work. This will show you your progression and, we hope, your improvement. At times, a static picture and quiet reflection by the moulage artist can reveal inconsistencies in technique as well as outright errors. In addition, this process will build a portfolio of your work as well as provide a reminder of past solutions to moulage challenges.

- Generally it is easier to produce more realistic results.
- Makeup blends more easily and consistently.
- Most human-approved adhesives work better.
- SPs can be taught to care for or refresh the makeup, shortening the reset time between encounters.
- They can assist with cleanup and removal of appliances.

Some drawbacks to working with live actors are that:

- They move (sometimes a lot).
- They have to go to the restroom (sometimes a lot).
- They may have allergies.
- They are sometimes fussy.
- It is sometimes difficult to get them to sit still for hours.

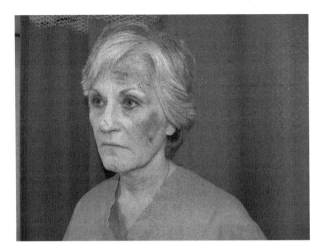

FIGURE 9.2 The application of moulage to a live person will produce more satisfactory results. The makeup blends better on the skin of the actor, allowing for more natural coloration and appearance.

It can be frustrating for the moulage artist if, after an hour of constructing a realistic wound, the patient returns from the restroom and states that the wound "just fell off." Patience is one other key ingredient that should be stocked in any makeup case (Figure 9.2).

MANNEQUINS AND MAKEUP: MOULAGE FOR HPs

Applying moulage to mannequins can be quite a challenge and produce widely varied results, especially when one compares the results achieved with live actors. The variation of the types of plastics that are found in the construction of most mannequins makes it difficult to have a standard approach to the application of makeup or appliances. Some of the issues encountered when working with mannequins and makeup are

- Blending of the makeup is more difficult and the results look less realistic at times.
- Some types of makeup can stain easily; this calls for all newly used makeup to be tested on a sample mannequin part or hidden area in advance. Generally, the softer and more porous the plastic, the greater the chance that staining may occur.
- When attaching appliances, some may not fit well unless specifically made for use with the mannequin in question.

SIMULATION TEACHING TIP 9.5

Recycling of old mannequin arms, legs, and so on, can produce parts with wounds that can be swapped out after the session. This can also help with the use of adhesives as well; if the limb will be reused to display similar wounds, permanently bonded appliances can be left in place.

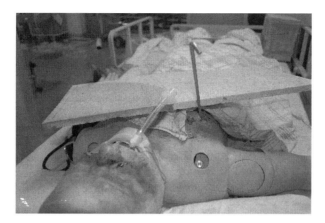

FIGURE 9.3 The Drexel University simulation lab.

Courtesy of Drexel University College of Nursing of Health Professions.

A concern that many people have when using makeup on mannequins is the fear that it will stain or permanently mark the mannequin. Although this is a valid concern, much of the higher quality makeup is useable with mannequins. Of course, the mannequin's manufacturer recommendations should be followed to take the most care. Cautious testing in an area that would not be seen if there is staining can produce favorable results and show which makeup can best be used (Figure 9.3). Testing on the reverse of the mannequin's chest skin or behind a removable leg pad or skin and then cleaning the area not only lets you know how the makeup behaves on the plastic, but also what is the best product to use for cleanup.

Another problem is the compatibility of the plastics with both the makeup that you are using as well as with the different types of plastics and adhesives that are used together. Care must be taken when combining plastics of different types, as some will inhibit the curing of some adhesives, leaving the appliance sliding off the mannequin. In addition, not all adhesives are created equal and do not stick to all plastics. One solution is to use a sheet of plastic material as a base, especially if it has some adhesive properties; a clear occlusive dressing comes to mind. At times, the challenge is finding an adhesive that has good sticking ability to keep wound appliances in place, but not so good that it forms a permanent bond or else you may end up with an unintentionally dedicated trauma mannequin.

Some mannequin manufacturers will produce wound sets that will fit onto their mannequins. These may not look as realistic as they should, and there is expense involved, but the ease of use may outweigh the investment. The realism can be enhanced with some makeup and a drizzle of blood. And if the part is repeatedly used in the same type of scenario, minimal staining may not be an issue. As with all moulage, some experimentation is needed to be sure what you implement is what you intended.

SPECIAL EFFECTS BASICS: CREATING PROPS AND SETTING THE STAGE

Many items needed for a simulation may be created as well as purchased. One is only limited by resources and imagination. Sometimes simply changing the mannequin's clothes, moving it from a bed to a stretcher, and adding a code cart will add the impression that care is being delivered in an emergency department. In the movie industry, this is called *setting the stage* or *dressing the set*. This should not be a daunting task or involve a great expense. Most often, the supplies that you need you can find in your environment or around you with only a bit of looking. A good source of wardrobe items for your mannequins may be only as far away as the local thrift store or an email to your faculty and staff requesting old cast-off clothing. Perhaps a short trip to a local beauty-supply store or wig shop for some new hair will really change the character of the patient: add a pair of glasses, a sweater, and a purse, and Mrs. Jones begins to emerge.

Empty cardboard boxes painted gray and black can make passable cinder blocks that can be used for the wall that will fall on the SP at the end of the disaster, providing yet one more victim; the best part is that they fold flat for storage, ready for use in future scenarios. Foam blocks painted gray will work as well but are more challenging to store. Making props and scene decorations can be fun and creative. Using props to add realism to the scenario makes it a much richer experience for the learners. All components should support the story and be logical additions that reinforce the reality for the learners. Props, however, should not get in the way or cause distractions, causing the learners to commit errors due to the incorrect representation of the scene. Therefore, it would seem that we need to construct completely realistic environments that use only real equipment and materials. That is not necessarily true; a fabricated prop can be valuable and inexpensive as long as it gives the proper and correct clue to the learner in the simulation. A cardboard box with the image of the front panel of a fetal monitor and actual monitoring strips pulled from the opening can assist the suspension of disbelief and provide information that the learner needs to navigate through the scenario. With props, as with moulage, if the learner spends more time trying to guess what he or she is looking at than getting useful information to use in the scenario, you have missed the mark.

> **SIMULATION TEACHING TIP 9.6**
>
> When designing the scenario, the character of the room should not be forgotten; it is as important to moulage the room as it is to moulage the patient.

STRIKING THE SET: CLEANUP AND RESETTING

The session is not over until the cleanup is done, and this can be one of the more challenging aspects of using moulage. It is wise to check materials used in moulage beforehand for ease of cleanup (Figure 9.4). Essentially, *striking the set* is a theater term that means to put the performance space back to the condition in which you found it. This means not only cleaning the mannequin and the simulation space, but also putting all the appliances and props away. If a logical and protective system is designed to store these materials when not in use, it will extend the useful life of the items. For example, the useable life of silicone- or latex-molded wounds can be extended if they are cleaned properly, removing excess adhesive and makeup, and stored in an air-tight container with a light dusting of talcum powder. Proper care of moulage supplies will ensure they will be available for many more uses. Props and wardrobes of both the mannequin and the SP should be stored in a way that will make them easily accessible for the next session. One method is to create a scenario container to house all the essentials for that scenario; this will help to keep all materials in one place, and if the storage container is portable, it may be taken to the location of the mannequin or actor during setup.

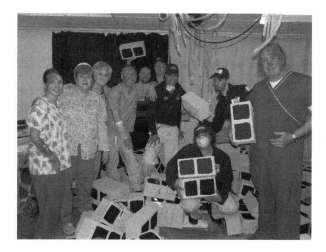

FIGURE 9.4 Striking the set; cleanup and resetting the scene.

Cleaning materials needed for after the sessions are not much different than those needed for daily cleanup in the simulation laboratory. Sponges and non-bleach-containing wipes are staples. Attention should be paid to items that can be used on humans, gentle cleansing wipes and makeup remover, cold cream, and the like. Mannequins may need some additional help, adhesive removers and alcohol, for instance. Some common needs for cleanup are as follows:

- **Baby wipes**: These are particularly helpful when working with actors and for keeping your hands clean during the makeup process.
- **Alcohol**: Any strength is good, but if you are working with liquid silicone compounds, you will need at least 90% as it does a better job of cleaning up the unreacted material.
- **Adhesive removers**: When using adhesive removers, start with the mildest form before using the acetone-based removers, as these may remove the coloring in the mannequin.
- **Makeup remover or cold cream**: This does work best on SP actors, and they can help with the cleanup. Some products can be used on mannequins as well.

It is important to follow the mannequin manufacturer's guidelines on products used for cleanup. And it is always a good practice to test all cleaning materials on a small nonobvious area of the mannequin before large-scale use. Sometimes it is a good idea to put a barrier material on the mannequin to make cleanup of makeup easier. Plastic wraps or adhesive clear dressings work well. Some experimentation may be needed to see what method fits your expertise and budget.

SUMMARY

Moulage is a great art to add to simulation and to encourage realism. Moulage is an art that calls for creativity, practice, and developing authenticity. Moulage can be applied to both the human simulation instrument and the environment to better assist healthcare learners to understand patient care.

> **CASE STUDY 9.1**
>
> You are setting up a trauma scene for interprofessional healthcare providers. You need to transform a large room into a car-accident scene in which four teenagers are involved. One is thrown from the car and has a compound femur fracture. The driver has a head injury. The third has an abdominal wound, and the fourth has a lacerated arm. What materials would you use to set the stage? How would you develop the wounds to produce realism? Where would you place the victims in the environment?

> **CASE STUDY 9.2**
>
> You are asked to develop a scenario in which several patients have been exposed to irritating chemicals due to an explosion at a rail yard. There were two workers who were close to the blast who have traumatic wounds secondary to flying shrapnel as well as the more severe chemical burns. There are three who were walking near the railroad crossing and contacted with airborne chemical particles. What materials would you use to set the stage? How would you develop the wounds to produce realism? Where would you place the victims in the environment? What wardrobe would you consider for the railroad workers?

■ PRACTICE QUESTIONS

1. When considering to use moulage in a simulation scenario, which is the most effective use of time and effort when preparing the moulage for a simulation session?

    A. Concentrate on the wounds or representation of the illness to save time and reduce the cost of the simulation.
    B. Strike the best balance between effort on the principal illness or wounds wardrobe and the scene staging to provide the best authenticity.
    C. Concentrate on the patient, clothing, and monitor settings as that is all the student will focus on.
    D. Spend most of the time and effort on developing charting materials and wound characteristics that can be documented.

2. The degree to which the moulage in a simulation scenario is important to how the learner performs because authenticity will

    A. Shock or jar the learner into paying attention to the simulation and give cues for use in the simulation.
    B. Resonate with the learner and his or her sense of fun and playing along with the simulation.
    C. Keep the learner on her or his toes and thinking ahead to the next realistic surprise.
    D. High levels of authenticity have an impact on the learners emotional arousal and engagement in the learning activity.

3. It is important to teach the standardized patient to protect/preserve the moulage because

    A. It is extremely expensive.
    B. It has to be perfect.
    C. It is very time-consuming to apply.
    D. It is a work of art.

4. Two advantages of using moulage on standardized patients (SPs) are

    A. Most standardized patients see moulage as fun and make the day of simulation more enjoyable and they don't mind coming in early to prepare.
    B. The SPs can be taught to care for and protect the moulage before and during the session as well as assisting with cleanup after the session.
    C. The anatomy of the SPs is very similar to the mannequins so appliances fit well and the adhesives work better on the SPs.
    D. SPs usually don't move much so the appliances tend not to fall off and the dyes in moulage do not stain the SPs.

5. When starting out working with moulage the best type of kit to begin with is one that

    A. Contains one of each of the most commonly used makeups as well as a varied assortment of application tools
    B. A professionally designed set with an organized case to carry and separate moulage used for mannequins from supplies used on standardized patients
    C. A kit assembled from the sale items at the makeup shop to keep the cost down in spite of the quality
    D. Matches the expertise of the user and provides enough variation to meet the objectives of the simulation while growing with the increased experience of the moulage artist

6. The most accurate statement regarding odors is

    A. They are always required as they help to involve all the senses in a simulation.
    B. They are wild an uncontrollable and must be used with caution only as the scenario dictates.
    C. They are easy to find in the correct quantity and quality so that anyone can apply them during the scenario.
    D. Involving multiple senses does not affect learner engagement so odors are not necessary.

7. When considering the recipe for vomit the moulage artist should

    A. Include some real food products as they can increase the gag factor and do not have any cautions to worry about
    B. Choose the visual representation to match the simulation learning points and carefully clean up to minimize unwanted growth and contamination in the lab
    C. Pay attention to the liquid content so that the resulting mixture is soupy and will run easily down the mannequin's face and neck
    D. Consider that it could possibly block the airway and choke the mannequin

8. Which items and materials that are found in the kitchen are good for use in moulage?

    A. Chocolate syrup
    B. Cherry pie filling
    C. Clear gelatin
    D. All of the above

9. Which would be the best choice of material to make a bruise on a mannequin?

    A. Oil-based makeup with high concentrations of red dye
    B. Wax crayons heated to soften them
    C. Cream-based theatrical makeup
    D. Blue and purple crushed grapes

10. What is the best source to acquire makeup for your kit?

    A. Local drug store
    B. Local grocery store
    C. Local theater supply store
    D. National department store

REFERENCES

Garg, R. (2009). *Modeling and simulation of two-phase flows* (Doctoral dissertation). (Paper 10657). Graduate theses and dissertations. Retrieved from http://lib.dr.iastate.edu/etd/10657

Mould, J., White, H., & Gallagher, R. (2011). Evaluation of a critical care simulation series for undergraduate nursing students. *Contemporary Nurse: A Journal for the Australian Nursing Profession, 38*(1/2), 180–190. doi:10.5172/conu.2011.38.1-2.180

Riva, A., Conti, G., Solinas, P., & Loy, F. (2010). The evolution of anatomical illustration and wax modelling in Italy from the 16th to early 19th centuries. *Journal of Anatomy, 216*(2), 209–222, doi:10.1111/j.1469-7580.2009.01157

Society for Simulation in Healthcare. (2018). *Certified Healthcare Simulation Educator Examination Blueprint, 2018 Version.* Retrieved from http://www.ssih.org/Portals/48/Certification/CHSE_Docs/CHSE_Examination_Blueprint.pdf

Stokes-Parish, J. B., & Duvivier, R., Jolly, B. (2017). Does appearance matter? Current issues and formulation of a research agenda for moulage in simulation. *Simulation in Healthcare, 12*(1), 47–50. doi:10.1097/sih.0000000000000211

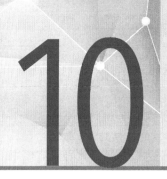

Simulation Principles, Practice, and Methodologies for Standardized Patient Simulation

LINDA WILSON, H. LYNN KANE, AND SAMUEL W. PRICE

All we got is all we need.

—Philadelphia Eagles

This chapter addresses Domain II: Healthcare and Simulation Knowledge/Principles (Society for Simulation in Healthcare, 2018).

[LEARNING OUTCOMES]

- Discuss the history of standardized patient (SP) simulation.
- Describe the process for SP simulation case development, SP training, implementation, and evaluation.

SPs were introduced into medicinal training in a limited fashion in the 1960s, but it took almost 30 years for the concept to enter the fields of nursing education and research (Barrows, 1993; Bolstad, Xu, Shen, Covelli, & Torpey, 2012). Initial objections toward using SPs included the high cost of implementation (hiring and training SPs, videotaping experiences); the so-called "Hollywoodization" of the hard sciences; and a skepticism that an actor, not a trained healthcare professional, could correctly help assess a learner's skills (Bolstad et al., 2012; Wallace, 1997). Yet, SPs are not necessarily all trained actors and have been found to have lower levels of unreliability and bias than nursing instructor observation or preceptor input (Bolstad et al., 2012). Overcoming this original skepticism and proving their usefulness, reliability, and consistency in a healthcare education setting, SP experiences have greatly increased in popularity, and for good reason, because they offer a safe environment for learners.

The realism of the SP encounter relies on effective case writing by the Certified Healthcare Simulation Educator™ (CHSE™) and precise training by either the CHSE or the specific SP trainer. The training is based around measurable learning outcomes, but not every single question or reaction that the SP might encounter during a day of work can be preemptively trained for, but an SP can be given guidelines, direction, and may even use his or her own personal background in some situations. A well-trained SP will react naturally, determined by the role he or she is playing that day. It is also important that the CHSE keeps the personality, attributes, and capabilities of the SP in mind when writing the scenario. It would not make much sense to write the case with a gender-specific problem if the available SPs are not all the same gender.

Flexibility is another benefit of working with SPs. During an SP experience, learners practice communication, history taking, and physical examination skills (Rutherford-Hemming & Jennrich, 2013). Different cases may emphasize certain illness manifestations, complications, or ethical challenges. The SP can even be instructed to emphasize his or her attitudes toward health professionals (Wallace, 2007). This attitude could range from a healthy skepticism to mild verbal aggression to contempt. The SP can be trained to propose a number of challenging situations that the learner might face with a real patient, and the entire group of learners can undergo the same experience because of the consistency and standardization provided by the SP.

SP CASE DEVELOPMENT

The SP case development begins with the identification of the simulation objectives or educational goals and setting for the simulation scenario (International Nursing Association for Clinical Simulation and Learning [INACSL] Standards Committee, 2016; Alexander et al, 2015; Olive, Elnicki, & Kelly, 1997). It is very important to be clear on the setting of the scenario to help the learners understand their role and what is expected of them during the simulation scenario. In an SP simulation scenario, the SP can have the role of a symptomatic patient, a nonsymptomatic patient, a psychiatric patient, an emotionally hysterical patient, a severely depressed patient, or any type of patient you need; the SP can also portray a family member; the sky is the limit because of the SP being a real person—anything is possible (Gorter et al., 2000; Wilson & Rockstraw, 2012). A well-written simulation scenario includes clear objectives; training materials, including a detailed script; and clear descriptions of medical details that are appropriately described for the SP's use, along with enough background to describe the complexity of the patient (Wallace, 2007).

TIMING OF THE SIMULATION SCENARIO

When planning the simulation scenario, you must consider the timing of the scenario. This is important for planning and scheduling the participant for the experience. The entire simulation encounter includes the following: (a) presimulation briefing; (b) total time the student has to work with the patient; (c) time for the patient to complete the student observation checklist; (d) time for the patient to provide feedback to the student; (e) time after the encounter if you want the participant to do documentation, or a survey, or a posttest; and (f) time for the SP to prepare for the next student. Many SP simulation scenarios do not include anything after the encounter. So, for example, if you are planning 15 minutes for the prebrief, planning for the learner to be with the patient for a maximum of 15 minutes, and you are going to allow 5 minutes for the SP to complete the checklist, 7 minutes for the feedback session, and 3 minutes for the patient to prepare for the next student—each total encounter will take 45 minutes.

Example 1: Prebrief = 15 minutes
Time with patient = 15 minutes
Checklist time = 5 minutes
Feedback time = 7 minutes
Turnaround time = 3 minutes
Total encounter time = 45 minutes

Example 2: Prebrief = 15 minutes
Time with patient = 30 minutes
Checklist time = 10 minutes
Feedback time = 15 minutes
Turnaround time = 5 minutes
Total encounter time = 75 minutes

This will assist you with planning the scheduling of the simulation experience, also taking into consideration the number of simulation rooms you have available and the number of learners who have to complete the simulation experience.

IDENTIFY THE SETTING

The setting is a very important part of scenario planning. Where is your scenario taking place? Is it taking place in a physician's office, in an ED, in a medical–surgical unit, in a critical care unit, in the community, in a patient's home, in a clinic, or in a surgical family waiting room? Ideally, the simulation room should depict this environment or, if that is not possible, a sign should be clearly posted to remind the student of the environment where the scenario is taking place.

SP ROLE

The role of the SP must be clearly identified. The SP can portray a patient, a family member, a student, or any other role imagined.

SP POSITION AND ATTIRE

As part of the scenario development, you must also identify the position of the patient when the student enters the room and the attire the patient should be wearing.

Position examples:

- Sitting in the chair
- Sitting on the exam table
- Walking back and forth in room
- Pacing anxiously in room

Attire examples:

- Wearing a patient gown, with underwear on
- Wearing a patient gown, no underwear on

- Wearing regular clothes
- Wearing a gown with pants on

> **EVIDENCE-BASED SIMULATION PRACTICE 10.1**
>
> Hawk, Kaeser, and Beavers (2013) used SPs to increase confidence in chiropractic learners when they had to confront patients about smoking cessation. Using SPs to demonstrate the interaction needed to put the five "A's" of smoking cessation (ask, advise, assess, assist, arrange) in place, 81% of learners (N = 68) said it increased their confidence, and 77% said they would now be comfortable using it in future practice.

STUDENT ROLE

The role of the learner should also be very clear. Is the learner working in a new graduate nurse role, a physician role, a physician assistant role, or an advanced practice nurse role? The students should be reminded of their roles in the simulation instructions and to observe the door sign so that they function within their scope of practice.

IDENTIFY THE FOCUS AND OBJECTIVES

The SP simulation scenario has to have a clear focus and objectives. Is the scenario going to be based on a specific medical diagnosis (asthma, congestive heart failure, shortness of breath, abdominal pain), a mental illness (psychosis, hearing voices), psychosocial challenges (depression, anxiety), ethical situations (do not resuscitate [DNR], organ donation, assisted suicide), or another scenario? This selection will be the basis for writing your case. It is important to include clear information about the selected condition/situation highlighted in the case for the education of the SPs.

Next, what are the objectives or educational goals for the learner completing this scenario? For example, if you are working with undergraduate nursing students, objectives could include the following:

1. Obtain a complete history from the patient.
2. Complete a focused physical exam based on the patient diagnosis.
3. Provide patient education based on educational needs identified during the time with the patient.

Another example, if you are working with medical students or advance practice nurses, objectives could include the following:

1. Obtain a complete history from the patient.
2. Complete a focused physical exam based on the patient diagnosis.
3. Identify the patient diagnosis.
4. Order diagnostic tests as appropriate.
5. Provide the patient with appropriate information and plan of care.

The objectives are also linked to the specific course, educational program, or clinical unit of the learner. It is important that the learner be aware of the required objectives or educational goals for the simulation experience.

SP QUESTIONS AND ANSWERS

The SP case should also include any questions the learner may ask during the scenario and the response the patient is supposed to provide to the learner. Any questions specific to the diagnosis or condition of the patient will need a specific answer, such as symptoms and medications, for example. For other questions that do not have a direct impact on the direction of the scenario, you may have the patients use their own information and not require a specific answer. Depending on the complexity of the case, one must be realistic as to how many specific lines or questions the SP can memorize and portray.

DOOR SIGN

The door sign is the sign that will be posted outside the simulation room to provide information to the student (Exhibit 10.1). The door sign should include the following:

- Information about the scenario
- What you expect the learner to do in the scenario
- How much time the learner has to complete the scenario
- Reminder to refer to the patient chart if one is included as part of the scenario

---

EXHIBIT 10.1

Door-Sign Examples

DOOR-SIGN EXAMPLE 1
Mr./Mrs. Pat Foles came to the emergency room with complaints of increased thirst, increased urination, and hunger and is now admitted to the medical–surgical unit. You have 45 minutes to complete a history, focused physical exam, and appropriate patient teaching.

DOOR-SIGN EXAMPLE 2
Mr./Mrs. Pat Wentz came to the emergency room with complaints of a severe headache and is now admitted to the medical–surgical unit. You have 45 minutes to complete a history, focused physical exam, and appropriate patient teaching. Please refer to the patient chart for additional information.

DOOR-SIGN EXAMPLE 3
Mr./Mrs. Fran Victorino has been in the hospital for the past week and was diagnosed as having HIV. The patient is preparing to be discharged from the hospital. You are to give the patient discharge instructions, including the important steps to prevent transmission of HIV to others, such as measures for safe sex, and so on. The discharge instructions have already been prepared for you by the doctor and are provided in the patient chart. You have 15 minutes to complete this encounter.

EVALUATION CHECKLIST

The evaluation checklist is a detailed checklist of what you expect the learner to do during the scenario. In most institutions, this checklist is completed by the SP immediately after the completion of the scenario and before the patient provides feedback to the learner. Depending on how you decide to design your checklist, you can choose to separate the checklist items by categories, such as communication, physical exam, patient teaching, diagnostic tests, or other categories. If a checklist item is subjective, it can be helpful to put a descriptor to provide information on how to evaluate that checklist item. For example, in Table 10.1 you will see a checklist item "good eye contact," and the descriptor explains that if the learner has good eye contact at least half of the time, he or she will get credit for that checklist item. It is also important to remember—the longer the checklist, the longer time you have to allow for the SP to complete the checklist.

> **SIMULATION TEACHING TIP 10.1**
>
> If there is a checklist item that has more than one part—where a student could possibly do one part correctly and one part incorrectly, such as listening to the lungs—it is helpful to separate that into two separate checklist items as you will see in the example checklist in the following text.

TABLE 10.1

Example Evaluation Checklist Items

COMMUNICATION	PHYSICAL EXAM
Introduced self (name and title) Checked patient's ID band Good eye contact (50% or greater of the time) Speaks clearly in terms the patient can understand Active listener Asked patient's age or date of birth Asked about patient's marital status Asked about patient's work history Asked about previous hospitalizations Asked about allergies Asked about past medical history Asked about current medications Asked about a history of chest pain Asked about a history of palpitations Asked about smoking history Asked about alcohol history Asked about diet Asked about exercise Asked about stresses in life Created an atmosphere that put the patient at ease	Washed hands before examination Explained to me what she or he was doing with each step of exam Helped to position me Was professional in manner Maintained modesty during exam Checked blood pressure in both arms Checked blood pressure sitting or lying down Checked blood pressure standing Counted my pulse Counted my respiratory rate Listened to my heart in at least four places on skin Listened to my lungs in at least four places (two pairs) anterior and posterior on skin

STUDENT EVALUATION CRITERIA AND PASSING SCORE

There are many ways to evaluate the student checklist items. Some of the common evaluation methods include:

- Done/Not Done/NA
- Done/Not done/Done but not correctly
- Likert scale rating

Your simulation program may select one way to evaluate all of your simulation experiences or they may be different based on a specific program or course.

If the simulation is a "high-stakes testing" simulation in which the student has to achieve a specific score to pass, you must also pick a passing score. Many programs will pick the lowest score for a full grade of "C" at their school. Or the specific score might be mandated by your licensing agency.

Another aspect to consider is the value of each checklist item. Is each checklist item of equal value, or are some checklist items worth more points than others? You can also identify specific patient safety checklist items that are critical—if the learner misses that checklist item, he or she automatically fails or has to repeat the experience—such as verifying the patient's identity or checking the ID band.

Exhibit 10.2 demonstrates two SP simulation cases, including the evaluation checklist. The first case is an ethical dilemma case and the second case is a hypertension case.

EXHIBIT 10.2

SP Simulation Cases and Student Checklists

Case 1
Case: DNR (Do Not Resuscitate) Ethical Dilemma—Mini Case—Passing Score 76%

Length of time for the encounter: 15 min
Checklist time: 5 min
Feedback time: 7 min
Turnaround time: 3 min

NAME: Mr./Mrs. Fran Victorino

SETTING: Inpatient room on a medical–surgical unit

SCENARIO: Your mother, Isabelle Victorino, is 86 years old, has metastatic liver cancer, and was found unconscious on the floor at home.

DOOR SIGN: The person in the room is the daughter/son of your patient. This family member is very upset by the information received from the other nurse, who told them their family member is a DNR. The family member wants to speak with you since you are the current nurse for the patient. Your assignment is to talk with this family member. You have 15 minutes for the encounter.

OPENING LINE: "I'm so glad you're here. I need to talk to you about my mother. What does 'DNR' mean? The other nurse just told me my mom has been made DNR. Exactly what does that mean?"

You have been out of town and your sister, who lives with your mother, called you this morning and told you your mother had to be taken to the hospital. You are now at the hospital in the intensive care unit's waiting room after seeing your mother. You just found out from the

(continued)

EXHIBIT 10.2 *(continued)*

other nurse that your mother has a DNR order, which was given by your sister. You do not understand what "DNR" means and want "everything done" for your mother. You are a little bit anxious, a little upset, and are pacing a bit in the room. When the nurse arrives, you ask the nurse, "What does 'DNR' mean anyway? Who made my mother a DNR?" You add, "My mother, if she could speak for herself, would want everything done . . . she wants to live!"

TRAINING QUESTIONS:

What do you think "DNR" means? It means you do not do anything. Right?

Do you understand what it means to resuscitate someone in your mother's advanced age and deteriorated condition? Not really.

Do you understand what is involved in the resuscitation? No.

Have you ever discussed this topic (DNR) with your mother? No, but I am sure she would want to live. I'm sure she would want everything done.

Do you know whether or not your mother has a living will? I'm not sure.

Do you understand what a "living will" is? No.

Do you have power of attorney over your mother's medical conditions? No, my sister does.

Have you spoken to your sister? No.

Do you think it would be wise to talk to your sister? Yes, perhaps I need to.

Would you like to speak to your mother's physician? Yes.

Would you like us to arrange a family meeting? Yes.

Would you like to speak to a hospital counselor or a clergy member? Yes, could I see a clergy member?

Challenge Question: "Are you sure this DNR is for my mom? I can't imagine my sister would do something like that."

Evaluation Checklist (Done/Not Done/NA)

Introduced self (name and title)
Checked patient's ID band
Good eye contact (50% or greater of the time)
Speaks clearly in terms the patient can understand
Active listener
Allowed you to speak without interruption
Explained DNR in a sensitive, informative way
Examined your perceptions, for example, what do you think DNR is?
Acknowledged your emotions
Has a professional manner
Exhibited comforting body language
Asked about your support system
Explained what DNR means
Verified the DNR order in the chart
Explained how a DNR order is obtained

(continued)

EXHIBIT 10.2 *(continued)*

Suggested speaking to your sister or suggested a family meeting
Offered to call the primary doctor to discuss the situation
Offered to call someone for you for support

SP will also provide feedback.

Case 2
Case: Hypertension—Passing Score 76%

Length of time for the encounter: 40 min
Checklist time: 7 min
Feedback time: 10 min
Turnaround time: 3 min

NAME: Mr./Mrs. Fran Jackson

SETTING: Medical–Surgical Unit (inpatient hospital room)

SCENARIO: The patient has a 2-day complaint of severe headache. On arrival to the emergency room, the patient was diagnosed with severe hypertension. The patient's initial blood pressure (BP) in the ED was 200/120. BACKGROUND: The patient had been to the ED about 6 months ago with a similar complaint and was diagnosed with hypertension at that time. The patient was given a prescription for a hypertension medication: Lopressor. The patient was taking the medication as prescribed until he or she went to a health fair at the church about 1 week ago. The BP at the health fair was "normal." Because the BP was normal and the patient was feeling great, the patient decided to just stop taking the medication. Plus, the medication was very expensive and the patient can certainly use that money for something else. The patient started getting a severe headache about 2 days ago and thought he or she should get checked at the ED. Patient is pleasant and talkative.

DOOR SIGN: Mr./Mrs. Fran Jackson was admitted to the medical–surgical unit from the ED that day. The patient has a 2-day complaint of severe headache. On arrival at the emergency room, the patient was diagnosed with severe hypertension. Do a complete history, focused physical exam, and appropriate patient teaching. You have 40 minutes for the encounter.

OPENING LINE:
"I thought my blood pressure was fixed!"

CHALLENGE QUESTIONS:

Q: The BP medicine that the doctor had me on . . . can you tell me how that medication works?
A: The medication acts on certain receptors in the body and decreases BP and heart rate.

Q: Why was my BP normal at the health fair?
A: The medication was working or was in you system so that made your BP within normal range when you went to the health fair.

(continued)

EXHIBIT 10.2 (continued)

TRAINING QUESTIONS:

What is your date of birth? Use your own.

Are you married? Use your own.

Occupation? Worked in a factory (or store, or office, etc.), left on disability due to back injury. Currently under a lot of stress because having a difficult time making "ends meet" on the income you are receiving.

When did the severe headache start? It began two days ago.

Does anything make it worse? No. I don't think so.

Does anything make it better? No. I tried the usual over-the-counter medication that I take for headache but it did not help at all.

Have you had any fever or chills? No, not that I know of, but I haven't taken my temperature.

Have you ever had anything similar in the past? Yes, I came to the ED about 6 months ago with a similar headache. At that time, they said I had high BP. They gave me a prescription for a BP medication called Lopressor.

Have you ever used any recreational drugs? No.

Have you ever been hospitalized? No (or use your own history if necessary but nothing related to current complaint).

Have you ever had surgery? Answer as for yourself.

Have you ever been pregnant? Answer as for yourself.

Do you have any chronic illnesses? Yes, I guess the high BP could be considered a chronic illness, but I did not think I had it anymore.

Are you taking any medications? Yes, I was taking a medication after my last visit to the ED. It was a medication for my high BP. I stopped taking the medication after I had my BP checked at the health fair at church. My pressure was normal when they took it there; so I knew I did not need the medication any longer. I also felt great! Plus that medication was very expensive!

How is your father? Died from a stroke a few years ago. Father also had hypertension.

How is your mother? Alive if appropriate, or answer as deceased.

How is/are your sibling(s)? Healthy.

Past health history (none or use your own)

Neurological (none)

Cardiovascular (high BP)

Respiratory (none)

Gastrointestinal (none)

Genitourinary (none)

Gynecological (none)

Obstetrical (use your own)

Diet I eat anything I want. I love potato chips, dill pickles, I love anything that tastes salty.

Medications
Prescription medications (I was taking Lopressor once a day when I had the high BP, but prior to coming to the ED today, I was not taking any medications.)

Over-the-counter medications (none or use your own)

Medication allergies (none)

Seasonal allergies (use your own)

(continued)

EXHIBIT 10.2 (*continued*)

Psychosocial history

Smoking history (Yes, I've smoked one pack a day for as long as I can remember.)

Alcohol history (I like to have a few beers with my friends on the weekend or sometimes a margarita with extra salt.)

Recreational drug history (none)

Sexual history (Use your own.)

Stressors—(I am stressed about finances; it is difficult making ends meet on the disability salary.)

You should be in a hospital gown, bra and underwear are okay, sitting on the edge of the table.

STUDENT CHECKLIST (Done/Not Done/NA)

COMMUNICATION

Introduced self (name and title)

Verified patient's identity

Good eye contact (50% or greater of the time)

Spoke clearly in terms I could understand (Use three-strikes rule.)

Active listener

Asked patient's age or date of birth

Asked about patient's marital status

Asked about patient's work history

Asked about previous hospitalizations

Asked about allergies

Asked about patient's past medical history

Asked about patient's family's past medical history

Asked about current medications

Asked about a history of chest pain

Asked about a history of palpitations

Asked about smoking history

Asked about alcohol history

Asked about patient's diet

Asked about exercise

Asked about stresses in life

Created an atmosphere that put the patient at ease

Answered patient's question about BP medication: Lopressor

Answered patient's question about why BP was normal at the health fair

PHYSICAL EXAM

Washed hands before examination

Explained to me what she or he was doing during each step of the exam

Helped to position me

Was professional in manner

(*continued*)

> **EXHIBIT 10.2** (*continued*)
>
> Maintained modesty during exam
> Checked BP in both arms
> Checked BP sitting or lying down
> Checked BP standing
> Counted patient's pulse
> Counted patient's respiratory rate
> Took patient's temperature
> Listened to patient's heart in at least four places anterior on skin
> Listened to patient's lungs in at least four places (two pairs) bilateral anterior on skin
> Listened to patient's lungs in at least four places (two pairs) bilateral posterior on skin
>
> **PATIENT TEACHING**
>
> Discussed the importance of taking meds as prescribed
> Discussed the importance of a low-salt diet
> Discussed the importance of exercise
> Offered information or suggested some options for stress management
> Offered information or suggested some options for smoking cessation
>
> ***SP will also provide feedback.****

■ SP FEEDBACK

Another important aspect of the case development is planning for the SP feedback at the end of the simulation experience. A common type of feedback is for the patient to provide interpersonal feedback on how the student made him or her feel as a patient. The feedback can be either very specific or general (see Chapter 18 for extensive information on SP feedback).

Examples of an SP case template and a blank SP case template are provided in Exhibit 10.3.

> **EXHIBIT 10.3**
>
> **Standardized Patient Case Template**
>
> Title of case:
>
> Patient name:
>
> **Length of time for the encounter** (Maximum time student can be in the room is 15 min/30 min/45 min.):
>
> Checklist time:

(continued)

EXHIBIT 10.3 (*continued*)

Feedback time:

Turnaround time:

Setting:

Overview of scenario/scenario background for patient:

Instructions/door sign (Information for student to see prior to experience that includes what is to be done during the experience and ends with how many minutes the student has to complete the experience.):

Mr./Mrs. . . . . . . came to the . . . . . . for . . . . . .
You have . . . . . . minutes to . . . . .

Opening line (What you want the patient to say at the beginning of the experience.):

Patient position at start of scenario (sitting on table/sitting in chair):

Patient dress at start of scenario (regular clothes/patient gown):

Challenge question (The question the patient is to ask the learner during the experience plus the answer to the question.):

Questions during the experience (training questions) (Identify questions the learner may ask during the experience that *require a specific answer*. List the question below and the answer to the question. For all other questions, the patient can use his or her information.):

Please delete/change/add to the list below.

What is your age?
Are you married?

(*continued*)

EXHIBIT 10.3 (*continued*)

Occupation?
Have you ever had anything similar in the past?
Have you ever used any recreational drugs?
Have you ever been hospitalized?
Have you ever had surgery?
Have you ever been pregnant?
Do you have any chronic illnesses?
Are you taking any medications?
How is your father?
How is your mother?
How is/are your sibling(s)?
Past health history:
Are immunizations up to date?
Diet/activity/exercise:

Medications
Prescription medications:
Over-the-counter medications:
Medication allergies:
Seasonal allergies:

Psychosocial history:

Checklist items (Items used to evaluate the learner during the experience—each of these items will be marked with one of the following: Done/Not done/NA):
Passing score:

Communication
1. Introduced self (name and title)
2. Verified patient identity
3. Good eye contact (at least 50% of the time)
4. Was professional in manner
5. Spoke clearly in terms I could understand (Use three-strikes rule.)
6. Active listener
7. Asked about
8. Asked about
9.
10.

Physical Exam
1. Washed hands before the exam.
2. Explained to me what he or she was doing with each step of the exam.
3.
4.

(*continued*)

> **EXHIBIT 10.3 (*continued*)**
>
> 5.
> 6.
> 7.
> 8.
> 9.
> 10.
>
> **Patient Education**
>
> 1. Discussed the importance of
> 2. Discussed the danger signs of
> 3. Offered information or suggested some options for
> 4.
> 5.
> 6.
> 7.
> 8.
> 9.
> 10.
>
> ***SP will also provide feedback.****

ORIENTATION, EDUCATION, AND TRAINING OF SPs

The SP case scenario written by the CHSE is explained to the SPs during the SP training session prior to the simulation experience, and ideally in advance of the day of the simulation experience. If the training is taking place on the day of the simulation experience, it is important that the learners do not interact with the SPs before the experience to keep the level of realism as high as possible.

Depending on the type of SP experience the instructor has crafted, "Training for a standardized patient involves, for example, learning what history questions to listen for or how the physical examination should be done" (Errichetti, Gimpel, & Boulet, 2002, p. 627). Along with describing the direction that the case is supposed to take, the CHSE will also explain the objectives of the scenario.

The training of the SP begins with the specifics of the simulation case, including the following:

- Name of the patient
- Role of the patient (patient, family member, etc.)
- Setting of the scenario (e.g., medical–surgical unit, ED, etc.)
- Background of the scenario (i.e., why the patient came in)

> **SIMULATION TEACHING TIP 10.2**
>
> If you are new to writing SP case scenarios, when you have finished your first case, and start your next case, just do a "save as" and start with your original case as a baseline.

- The information the learner will know before beginning the scenario (such as the door sign)
- An opening line or lines to use to begin the scenario (if included in the scenario)
- Challenge questions (i.e., a specific question about the condition or chief complaint about the SP's condition if included in the scenario)
- Training questions (questions the students might ask and what answer is required)
- Checklist items
- Feedback

Along with the education about the case itself, the SP must also be clear on the learner checklist and how it should be completed. After the scenario, the SP will complete the learner checklist prior to the feedback session. Through observation, the SP completion of the checklist contributes to the learner evaluation, which is formally done by the CHSE.

> **SIMULATION TEACHING TIP 10.3**
>
> When using SPs for simulation learning experiences, it is best to use a consistent set of actors who work routinely at your institution because they become part of the "culture of learning" at your educational organization.

After reviewing the case and the checklist, the SPs can ask questions, discuss strategies, or practice through role-playing. The goal of the SP's training and education on the case is that the SP enters the role "so carefully coached . . . that the simulation cannot be detected by a skilled clinician" (Barrows, 1993, p. 444).

SP'S ROLE IN LEARNER EVALUATION AND FEEDBACK

For an SP scenario, the SP can be clearly instructed on how to complete the learner checklist. The SP's training is directly related to the accuracy of the SP's completion of the checklist (Wallace, 2007). In addition, for the results of the checklists to be valid, how the checklist is created is crucial to the validity and reliability of the checklist (Gorter et al., 2000). As mentioned previously, the SP's completion of the checklist contributes to the learner evaluation, which is formally done by the CHSE.

SPs have a unique role in postscenario feedback. The feedback time can be a heightened time of awareness for the learner, and information provided to the learner at that time can make a lasting impression. Many learners, after completing the SP simulation experience, state, "I will never forget what that patient told me!" or "The SP feedback was the best part of the experience." The role of SPs in healthcare simulation education is depicted in Figure 10.1.

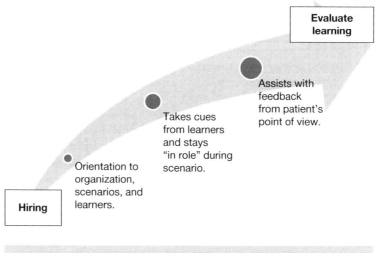

FIGURE 10.1 SP's role in healthcare simulation education.

■ HYBRID SIMULATION USING SPs AS CONFEDERATES

Many simulation scenarios find it optimal to combine both the human patient simulator (HPS) and SPs in a simulation scenario. When SPs are used in this fashion, it is referred to as *hybrid simulation* or the SP can be referred to as a *confederate* in the simulation scenario (see Chapter 11 for extensive information on hybrid simulation).

■ SUMMARY

SPs are a very important aspect of healthcare simulation education. To have a successful SP simulation experience, the case development must be accurate and comprehensive. In addition to the carefully developed case scenario, SP training is equally important. The SP's completion of the checklist must be accurate and consistent. The SP feedback has to be carefully structured because it can have a lasting impression on the student. SP simulation provides the opportunity for the most realistic simulations in a safe environment. In the future, SP simulation will be an expected standard in every simulation program.

> **CASE STUDY 10.1**
>
> A medical learner during an SP simulation scenario leaves the examination room without fully interviewing the SP. The learner comes out and tells the CHSE that this is difficult for her because the SP "looks exactly like" her mother who died less than a month ago. The SP also leaves the examination room and comes out to the desk to discuss the situation with the CHSE. How would the CHSE best handle this specific situation?

PRACTICE QUESTIONS

1. A simulation educator is planning a simulation to practice therapeutic communication. What type of simulation is most effective for the focus of this scenario?

   A. Human patient simulator (HPS) simulation
   B. Computer-based simulation
   C. Standardized patient (SP) simulation
   D. Virtual reality

2. A simulation educator has hired a new group of standardized patients (SPs) who have minimal or no previous experience. During the training session the majority of the SPs state they are not comfortable with providing feedback. The simulation educator should

   A. Provide videos for the SPs to review from previous simulations
   B. Provide each SP with a book and feedback methods
   C. Provide the SPs extra time to practice and role play
   D. Provide an education and training session on feedback methods for the SPs

3. When developing a standardized patient (SP) simulation scenario, the SP can portray what types of roles?

   A. Patient
   B. Family member
   C. Health professional
   D. All of the above

4. What is the required length of time for the standardized patient (SP) training session?

   A. 1 hour
   B. 2 hours
   C. 4 hours
   D. The specific training time is based on the complexity of the case

5. During a simulation scenario, the learner, completing the assessment, proceeds to gag the patient with a tongue depressor. The patient should

   A. Not do anything
   B. Run out of the exam room
   C. Scream
   D. State, "I do not want you to do that to me"

6. During a standardized patient (SP) scenario, the SP notices the learner chewing gum. The SP should

   A. Do nothing
   B. Make a note on the student checklist
   C. Ask the learner why he or she is chewing gum
   D. Notify the simulation educator

7. An educator is interested in learning how to write a standardized patient (SP) scenario. What is the best method for the simulation educator to use to provide this training?

A. Give the educator a book on SP simulation
B. Give the educator a simulation case they can copy
C. Provide the educator with a book, a sample case and meet with the educator
D. Provide the educator with some helpful websites on SP simulation

8. The standardized patient (SP) is reviewing the list of learners assigned to the room prior to the simulation experience. The SP notices that one of the names on the list is someone he or she might know personally. The SP should

   A. Do nothing
   B. Put a note on the checklist
   C. Notify the simulation educator after the simulation
   D. Notify the simulation educator immediately

9. At the completion of an assisted suicide simulation, the simulation educator notices several of the learners are crying. The simulation educator should

   A. Gather the learners together for a debriefing session
   B. Do nothing
   C. Notify the primary contacts for the learners
   D. Revise the scenario

10. Following a simulation experience a learner comes out of the room and appears very upset. The simulation educator should

    A. Escort the learner out of the simulation lab
    B. Notify the primary contact for the learner
    C. Take the learner aside and speak to them privately.
    D. Speak to the standardized patient

REFERENCES

Alexander, M., Durham, C. F., Hooper, J. I., Jeffries, P. R., Goldman, N., Kardong-Edgren, S., … Tillman, C. (2015). NCSBN simulation guidelines for prelicensure nursing education programs. *Journal of Nursing Regulation*, 6(3), 39–42. doi:10.1016/S2155-8256(15)30783-3

Barrows, H. S. (1993). An overview of the uses of standardized patients for teaching and evaluating clinical skills. *Academic Medicine*, 68(6), 443–451. doi:10.1097/00001888-199306000-00002

Bolstad, A. L., Xu, Y., Shen, J. J., Covelli, M., & Torpey, M. (2012). Reliability of standardized patients used in a communication study on international nurses in the United States of America. *Nursing & Health Sciences*, 14(1), 67–73. doi:10.1111/j.1442-2018.2011.00667.x

Errichetti, A., Gimpel, J., & Boulet, J. (2002). State of the art in standardized patient programs: A survey of osteopathic medical schools. *Medical Education*, 102(11), 627–631.

Gorter, S., Rethans, J. J., Scherpbier, A., van der Heijde, D., Houben, H., van der Vleuten, C., & van der Linden, S. (2000). Developing case-specific checklists for standardized-patient-based assessments in internal medicine: A review of the literature. *Academic Medicine*, 75(11), 1130–1137. doi:10.1097/00001888-200011000-00022

Hawk, C., Kaeser, M. A., & Beavers, D. V. (2013). Feasibility of using a standardized patient encounter for training chiropractic students in tobacco cessation counseling. *Journal of Chiropractic Education*, 27(2), 135–140. doi:10.7899/JCE-13-2

INACSL Standards Committee. (2016). INACSL standards of best practice: Simulation SM Simulation design. *Clinical Simulation in Nursing*, 12(S), S5–S12. doi:10.1016/j.ecns.2016.09.005

Olive, K. E., Elnicki, D. M., & Kelley, M. J. (1997). A practical approach to developing cases for standardized patients. *Advances in Health Sciences Education*, 2(1), 49–60. doi:10.1023/A:1009704030279

Rutherford-Hemming, T., & Jennrich, J. A. (2013). Using standardized patients to strengthen nurse practitioner competency in the clinical setting. *Nursing Education Perspectives*, 34(2), 118–121. doi:10.1097/00024776-201303000-00010

Society for Simulation in Healthcare. (2018). *Certified Healthcare Simulation Educator Examination Blueprint, 2018 Version*. Retrieved from http://www.ssih.org/Portals/48/Certification/CHSE_Docs/CHSE_Examination_Blueprint.pdf

Wallace, P. (1997). Following the threads of an innovation: The history of standardized patients in medical education. *Caduceus*, 13(2), 5–26.

Wallace, P. (2007). *Coaching standardized patients*. New York, NY: Springer Publishing.

Wilson, L., & Rockstraw, L. (2012). *Human simulation for nursing and health professions*. New York, NY: Springer Publishing.

11

Hybrid Simulation

ANTHONY ERRICHETTI

The whole is greater than the sum of its parts.

—*Aristotle*

> This chapter addresses Domain II: Healthcare and Simulation Knowledge/Principles (Society for Simulation in Healthcare, 2018).

[LEARNING OUTCOMES]

- Discuss an overview of patient simulation modalities.
- Compare hybrid patient simulations—varieties and possibilities.
- Describe how to develop mannequin-based and human hybrid simulations.
- Describe documents to create mannequin-standardized participant scenarios.
- Discuss preparing the standardized participant for hybrid simulations.
- Discuss issues of simulation fidelity.

Aristotle's maxim about how complexity is created from simplicity holds true for hybrid patient simulations, the use of two or more patient simulation modalities simultaneously or sequentially. For example, when mannequin simulators are combined with standardized patients (SPs), there is an advantage gained that neither of the two could offer alone. Hybrid patient simulations combine a mixture of simulation modalities, learning strategies, and professionals into a powerful platform for teaching and assessing clinical competencies. However, the complexity of combining multiple simulation modalities—from the artificial to the human—requires planning and cooperation.

Simulation is an aid to the imagination for both the educator and learner. "It allows us to create, populate and activate possible futures, and explore ramifications of these developed scenarios" (Vincenzi, Wise, Moulana, & Hanock, 2009, p. ix). The "willful suspension of disbelief," a concept described by the poet Samuel

Taylor Coleridge (1817), is directly applicable to simulation learning. If writers could combine "human interest with a semblance of truth" (Coleridge, 1817, p. 2), then readers could overlook a story's implausibility (Barth, 2001). Indeed, the first task for simulation educators is to get learners to "buy into" a scenario that all know is a construction, a representation of reality. Hybrid patient simulation is an approach that combines various elements of "constructed reality"—live, computerized, and mechanical—used in an environment that looks and sounds real. Live participants can be incorporated into a scenario and be given distinct roles to create that "semblance of truth" (Coleridge, 1817, p. 2), which makes learning compelling.

FOUNDATIONS OF PATIENT SIMULATIONS

The use of simulation to teach essential skills is widespread and deeply embedded into human culture. We seem to be "hardwired" to substitute the authentic with constructed reality. From infancy, we practice sucking and rooting reflexes through a pacifier, essentially a part-task trainer that simulates a mother's nipple (Moroney & Lilienthal, 2009).

The military has used war simulation for millennia. The ancient Hindu game *Chaturanga* and the Chinese *Go* were used to practice strategic thinking, and large-scale "war games" replicated battlefield conditions (Allen, 1987). The Roman Jewish historian Flavius Josephus (1981) notes that the Roman general Tiberius conducted war games that were "bloodless battles" to prepare for actual battles that were "bloody drills" (Josephus, 1981, book 3.5.1).

Aviation has long been at the forefront of using simulation to teach core competencies in our era, and its use has been a model for healthcare simulation (Friedrich, 2002; Gaba & DeAnda, 1988). The Wright Brothers used a "kiwi bird" simulator in 1910 to teach flight control using a defunct Wright Type B Flyer (Bernstein, 2000). The Antoinette trainer (*ca.* 1910; Figure 11.1) was a barrel split in half with short wings, allowing students to practice banking and turning while an instructor,

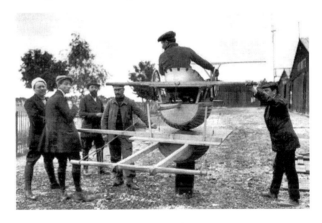

FIGURE 11.1 Antoinette trainer.

Source: Used with permission from flightsimulationmuseum.org

pushing or pulling on the wings, simulated turbulence. Such simulators were hybrids combining task trainers with an instructor acting as a "standardized participant," that is, an individual who plays a role in a simulation to add realism and to move critical action forward.

Human patient simulation today has two roots: computerized mannequins and SPs. SimOne, the first computer-controlled mechanical patient simulator was developed at the University of Southern California in 1967 by a team led by Stephen Abrahamson and Judson Denson (Abrahamson, 1997). In the late 1960s, the Harvey simulator, a hybrid between a cardiac task trainer and computer-enhanced mannequin simulator, integrated the bedside findings and realistically reproduced both common and rare cardiac diseases (Gordon, 1974).

SPs, introduced by Howard Barrows in 1963 at the University of Southern California, have long been used to teach clinical skills and are the foundation for performance-based assessment (Harden & Gleeson, 1979).

> **EVIDENCE-BASED SIMULATION PRACTICE 11.1**
>
> Downar et al. (2017) studied the effects of using standardized patient simulation compared to didactic learning for improving skill and patient comfort in medical students ($N = 94$) using a single-blind, randomized, controlled design. Finding supported simulation improved communication skills and empathy when compared to didactic learning alone.

TYPOLOGY AND MODES OF SIMULATION

Simulations can be divided into four types (Andrews, Brown, Byrnes, Change, & Hartman, 1998).

1. *Live*—Learners interact with real systems or people, for example, evaluating patients as SPs or customer exercises in which actors, playing patients, assess reception office staff.

2. *Virtual*—Learners interact with simulated systems, for example, training on a computer-based virtual reality (VR) surgical simulation (Gallagher et al., 2005).

3. *Constructive*—Learners interact with simulated systems and simulated people, for example, operating room team training using VR in which simulated participants substitute for actual participants (Baydogan, Belfore, Scerbo, & Mazumbar, 2009).

4. *Hybrid*—Combines live, virtual, and constructive modes of simulation in different combinations.

There are four kinds of simulated patients used by healthcare educators for teaching and skills evaluation:

1. Part-task trainers
2. Humans (SPs and standardized participants)
3. Computerized mannequins
4. Virtual (computer-based) patients

> **EVIDENCE-BASED SIMULATION PRACTICE 11.2**
>
> Bennett, Rodger, Fitzgerald, and Gibson (2017) completed a literature review ($N = 57$) about the use of different types of simulation used for occupational therapy (OT) education and found that within OT curricula educators have used the full scope of simulation modalities, including written case studies (22), standardized patients (13), video case studies (15), computer-based and VR cases (7), role-play (8), and mannequins and part-task trainers (4). Ten studies used hybrid simulation learning experiences. The review indicated that simulation was being used effectively in OT education.

The following summarizes their utilization and features, with examples of combining the modes into hybrid simulations.

Part-Task Trainers

Resusci Anne, a plastic mannequin, was introduced in 1960 to teach cardiopulmonary resuscitation (Grenvik & Schaefer, 2004), and thus began the advent of commercially available part-task trainers. Today, a wide variety of trainers is available to practice airway management, vascular access, echocardiography, cardiovascular assessment, and many others tasks.

Part-task trainers replicate the anatomy, for example, the skin, head, upper and lower extremities, esophagus, and thorax; and in some cases, the physiology of a part of the human body. This allows learners and professionals to practice specific tasks or technical procedures (Aggarwal, Moorthy, & Darzi, 2004) without harming or hurting an actual patient. Parts of the whole task are used to prepare the learner for the whole task (Sinz, 2004). Part-task procedures can improve learning efficiency because a specific skill can be practiced multiple times until mastered. They can also reduce training costs because the learner would not participate in a full simulation exercise until a particular skill is mastered. Examples of part-task trainers, which are hybrids, are the following:

> **SIMULATION TEACHING TIP 11.1**
>
> Part-task procedures can also be practiced using common objects, for example, using an orange to practice injection or using a pig's foot to practice suturing.

- Starting an intravenous (IV) line on an arm attached to an SP
- Suturing a leg wound attached to an SP
- Using a pelvic trainer with an SP
- Performing a urinary catheterization on a part-task trainer with an SP
- Doing a rectal exam on a part-task trainer with an SP

Human Patient Simulations

Although SPs are used mostly to teach and assess individual clinician competencies, they can be combined with standardized participants, sometimes referred to as *confederates*, who portray nonpatient roles. Also, standardized participants are increasingly incorporated into mannequin-based hybrid scenarios. They are scripted into a simulation to add realism and provide additional challenges and information to learners. They can portray, for example, a patient's (mannequin) family member, a healthcare team member, or any other role required by the scenario. They can be "programmed" to portray distinct personality "types" and emotionally complex and nuanced roles that correspond to the learning objectives of a learning module. Standardized participants can also be used to assess skills (e.g., to determine whether procedures are used in a correct and timely manner, assess team communication) and provide feedback during the postencounter debriefing. Standardized participants, like SPs, require training for whatever roles they take on. Examples of how to use SPs or standardized participants with hybrid simulation are the following:

- Learner interacts with an SP, and a standardized participant is a healthcare team member
- Learner must provide "bad news" to a distraught family member after examining an SP who portrays an end-of-life patient

Mannequin-Based Simulations

Mannequin-based simulations are used primarily for training and assessing healthcare teams. Depending on the model, these computerized, mechanical high-fidelity mannequins represent patients at various developmental stages (infant, child, adult) and are used for different purposes (e.g., anesthesia training; birthing simulations; and with programmable cardiovascular, respiratory, and neurological responses to clinical interventions). Depending on the model, the ingenuity of the simulation technician, and the condition of the patient, all mannequins can have a "voice." Talking through a microphone and listening though headphones, the patient's voice is usually that of a standardized participant placed at a distance, for example, behind a one-way mirror, and whose role is to answer questions as a patient would. Examples of SPs or standardized participants with hybrid mannequins are as follows:

- Learners interact with both the SP and the mannequin because they are portraying the same patient
- Standardized participants are used as
  - Mannequin's voice
  - A family member
  - A healthcare team member

VR and Computer-Based Simulations

Computer-based simulations using videos, drawings, and animation used to represent the patient have shown promise in developing clinical reasoning skills (Cook & Triola, 2009). Learners interact with the patient by asking questions (typing or speaking); by viewing data from monitors, labs, or x-rays; and by performing diagnostic or therapeutic actions (typically by making choices with the mouse).

At a much higher technology level, VR systems allow learners to become immersed in a computer-generated environment with individuals or groups of individuals (Schmorrow et al., 2009). One purpose of VR is to immerse the user in a computer-generated environment (Pimentel & Teixeria, 1992). The cost of VR systems, however, is high, making their use impractical at this time for most users. Below are examples of hybrid VR, and Chapter 13 provides in-depth information on VR.

- A computer program simulates a living condition of a patient before the learner interacts with the SP or mannequin in the simulation laboratory
- Use of real-time VR with a group of learners and multiple SPs

THE ROLE OF THE SIMULATION EDUCATOR IN HYBRID SIMULATION

Arguably, the most common hybrid simulation involves mannequins and standardized participants. Such hybrids involve four simulation education roles. However, there is a great deal of overlap in the following functions that may be performed by one or more people with multiple responsibilities.

1. **Mannequin–patient simulation specialist**: Preferably an individual with a clinical background, for example, physician, nurse, or paramedic. This individual designs healthcare team educational and assessment programs, constructs mannequin–patient scenarios, and participates in debriefing and feedback.
2. **Mannequin–patient technician**: An individual with both mechanical and computer skills is desirable. The technician works with the specialist to prepare the mannequin for the encounter, troubleshoots mannequin technical/mechanical problems, keeps the mannequins in good repair, and occasionally functions as the mannequin voice or standardized participant. Often, the specialist doubles as the technician.
3. **SP educator**: Working with the simulation specialist, the SP educator advises how to use people effectively in a scenario, writes standardized participant training notes, and trains them for the scenario.
4. **Psychometrician**: Designs assessment rubrics and collects, analyses, and reports performance data.

Simulation educators have a number of functions in this resource-intensive process, which are outlined here.

Stakeholder Education

One of the most important roles is to educate stakeholders (e.g., learners and clinical faculty) about how patient simulations are used as an educational strategy. Learning topics include:

- Simulation as an educational strategy
- Adult learning principles
- Simulator applications
- Logistics
- Developing scenarios
- Assessing performance validly and reliably
- Debriefing and feedback

Faculty development can take many forms, for example, seminars, webinars, and discussion of articles. One of the most powerful ways to educate faculty about how simulation works is to take them through actual encounters, experiencing the simulation, assessment, and debriefing process as the learner would. This step helps faculty to understand the needs of learners and the strengths and limitations of simulation learning. Faculty need to understand the curricular, technical, and logistical issues involved in developing simulations to facilitate effective educational programs. These issues become more complicated when developing hybrid scenarios.

Simulation Venues

Where patient simulation takes place dictate different processes and expectations. If simulations take place in a clinical education setting, for example, in a medical or nursing school, the learner and faculty time in the lab is scheduled; learners can participate and be debriefed in cohesive groups; interprofessional activities can be built into the curriculum; and learner retraining can be required before moving to the next learning level. Hospital-based simulation requires extreme flexibility. The learners are working clinicians; scheduled programs can be cancelled or cut short if staff is called; "just-in-time" training can be scheduled quickly and in a timely manner; and the assessment of skills is less reliable than the "standardized" performance testing possible in school-based programs.

Curriculum Development

Development of the educational curriculum with its various goals, objectives, methods, and intended outcomes is the first step in developing a program. Done in conjunction with clinical faculty, educators determine what skills are best taught and practiced through simulations and at the appropriate learner level. They have to decide what simulation modalities are best suited to the educational plan and be creative when the desired modality is not available, lacks fidelity, or is in short supply.

Scenario Development

Simulation scenarios are vehicles for assessing skills. All simulations are an opportunity to provide learners a formative or summative assessment and help faculty self-assess the quality of their clinical education. The patient simulation scenario is a plan indicating how a program will unfold, how the mannequin will be programmed or operated remotely, and how standardized participants will be part of the scenario. An example of information supplied to a standardized participant to prepare for role portrayal is shown in Table 11.1.

Standardized Participant Training

Standardized participants can have a number of functions that require preparation, training, and rehearsal. Scenario notes that guide role portrayal, like SP cases, must be written down and modified as needed. Training "on the fly" should be avoided, especially when assessing and comparing the performance of groups. All simulation scenarios have the ability to be "standardized" (as in standardized test) if the conditions of testing are standardized.

- Training objectives
- Setting, scenario (the vehicle for assessing skills)
- Types of simulators used
- Timing
- Equipment
- Performance assessment and debriefing/feedback

The following list is an outline of required training for standardized participants, depending on how extensive their role will be in the simulation.

TABLE 11.1
Hybrid Mannequin With Standardized Participant

SCENARIO SUMMARY
1. Scenario name
2. Patient's name, age, gender (mannequin)
3. Scenario setting
4. Condition of the patient at scenario start
5. Educational plan
   - Learner level
   - Program goals
   - Program learning objectives
   - Methods—e.g., types of simulators used
   - Intended outcomes
   - Challenges to the learner

Standardized Participant Information
1. Standardized participant's name(s) and relationship to the patient.
2. Narrative—Describe the scenario, what the standardized participant will know about the patient's condition at the start of the scenario, how the SP will interact with the healthcare team, and how the SP will act.

Patient Information (Mannequin)
List information the family member(s) will be able to give team members if requested.
NOTE: Write the answers to the following information, as the family member would give it. Avoid jargon.
- Patient's overall health
- Past medical history
- Patient's medications and why taken
- Past surgical history
- Health risk behaviors
  - Exercise
  - Diet
  - Tobacco use
  - Alcohol use
  - Substance use
- Other pertinent information

- *Portraying a nonclinical role*: Standardized participants can be trained for a number of roles, such as patient (as part of a two-part sequential simulation [e.g., a live patient who "becomes" a mannequin patient]) a family member, or other auxiliary role required of the scenario (e.g., a bystander in a simulation taking place in the field).

- *Portraying a clinical role*: A clinician can enter a simulation as a standardized participant playing a clinical role he or she can perform with credibility. This adds verisimilitude to the simulation because the clinician can realistically participate and further the action from the inside out. Standardized participants can also "fill in" as simulated team members or clinicians, but their participation will be limited to whatever part they can play realistically.

- *Skills assessment*: Standardized participants, both clinical and nonclinical, can be trained to document when procedures are done in a timely and correct manner (e.g., correctly intubating a mannequin patient or part-task trainer). It is recommended that all charged with this task practice the skill being assessed until mastered, and practice observing, assessing the skill, and remembering it for later documentation during practice encounters. Clinical experience and performance assessment experience are two separate skill domains.

- *Assessing team communication skills*: Standardized participants are arguably in the best position to assess team communication because they are participating from within. Their roles may also require them to challenge learners, for example, to be a demanding family member or an incompetent team member. Such challenges are dictated by the training objectives. They are therefore part of their training notes, and they can then judge how well the learners respond to their challenges. Team communication is best assessed through the use of an assessment rubric.

- *Debriefing and feedback*: Standardized participants, who are clinicians, as well as simulation specialists/facilitators, are in the best position to explore clinical decision-making issues and identify "performance gaps" during debriefing (Rudolph, Simon, Rivard, Dufresne, & Raemer, 2007). Their clinical knowledge and understanding of the teaching objectives can create a climate of trust and learner engagement. Both clinical and nonclinical standardized participants who have been charged with assessing communication have a role in debriefing communication. Their role may be to challenge learners to maintain both interpersonal and team communication throughout the encounter.

Issues of Hybrid Simulation and Patient Fidelity

Simulation fidelity refers to the extent to which a simulation or device replicates the environment or a patient's physiological condition (Alessi, 1988). All simulation modalities have "fidelity issues," that is, they are more or less realistic, possessing a "degree of similarity" to actual patients (Hays & Singer, 1989). In general, the more "standardized" or replicable the simulation is, the less realistic it may seem because of the need to standardize testing conditions for all. One advantage of hybrid simulations is that higher fidelity simulators (e.g., high-end mannequins and SPs) can balance out the less realistic, low-fidelity simulators.

But the so-called "high-fidelity" mannequin simulators only come alive when used with human simulations, for example, by adding a human voice or using standardized participants.

Applying the general simulation fidelity classifications of Yaeger et al. (2004), hybrid simulation can be labelled in the following manner:

- *Low-fidelity* simulations using part-task trainers that focus on single skills and permit learners to practice in isolation
- *Medium-fidelity* simulations that employ "full-body" mannequins, hybrid simulations, or SPs, but in a setting that lacks sufficient cues for the learner to be fully immersed in the situation
- *High-fidelity* simulations that allow for full immersion in settings that could potentially be used for actual patient examination or treatment

The preceding items focus on mechanical or "physical fidelity," that is, how closely a simulator resembles the thing being simulated physically and kinesthetically (Salas, Bowers, & Rhodenizer, 1998). By this definition, SPs have the highest fidelity. But from a training perspective, the issue is more complex. A training system is a series of episodes or experiences that systematically build key skills from basic to more complex adaptive skills (Kozlowski, 1998). Low-fidelity simulation, therefore, can be a building block toward higher level functioning that can be practiced and assessed through higher fidelity hybrid simulations.

> **SIMULATION TEACHING TIP 11.2**
>
> Combining simulators and manipulating the environment, when done well, has the potential to add realism to a scenario and deflect artificiality.

One goal of simulation training, regardless of the simulators used, is to achieve "psychological fidelity," that is, a situation in which the risks and rewards of learner participation correspond in a convincing way to real-world risks and rewards (Ranney, 2011). Indeed, patient simulations reach their full potential as teaching and assessment opportunities when learners suspend disbelief, immerse themselves in the scenario, and perform as they would in a real-world situation. This can only be achieved with the expertise of the simulation educator who has the ability to construct a realistic work setting from simulation devices, humans, hybrids, environmental cues, and the judicious use of imagination.

SUMMARY

Hybrid simulation is limited only by the imagination. It requires the simulation educator to be proficient in human and mannequin-based simulations and practices. Combining the best methods of simulation to achieve the learning outcomes is the goal of simulation educators. Assessment of learners from within, that is, by utilizing standardized participants, has distinct advantages over assessment done by external or remote educators. Hybrid simulation methods provide flexibility and realism to help learners achieve their learning outcomes.

> **CASE STUDY 11.1**
>
> As an experienced simulation educator, you would like to teach fourth-year healthcare students the following learning objectives:
> - Discuss methods of attaining sobriety with the patient and family.
> - Recognize the symptoms of alcohol withdrawal.
> - Implement treatment measures to minimize the effect of alcohol withdrawal.
> - Communicate the prognosis of esophageal cancer that has metastasized to other organs.
>
> Choose two different hybrid methods that could be used to accomplish these learning outcomes and explain how to do it.

PRACTICE QUESTIONS

1. One assessment advantage afforded though hybrid simulation is:

   A. It combines interprofessional groups in a single training program.
   B. It is primarily used for formative versus summative assessment.
   C. Assessment can be done by a trained standardized participant.
   D. Debriefing is optional because scores are given by the standardized participant.

2. The simulation venue:

   A. Is the best place to conduct debriefing
   B. Generates different processes and expectations
   C. Dictates the types of scenario used
   D. Always utilizes standardized participants

3. Psychological fidelity occurs when:

   A. The risks experienced through the simulation closely approximate what is experienced in real life.
   B. Patient safety measures are ensured.
   C. The learners experience "psychological safety."
   D. The simulation educator adheres to the training objectives.

4. A standardized participant:

   A. Can be a faculty member who plays the part of a clinician in a scenario
   B. Is another term for *standardized patient*
   C. Is a simulated patient participating in a standardized examination
   D. Cannot reliably assess skills because they are too involved with the scenario to pay attention to the learners

5. Physical fidelity is compromised when:

   A. The raters are not adequately trained.
   B. When the simulation is cut short.
   C. The learners are required to take excessive risks.
   D. A patient condition cannot be realistically simulated.

6. To assess skills, it is recommended that the raters:
   A. Develop the clinical-skills checklists to be used.
   B. Always participate in the scenarios.
   C. Know how to perform the skill being assessed, and practice assessing it.
   D. Develop quality-assurance practices.

7. Which one of the following is not a role for standardized participants:
   A. Standardized patient
   B. Standardized family member
   C. Standardized test developer
   D. Simulated clinician

8. Hybrid simulation requires the simulation educator to:
   A. Be proficient in all modes of simulation
   B. Understand the principles and practices of test development
   C. Debrief the learners after scenarios
   D. Manage all technical problems that may arise

9. A standardized patient educator:
   A. Manages the simulation scenario
   B. Services the mannequins
   C. Creates standardized patient (SP) cases and trains SPs to participate in hybrid simulation
   D. Analyzes performance assessment data

10. One of the best ways to educate faculty about how simulation works is to:
    A. Conduct ongoing faculty development webinars.
    B. Show videos of actual simulation sessions.
    C. Observe simulations.
    D. Participate in simulations.

■ REFERENCES

Abrahamson, S. (1997). SimOne: A patient simulator ahead of its time. *Caduceus, 13*(2), 29–41.

Aggarwal, R., Moorthy, K., & Darzi, A. (2004). Laparoscopic skills training and assessment. *British Journal of Surgery, 91*, 1549–1580. doi:10.1002/bjs.4816

Alessi, S. M. (1988). Fidelity in the design of instructional simulations. *Journal of Computer-Based Instruction, 15*(2), 40–47.

Allen, T. B. (1987). *War games*. New York, NY: McGraw-Hill.

Andrews, D. H., Brown, J., Byrnes, J., Chang, J., & Hartman, R. (1998). *Enabling technology: Analysis of categories with potential to support the use of modelling and simulation in the United States air force*. Mesa, AZ: Human Effectiveness Directorate, Air Force Research Lab.

Barth, J. (2001). *The symbolic imagination*. New York, NY: Fordham.

Baydogan, E., Belfore, L. E., Scerbo, M., & Mazumdar, S. (2009). Virtual operating room team training via computer-based agents. *International Journal of Intelligent Control and Systems, 14*(1), 115–122.

Bennett, S., Rodger, S., Fitzgerald, C., & Gibson, L. (2017). Simulation in occupational therapy curricula: A literature review. *Australian Occupational Therapy Journal, 64*(4), 314–327. doi:10.1111/1440-1630.12372

Bernstein, M. (2000). *Grand eccentrics: Turning the century: Dayton and the inventing of America*. Wilmington, OH: Orange Frazer Press.

Coleridge, S. T. (1817). *Biographia literaria*. Princeton, NJ: Princeton University Press.

Cook, D. A., & Triola, M. M. (2009). Virtual patients: A critical literature review and proposed next steps. *Medical Education, 43*(4), 303–311. doi:10.1111/j.1365-2923.2008.03286.x

Downar, J., McNaughton, N., Abdelhalim, T., Wong, N., Lapointe-Shaw, L., Seccareccia, D., ... Knickle, K. (2017). Standardized patient simulation versus didactic teaching alone for improving residents' communication skills when discussing goals of care and resuscitation: A randomized controlled trial. *Palliative Medicine, 31*(2), 130–139. doi:10.1177/0269216316652278

Friedrich, M. J. (2002). Practice makes perfect: Risk-free medical training with patient simulators. *Journal of the American Medical Association, 288*(22), 2808, 2811–2812. doi:10.1001/jama.288.22.2808

Gaba, D., & DeAnda, A. (1988). A comprehensive anesthesia simulation environment: Re-creating the operating room for research and training. *Anesthesiology, 69*(3), 387–394.

Gallagher, A. G., Ritte, E. M., Champion, H., Higgins, G., Fried, M. P., Moses G., ... Satava, R. M. (2005). Virtual reality simulation for the operating room: Proficiency-based training as a paradigm shift in surgical skills training. *Annals of Surgery, 241*(2), 364–372. doi:10.1097/01.sla.0000151982.85062.80

Gordon, M. S. (1974). Cardiology patient simulator. Development of an animated manikin to teach cardiovascular disease. *American Journal of Cardiology, 34*, 350–355. doi:10.1016/0002-9149(74)90038-1

Grenvik, A., & Schaefer, J. J. (2004). From Resusci-Anne to Sim Man: The evolution of simulators in medicine. *Critical Care Medicine, 32*, S56–S57. doi:10.1097/00003246-200402001-00010

Harden, R. M., & Gleeson, F. A. (1979). Assessment of clinical competence using an objective structured clinical examination (OSCE). *Medical Education, 13*, 41–54. doi:10.1111/j.1365-2923.1979.tb00918.x

Hays, R., & Singer, M. (1989). *Simulation fidelity in training system design: Bridging the gap between reality and training*. New York, NY: Springer-Verlag.

Josephus, F. (1981). *The Jewish war* (G. A. Williamson, Trans). New York: NY: Penguin.

Kozlowski, S. W. J. (1998). Training and developing adaptive teams: Theory, principles, and research. In J. A. Cannon-Bowers & E. Salas (Eds.), *Decision making under stress: Implications for training and simulation* (pp. 115–153). Washington, DC: APA Books.

Moroney, W. F., & Lilienthal, M. G. (2009). Human factors in simulation and training: An overview. In D. Vincenzi, J. Wise, M. Mouloua, & P. A. Hancock (Eds.), *Human factors in simulation and training*. Boca Raton, FL: Taylor and Francis CRC Press.

Pimentel, K., & Teixeria, K. (1992). *Virtual reality: Through the new looking glass*. New York, NY: McGraw-Hill.

Ranney, T. A. (2011). Psychological fidelity: Perception of risk. In D. L. Fisher, M. Rizzo, J. Caird, & J. D. Lee (Eds.), *Handbook of driving simulation for engineering, medicine and psychology*. Boca Raton, FL: Taylor and Francis CRC Press.

Rudolph, J. W., Simon, R., Rivard, P., Dufresne, R. L., & Raemer, D. B. (2007). Debriefing with good judgment. *Anesthesiology Clinics, 15*, 361–376.

Salas, E., Bowers, C. A., & Rhodenizer, L. (1998). It's not what you have but how you use it: Toward a rationale use of simulation to support aviation training. *International Journal of Aviation Psychology, 8*(3), 197–208. doi:10.1207/s15327108ijap0803_2

Schmorrow, D., Nicholson, D., Stephanie, J., Lackey, S. J., Allen, R. C., Norman, K., ... Peter, A. (2009). Virtual reality in the training environment. In D. Vincenzi, J. Wise, M. Mouloua, & P. A. Hancock (Eds.), *Human factors in simulation and training*. Boca Raton, FL: Taylor and Francis CRC Press.

Sinz, E. (2004). Partial-task-trainers and simulation in critical care medicine. In W. F. Dunn (Ed.), *Simulators in critical care and beyond* (pp. 33–41). Des Plaines, IL: Society of Critical Care Medicine.

Society for Simulation in Healthcare. (2018). *Certified Healthcare Simulation Educator Examination Blueprint, 2018 Version*. Retrieved from http://www.ssih.org/Portals/48/Certification/CHSE_Docs/CHSE_Examination_Blueprint.pdf

Vincenzi, D. A., Wise, J. A., Moulana, M., & Hanock, P. A. (2009). In *Human factors in simulation and training*. Boca Raton, FL: Taylor and Francis CRC Press.

Yaeger, K. A., Halamek, L. P., Coyle, M., Murphy, A., Anderson, J., Boyle, K., … Smith, M. D. (2004). High-fidelity simulation based training in neonatal nursing. *Advances in Neonatal Care*, 4(6), 326–331. doi:10.1016/j.adnc.2004.09.009

12

Part-Task Trainers

RUTH A. WITTMANN-PRICE AND DEBORAH S. ARNOLD

Practice does not make perfect. Only perfect practice makes perfect.
—Vince Lombardi

This chapter addresses Domain II: Healthcare and Simulation Knowledge/Principles (Society for Simulation in Healthcare, 2018).

[LEARNING OUTCOMES]

- Identify the principles behind choosing an appropriate part-task trainer.
- Compare different types of part-task trainers.
- Review practice questions as they relate to part-task trainers.

Part-task trainers (PTTs) are probably among the oldest types of healthcare simulations known to professions besides practicing skills on one another. PTTs have been used successfully for years to teach "healthcare skills" and are still a valuable part of simulation education.

Simulation education using PTTs allows learners to obtain and/or enhance clinical skills and processes in a safe learning environment. PTT can be incorporated into all levels of education from novice to expert. The ability to practice high-risk, low-volume skills can enhance the confidence of individuals and teams and assist them to think critically and respond appropriately individually as well as within a team (Brown, 2017). Practicing skills deliberately helps learners know how to respond when a complex emergency occurs (Issenberg et al., 1999). The comprehensive use and worth of PTT cannot be understated. Spooner, Hurst, and Khadra (2012) state, "Task trainers are fundamental in the teaching of anatomic landmarks and in enabling learners to acquire, develop, and maintain the necessary motor skills required to perform specific tasks" (p. 59).

Their vital impact on quality patient care and safety is likely to become more prominent as learners are able to demonstrate enhanced psychomotor and cognitive thinking skills. Choosing to use a PTT allows the faculty to validate a skill prior to performing a skill on a real patient. PTTs are affordable, easy to move, skill specific, and allow for standardization of a process.

SIMULATORS, FIDELITY, PTTs, AND COMPLEX TASK TRAINERS

Simulator refers to a physical object or a representation of the full or part task to be replicated. It is used by some specifically to refer to technologies that recreate the full environment in which one or more targeted tasks are carried out. This can also be called *fully immersive simulation* (Scott et al., 2016).

Fidelity means that a simulator is able to realistically imitate true physiological realism. *Fidelity* can be defined as the degree to which the appearance and capabilities of the simulator resemble the appearance and function of the simulated system. Low fidelity is the farthest from realism, showing no physiological change, movement, animation, or progression. High fidelity is the closest to realism, showing physiological change, movement, animation, and progression. Anatomical fidelity of PTT assists students in mastering skills (Woo, Malekzadeh, Malloy, & Deutsch, 2017).

PTTs are devices that replicate limited aspects of a task, but do not present an integrated experience (Rodriques et al., 2016). Examples of PTTs are provided in Exhibit 12.1.

EXHIBIT 12.1

Examples of Part-Task Trainers

Intubation mannequins

IV arms

Female pelvises

IV, intravenous.

PTTs are used in healthcare education and include the anatomical segment relevant to a particular procedural skill. Cost, size, and risk of simulation equipment is considered when selecting resources. They are used to teach novices the basics of psychomotor skills and allow for maintenance and fine-tuning of expert skills. PTTs can be used in situ in a real clinical environment or set up in a simulated learning environment. The benefit of portability adds value to just-in-time education, education that takes place in relation to a decrease in census and downtime. PTTs minimize wear and tear of high-fidelity mannequins and are more cost-effective when used for acquisition of skills.

PTTs range in complexity from using a piece of fruit to teach injections to using a torso to teach central-line placement and care. They typically do not include patient feedback. An important trend is the combination of PTTs with either standardized simulated patients (live actors) or full-mannequin simulators to allow for task completion in a more fully immersive environment (Brown, 2017).

It is often difficult to *suspend disbelief* with PTTs, but they are often used in hybrid formats to increase realism if that is essential to the learning outcomes (Muckler, 2017). An example is placing a task-trainer arm for an intravenous (IV) line in the shirt sleeve of a standardized patient while the actual arm is concealed under a hospital gown. This can prevent pain while the learner is practicing an

IV procedure on the task trainer. Chapter 11 explains the hybrid concept more completely.

Complex PTTs increase the fidelity in the learning experience by allowing the learner to use a PTT along with a computer-simulated environment or different evaluative or technological techniques (Oussi et al., 2018). Examples are provided in Exhibit 12.2.

EXHIBIT 12.2

Examples of Complex Part-Task Trainers

- Surgical skills
- Central-line catheterization
- Scopes, such as bronchoscopes
- Chest-tube insertion
- Ultrasound techniques

Complex task trainers represent both virtual reality and haptic technology in healthcare education using computer-based technology. This equipment tends to be more expensive. Complex task trainers work better in a simulated learning environment related to portability. *Haptic* refers to the sense of touch and the meaning of touch (Orledge, Phillips, Murray, & Lerant, 2012). This type of trainer allows the faculty to clearly see where the learner is applying touch and the amount of pressure applied as well as to assess whether a thorough exam has been done (Hagelsteen et al., 2017). Complex PTTs are used in combination with web-enhanced simulation programs so that physical interaction can occur within the virtual-reality environment. This may be referred to as box-type simulation trainers. They can be used for surgical techniques, such as laparoscopic surgery.

> **SIMULATION TEACHING TIP 12.1**
>
> Learners can often practice on part- and complex task trainers independently if the protocol for the procedure has been taught and is written out. This assists learners in providing self-directed deliberate practice and in being accountable for the learning before it is time for evaluation of knowledge.

An example used commonly is an IV PTT that is attached to a computer program. The learner must demonstrate knowledge of the correct procedure on the computer for the PTT to respond to the tourniquet and the arm vein to protrude to accommodate an IV insertion. This may also provide haptic simulation.

CURRICULUM DEVELOPMENT USING PTTs

Educational goals and simulation tools go hand in hand when thinking about the type of simulator equipment to use. The educator needs to have the end in mind. What will the learner achieve at the end of this learning encounter? The educator needs to identify whether there is financial value in using a high-fidelity mannequin for the placement of an IV line or practice of chest-tube insertion when the consumable costs are much higher with higher fidelity simulation equipment.

Faculty should weigh the benefits of using a PTT for individual educational encounters against the benefits of using a high-fidelity simulator to place a second line during a critical event in immersive team simulation training. Using technology to provide hands-on experience guided by proven educational principles, we can provide the very best evidence-based learning environment for our future caregivers (Brown, 2017).

PTTs are an invaluable asset when setting up a simulation experience for a group of learners. PTTs can be used as an "unmanned station" for learners to practice as long as they are properly prepared. Chapter 16 discusses setting up stations for learner practice in depth.

> **SIMULATION TEACHING TIP 12.2**
>
> There is increasing research using PTTs to promote better patient outcomes. Posner and Hamstra (2013) studied groups of medical students ($N = 145$) using a PTT (female pelvis) with and without a hybrid component (standardized patient). The study observed communication skills in randomized groups of students. The results showed no significant difference in communication skills, but technical skill was increased in the group that performed on the PTT without the standardized patient. This study indicates that PTTs are effective for skill practice.

Additional studies are needed that focus on the evaluation of a learned skill on a PTT and the performance of that skill in actual practice and their effect on communication and empathy (Bauchat, Seropian, & Jeffries, 2016).

> **EVIDENCE-BASED SIMULATION PRACTICE 12.1**
>
> Scott et al. (2016) developed a complex PTT to teach junior otolaryngology head-and-neck surgery residents. The PTT demonstrated epistaxis and the students learned (**N = 13**) two techniques of nasal packing (formal nasal pack and nasal tampon) for the management of epistaxis using the task trainer. Learners were videotaped and demonstrated a statistically significant increase in global rating scores ($p < .05$) in all items measured for both packing methods by practicing on the PTT.

■ ADVANTAGES OF PTTs

Of all the simulation methods, PTTs are probably the least expensive. Once the equipment is bought, it can usually be used over and over with very little maintenance.

Table 12.1 provides examples of PTTs developed as cost-effective teaching tools to assist healthcare learners reach their learning goals.

> **SIMULATION TEACHING TIP 12.3**
>
> Care of PTTs is important. Follow the manufacturer's instructions on cleaning and storing to increase the usability and shelf life of PTTs.

TABLE 12.1
Examples of PTT Use

AUTHOR	USE OF PTTs
Komasawa, Berg, and Minami (2017)	Used problem-based learning and task trainer for central venous catheter insertion training successfully with medical students.
Ruest et al. (2016)	Developed a PTT for penile corpus cavernosa aspiration practice and demonstration.
Ng, Plitt, and Biffar (2018)	Developed a PTT to teach medical students safe aspiration of peritonsillar abscesses, a common condition that presents in the EDs.
Dedmon et al. (2017)	Used a PTT to improve fine motor control of surgical residents for endoscopic ear surgery.

ED, emergency department; PTT, part-task trainer.

SUMMARY

PTTs are among the first-used simulation modalities and are still very effective for student learners when used alone and in a hybrid format. PTTs are cost-effective and can be used by learners independently as well as with the guidance of a simulation educator. Everyone working in the field of simulation should become broadly familiar with the technologies, pedagogies, and research methods in each domain to better inform strategies and tactics for application and diffusion of simulation in healthcare education, training, and research (Brown, 2017).

CASE STUDY 12.1

A learner is using an IV task trainer that is hybrid and uses a computer to run through the procedure.

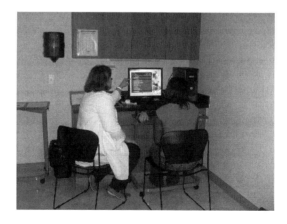

The learner does well on the IV insertion on the PTT, but states, "I know this is not how it is really going to be with patients." As the simulation educator, how would you respond?

PRACTICE QUESTIONS

1. The simulation educator is deciding on the modality of simulation to use to present a set of skills to interprofessional healthcare learners. The first consideration should be:

   A. The cost of the equipment needed
   B. The learning level of the students
   C. How the learning outcomes are met
   D. How the students responded during a previous simulation

2. A simulation educator would like to **increase fidelity** related to cardiac arrest response. The best simulation method to accomplish this would be:

   A. Using a part-task trainer (PTT) of a torso
   B. Using a standardized simulated patient
   C. Using a computer program in "real life"
   D. Using a mannequin that is fully equipped

3. The novice simulation educator needs further understanding when he states:

   A. "A part-task trainer (PTT) can only be used for simple procedures."
   B. "PTT can be used in hybrid form."
   C. "PTT are at times more durable."
   D. "PTT may jeopardize suspending disbelief."

4. A simulation educator is developing a haptic hybrid skill station. In order to do this, she will need:

   A. A part-task trainer (PTT) and a mannequin
   B. Two PTTs
   C. A PTT and a computer
   D. A PPT with the feel of real anatomy

5. An element to consider when using part-task trainers (PTTs) in the simulation laboratory is:

   A. They are always easy to move.
   B. They are usually less expensive.
   C. They may have to be replaced.
   D. They are usually durable.

6. To increase fidelity using a part-task trainer (PTT) the simulation educator may consider using a PTT with:

   A. A standardized patient
   B. Another PTT
   C. A high-fidelity mannequin
   D. A virtual environment

7. Part-task trainers (PTTs) are considered:

   A. High fidelity
   B. Low fidelity
   C. Midfidelity
   D. Are not classified

8. Simulation educators understand the usefulness of part-task trainer (PTT) mainly because they are:

    A. Easy to obtain and use
    B. Anatomically exact
    C. Travel well
    D. Have been around many years

9. Using part-task trainers (PTTs) decreases the risk of:

    A. Replacing expensive equipment
    B. Mistakes in procedures
    C. Simulation burnout
    D. Test anxiety

10. When a part-task trainer (PTT) needs repair the simulation coordinator should:

    A. Use special chemical to clean it well.
    B. Order a new one because they are inexpensive.
    C. Take it apart and check functionality.
    D. Read the manufacturer's instructions.

■ REFERENCES

Bauchat, J. R., Seropian, M., & Jeffries, P. R. (2016). Communication and empathy in the patient-centered care model—Why simulation-based training is not optional. *Clinical Simulation in Nursing, 12*(8), 356–359. doi:10.1016/j.ecns.2016.04.003

Brown, D. K. (2017). Simulation before clinical practice: The educational advantages. *Audiology Today, 29*(5), 16–24.

Dedmon, M. M., O'Connell, B. P., Kozin, E. D., Remenschneider, A. K., Barber, S. R., Lee, D. . . Rivas, A. (2017). Development and validation of a modular endoscopic ear surgery skills trainer. *Otology & Neurotology, 38*(8), 1193–1197. doi:10.1097/MAO.0000000000001485

Hagelsteen, K., Langegard, A., Lantz, A., Eklund, M., Anderberh, M., & Bergenfelz, A. (2017). Faster acquisition of laparoscopic skills in virtual reality with haptic feedback and 3D vision. *Minimally Invasive Therapy & Allied Technologies, 26*(5), 269–277. doi:10.1080/13645706.2017.1305970

Issenberg, S. B., McGaghie, W. C., Hart, I. R., Mayer, J. W., Felner, J. M., Petrusa, E. R., ... Ewy, G. A. (1999). Simulation technology for healthcare professional skills training and assessment. *Journal of the American Medical Association, 282*, 861–866. doi:10.1001/jama.282.9.861

Komasawa, N., Berg, B. W., & Minami, T. (2017). Hybrid simulation utilizing problem-based learning and task trainer for central venous catheter insertion training. *American Journal of Emergency Medicine, 35*(9), 1379–1379. doi: 10.1016/j.ajem.2017.03.068

Muckler, V. C. (2017). Exploring suspension of disbelief during simulation-based learning. *Clinical Simulation in Nursing, 13*(1), 3–9. doi:10.1016/j.ecns.2016.09.004

Ng, V., Plitt, J., & Biffar, D. (2018). Development of a novel ultrasound-guided peritonsillar abscess model for simulation training. *Western Journal of Emergency Medicine: Integrating Emergency Care with Population Health, 19*(1), 172–176. doi:10.5811/westjem.2017.11.36427

Orledge, J., Phillips, W. J., Murray, W. B., & Lerant, A. (2012). The use of simulation in healthcare: From systems issues, to team building, to task training, to education and high stakes examinations. *Current Opinion in Critical Care, 18*(4), 326–332. doi:10.1097/MCC.0b013e328353fb49

Oussi, N., Loukas, C., Kjellin, A., Lahanas, V., Georgiou, K., Henningsohn, L. . . Enochsson, L. (2018). Video analysis in basic skills training: a way to expand the value and use of BlackBox training? *Surgical Endoscopy*, 32(1), 87–95. doi:10.1007/s00464-017-5641-7

Posner, G. D., & Hamstra, S. J. (2013). Too much small talk? Medical students' pelvic examination skills falter with pleasant patients. *Medical Education*, 47(12), 1209–1214. doi:10.1111/medu.12280

Rodriques, S., Horeman, T., Blomious, M., Hiemstra, E., Dobbelsteen, J., Jansen, F. (2016) Laparoscopic suturing learning curve in an open versus closed box trainer. *Surgical Endoscopy*, 30(1), 315–322. doi:10.1007/s00464-015-4211-0

Ruest, A. S., Getto, L. P., Fredette, J. M., Cherico, A., Papas, M. A., & Nomura, J. T. (2016). A novel task trainer for penile corpus cavernosa aspiration. *Annals of Emergency Medicine*, 68, S126. doi:10.1016/j.annemergmed.2016.08.343

Scott, G. M., Roth, K., Rotenberg, B., Sommer, D. D., Sowerby, L., & Fung, K. (2016). Evaluation of a novel high-fidelity epistaxis task trainer. *Laryngoscope*, 126(7), 1501–1503. doi:10.1002/lary.25652

Society for Simulation in Healthcare. (2018). *Certified Healthcare Simulation Educator Examination Blueprint, 2018 Version*. Retrieved from http://www.ssih.org/Portals/48/Certification/CHSE_Docs/CHSE_Examination_Blueprint.pdf

Spooner, N., Hurst, S., & Khadra, M. (2012). Medical simulation technology: Educational overview, industry leaders, and what's missing. *Hospital Topics*, 90(3), 57–64. doi:10.1080/00185868.2012.714685

Woo, J. A., Malekzadeh, S., Malloy, K. M., & Deutsch, E. S. (2017). Are all manikins created equal? A pilot study of simulator upper airway anatomic fidelity. *Otolaryngology—Head & Neck Surgery*, 156(6), 1154–1157. doi:10.1177/0194599816674658

13

Virtual Reality

ROSEMARY FLISZAR

Unless you try to do something beyond what you have already mastered, you will never grow.

—Ralph Waldo Emerson

This chapter addresses Domain II: Healthcare and Simulation Knowledge/Principles (Society for Simulation in Healthcare, 2018).

[LEARNING OUTCOMES]

- Discuss the basic components of virtual reality (VR).
- Identify ways in which VR can be used to facilitate learning.
- Discuss the platforms used to design virtual learning (VL) activities.
- Discuss the feasibility of using VL and virtual simulation in designing classroom and clinical activities.

The healthcare environment of today is fast paced and, with the advancement of technology, is moving rapidly in the provision of patient care and learning environments. There is a large demand for clinical sites within the nursing field alone, and acute care facilities are not able to accommodate the large numbers of students seeking clinical placements. There has also been a proliferation of distance education programs that traditionally have been delivered in a two-dimensional environment with limited interaction between the learners and faculty member. In addition, the complexity of healthcare in today's world is moving toward interprofessional collaboration among healthcare providers, increased teamwork, enhanced critical thinking skills and clinical judgment, and time for skill practice. Changes are needed in the way learners are educated to meet the demands of complex healthcare settings.

Virtual worlds (VWs) are evolving as strategies to meet the demands of this changing environment, thereby changing the way nursing education is delivered (Billings, 2009; Farra, Miller, & Hodgson, 2015; Green, Wyllie, & Jackson, 2014; Walsh & van Soeren, 2012). This chapter begins with a description of virtual learning (VL) environments. The components of VL worlds are discussed, as well as the three-dimensional (3-D) platforms used to create these worlds. Advantages and disadvantages are presented with regard to VWs. Examples of application of virtual reality (VR) to areas of practice are presented. The chapter concludes with a case study and review questions.

VIRTUAL LEARNING

Several terms are used to describe VL, including *virtual reality simulation* (*VRS*), *VR*, *VWs*, *virtual patients* (*VPs*), and *multiuser virtual environments* (*MUVEs*). VR is a broad term that encompasses a wide range of technology. However, the common definition of *VR* is that learners immerse themselves in a multimedia, computer-generated, 3-D–simulated environment that simulates reality and allows learners to interact, practice skills, learn teamwork and collaboration, and manipulate medical equipment (Billings, 2009; Billings & Halstead, 2012; Farra et al., 2015).

Key features of the VR environment include the following:

- 3-D immersive experience
- The ability to interact with the virtual environment via an avatar
- Visual and auditory feedback
- Replicate real-world activities (Tiffany & Hoglund, 2014)

A VW is a 3-D computer-based simulated healthcare environment. The environment, or "world," provides an interactive experience based on teacher-designed case scenarios (Bai et al., 2012). VWs allow simulated interaction among a variety of individuals, including students, educators, patients, families, and multidisciplinary professionals (Green et al., 2014). Other benefits of VWs are that they:

- Provide dynamic feedback.
- Allow for learner experimentation.
- Allow for creativity.
- Provide opportunities for social networking and social interaction.
- Facilitate collaboration among participants.
- Lower learner anxiety.

The faculty and learners enter the VW, otherwise known as being "in world," by creating an avatar. An avatar is a digitized person created in 3-D, which represents the individual participating in the VW and is created by that person (Anderson, Page, & Wendorf, 2013; Second Life, n.d.). The participant creates the characteristics of the avatar, including eye and hair color, clothing, age, race, ethnicity, and gender. However, it is highly recommended that the learners create an avatar that mimics their own features and appearance. Avatars are two-dimensional in character when used in a game or VW (Anderson et al., 2013). Avatars interact with each other through online chat by typing messages or talking using a headset with a microphone and Internet or telephone connection (Billings, 2009). The avatar can function in the world, move around, perform skills, role-play, and participate in meetings and communicate with other avatars in the world such as patients, doctors, or nurses. The VW provides the learner the opportunity to simulate real-life experiences either synchronously or asynchronously and can be used in various settings in the learning environment. The virtual environment allows options for the development of social and professional relationships, especially in areas of distance learning. It also allows the learner to practice and demonstrate skills and knowledge without the fear of harming a live patient and can be used as an evaluative tool to determine whether learning has occurred. Examples of areas in which VWs have been created include:

- Classrooms
- Distance education
- Clinical agency
- Staff orientation
- Operating room (Patel, Aggarwal, Cohen, Taylor, & Darzi, 2013)
- Community settings
- Disaster training (Farra & Miller, 2013)
- Pediatric primary care clinic (Cook, 2012)
- Mental health education (Guise, Chambers, & Valimaki, 2012)
- Clinical reasoning and decision-making skills (Johnsen, Fossum, Vivekananda-Schmidt, Fruhling, & Slettebo, 2016; Koivisto, Multisilta, Niemi, Katajisto, & Eriksson, 2016)

> **SIMULATION TEACHING TIP 13.1**
>
> Avatars represent the individuals creating them and should be as realistic as possible.

VIRTUAL PATIENTS

A VP is an interactive computer-based simulation of a real-life clinical case scenario. Learners assume the role of the healthcare professional as an avatar, such as a nurse or doctor, and make judgments and clinical decisions based on the assessments made of the VP (Guise et al., 2012; Patel et al., 2013). Participants learn the role of the professionals they represent with regard to assessment, clinical diagnosis, treatment, and care of the patient, just as they would if interacting with a real-life patient. VP simulations are case-based educational computer games in which the user progresses through various steps and applies clinical knowledge and critical thinking skills in making judgments about the care and treatment of the VP (Guise et al., 2012). The pathway for clinical decision making may be preprogrammed or may have a branching structure, which allows for several alternative pathways depending on each action taken by the learner.

SERIOUS GAMES

The term *serious games* has loosely been defined in several contexts, including technology for professional use, interactive video simulation, avatars, and watching videos (dit Dariel, Raby, Ravuat, & Rothan-Tondeur, 2013). The serious game has as its primary purpose educational and professional goals and not entertainment (Hogan, Kapralos, Cristancho, Finney, & Dubrowski, 2011). Serious games are computer-based simulations and combine knowledge and skills development with video game-playing aspects, thereby enabling active, experiential, situated, and problem-based learning (dit Dariel et al., 2013; Johnsen et al., 2016).

In recent studies, Johnson et al. (2016) and Koivisto et al. (2016) developed a serious game to enhance the clinical reasoning and decision-making skills of nursing students in a realistic, safe environment.

Students enter the VW on a computer and can interact in a realistic environment to practice skills and develop different competencies. The learner-centered approach is used as the player controls the learning through interactivity (Ricciardi & DePaolis, 2014). The game can be designed so that as the student makes a choice, with regard to an action or intervention, it leads to another step based on the previous decision. This design fits nicely with Kolb's (1984) experiential learning theory.

The design of a serious game should be based on several key components (Billings & Halstead, 2012).

- Identify the content of the lesson.
- Identify the information the learner is to receive.
- Base the game on objectives and outcomes.

Several platforms have been identified for the serious games' simulation environment, also known as *MUVEs* (Wang & Braman, 2009).

- Second Life
- Task trainers
- vSim by Laerdal
- Twinity
  - Voki Avatar

Second Life is a serious game 3-D software platform, or framework, which delivers computerized virtual training and research environments (Tiffany & Hoglund, 2014). Scenarios can be constructed by the faculty to design simulations in which the student may practice skills, make decisions, try new ideas, and learn from mistakes in a safe and controlled environment. The creation of a serious game is more complex than a case study or a laboratory simulation designed for a classroom. The serious game is not linear in nature, but rather is a dynamic experience in which the player participates in the unfolding of a sequence of problems, and the interaction with the game influences the outcomes (dit Dariel et al., 2013). Serious games can be designed so that rules may be broken or the scenario changed based on the decisions made and actions of the learner (Charsky, 2010). Serious games may be designed as a means of summative evaluation based on specific outcomes or provide a means for formative evaluation to determine whether learning is occurring.

VL PLATFORMS

The Second Life platform allows faculty and students to perform some of the following activities (Second Life, n.d.).

- Build an avatar designed by the participant.
- Join or create groups.
- Develop one's own online community.
- Attend or organize events.

- Participate in forums.
- Use 3-D voice chats, gestures, language, and so on.

The Voki platform allows teachers and students to do the following (Voki, 2018):

- Build a customizable speaking avatar.
- Create a visual representation of a character.
- Post a lesson or case study (Anderson et al., 2013).
- Share on email, post on Facebook, Twitter, or personal website.

Task trainers are specific tools that are used to train the professional for a specific purpose. These may include:

- Intravenous (IV) arm for venipuncture
- Airway trainers
- Blood pressure skills
- Femoral artery access
- Intubation trainers
- Chest-tube insertion
- Neonatal procedures

> **SIMULATION TEACHING TIP 13.2**
>
> The simulation or scenario must be appropriate for the level of the learner.

THEORETICAL FRAMEWORKS

Serious games should be designed based on the objectives for the game, outcomes to be met by students, and processes that have a theoretical basis. Three main theoretical approaches include constructivist theory, Kolb's experiential learning theory, and Knowles's adult learning theory.

The constructivist learning theory states that learners construct knowledge based on their experiences in relation to an event (Keating, 2011). The constructivist theory supports the movement of the learner from the novice to advanced beginner level, and recognizes that actions by the learner may be determined by previous exposure to a situation as well as the knowledge base of the learner. According to Woolfolk (2010), there are five conditions for learning that are integral to the constructivist theory:

- The learning environment should provide a realistic and relevant learning experience.
- Social interactions and peer collaboration are essential to the learning process.
- It is important to support multiple perspectives of the experience, especially as the learner gains more knowledge and moves through more complex situations.
- Learners must be aware of their own beliefs and knowledge that shapes their learning and assumptions, which allows them to respect that others may have a different perspective of the scenario.
- Learners must assume ownership of learning and use multiple resources to enhance learning.

When designing a serious game using the constructivist theory, it is important to formulate objectives and outcomes prior to the development of the scenario for the game. The level of the learner must also be taken into consideration; for example, a scenario designed for a beginning nursing student may require the instructor to be more actively involved in the game based on limited knowledge of the learner. As the student moves through the curriculum, there is less involvement by the instructor, and eventually the student assumes total control of the decision making for the scenario. This type of design is termed *instructional scaffolding* (Keating, 2011).

Kolb's (1984) experiential learning theory provides a solid platform for the design of VL activities. Kolb described learning "as the process whereby knowledge is created through transformation of experience" (p. 41). Kolb suggests that a person learns through a concrete experience, which provides a basis for observation and reflection on the experience in the virtual simulated environment, and discovers new knowledge (Rogers, 2011). Kolb further proposes that reflections are then assimilated into abstract concepts and can be applied to a new experience. This in turn suggests that learning, which has occurred from a simulation in a virtual environment, can be applied to situations encountered in the real world (Rogers, 2011).

Green et al. (2014) postulate that Vygotsky's (1978) activity theory is important in the relationship of engagement in VWs. Vygotsky espoused that learning is a social experience and learners should be actively involved in their learning. Vygotsky proposed that social interactions are fundamental to the process of cognitive development, and that connections between people and how learners interact in shared experiences are essential to collaborative learning. The VW is ideal for social interaction with simulated environments (Green et al., 2014).

SIMULATION TEACHING TIP 13.3

The development of a serious game should be based on sound theoretical principles and designed around the purpose, objectives, and outcomes of the learning exercise.

Knowles's adult learning theory (1978) can also be applied to the VR environment and development of serious games. Knowles proposed that adults learn differently from children, and their learning is dependent on autonomy, life experiences, personal goals, and relevance of the experience. He termed this *andragogy*. This theory is applicable to the VR environment as the learners can apply theoretical principles to the situation and receive immediate feedback on their decisions and actions. Virtual environments can stimulate adult learners to apply their knowledge and experiences to concrete situations in a controlled environment, then consider the consequences of their actions and make changes to future choices. The learner is actively engaged in the learning process through simulated activities and can apply what is learned to real-life situations.

ADVANTAGES AND DISADVANTAGES OF VR LEARNING

The integration of VR learning is important in the learning environment in order to allow the learners an opportunity to immerse themselves in environments where they can practice skills, interact and collaborate with peers or other professionals, make decisions related to care and interventions, and manipulate equipment without fear of harming an individual. VL simulations can be used in any area of clinical practice, but is especially useful in environments where limited access to the experience is available such as disaster or perioperative nursing. Some benefits and limitations are described in Table 13.1.

TABLE 13.1

Advantages and Disadvantages of Virtual Learning Environments

ADVANTAGES/BENEFITS	DISADVANTAGES/CHALLENGES
Provide learning experiences in a safe environment to enhance experiential learning (Herold, 2012).	VR learning environments, such as serious games, are expensive to produce.
Provide interactive and innovative educational scenarios that simulate real-world experiences (Tiffany & Hoglund, 2014).	Educators and learners must be oriented on how to use the virtual game or task trainer.
Simulate clinical experiences, have a student-centered approach, and promote active learning (Rogers, 2011).	Time must be allotted for development of the scenario and creation of avatars (Billings, 2009).
Provide opportunities for learning, which are not readily available in clinical practice or situations that may be dangerous (Kilmon, Brown, Ghosh, & Mikitiuk, 2010).	Technological support must be available to users and designers.
Foster collaboration with peers and users from other disciplines, both locally and globally.	Scenario must be relevant for the learning community for which it is designed, and globally relevant if used in a multidisciplinary context (Hogan et al., 2011).
Engage students in role-playing in a more natural environment.	Educators and learners must keep an open mind and be willing to learn how to function within the virtual environment.
Manipulate equipment and perform procedures in a safe environment (Billings & Halstead, 2012).	Lacks a comprehensive theoretical framework to support and guide the use of simulation in nursing (Guise et al., 2012).
Incorporate a variety of problems and information the learner can use as part of the assessment phase and test solutions (Hogan et al., 2011).	Educators must have a firm understanding and grounding of pedagogical principles in educational theories appropriate for learning in virtual worlds (Green et al., 2014). There is a lack of empirical evidence on the impact of VL.

(continued)

TABLE 13.1

Advantages and Disadvantages of Virtual Learning Environments (*continued*)

ADVANTAGES/BENEFITS	DISADVANTAGES/CHALLENGES
Reflect on outcomes related to learner actions and propose new strategies or interventions for the situation.	Usability issues of serious games can negatively impact a user's experience and intended learning outcomes (Johnsen et al., 2016). Current research addresses teaching and learning in the affective domain or technological learning domain (Tiffany & Hoglund, 2014). Computer requirements for VL environments may not be available on entry-level computers (Billings & Halstead, 2012).
Evaluate student performance to determine whether learning outcomes have been met	
Provide opportunities for social interaction, facilitation, and collaboration (Green et al., 2014) Improve online and distance education by adding a real-life component to relationships between online learners in a virtual world (Tiffany & Hoglund, 2014) Communicate effectively across disciplines	
Useful in a multitude of disciplines and environments such as community health nursing, disaster preparedness, and perioperative areas (Kaplan, Holmes, Mott, & Atallah, 2011; Patel et al., 2013)	

VL, virtual learning; VR, virtual reality.

ENTERING AND DESIGNING A VIRTUAL SIMULATION

There are several issues that need to be considered in order to develop a simulation in the VW using a platform, such as Second Life, in order to enhance teamwork and problem solving for the simulated experience. In order to participate in the VW, the individual:

- Must be able to access the Internet through a high-speed connection.
- Creates an avatar the first time the platform is accessed.
- Participates in the simulation community through one of two ways:
  - Types messages as done in texting or online chats.
  - Communicates using a headset with a microphone or Internet telephone connection.
- Participates either synchronously (in real time) or asynchronously (virtual time; Billings, 2009).

Once the participant enters the simulation or serious game, the participant is able to interact in the environment created in the VW. This may include role-playing, practicing skills, decision making, or participating in conferences or classroom activities.

Several steps should be taken in designing the MUVE (Rogers, 2011, p. 612).
- Briefing stage
  - Learners create their avatar and familiarize themselves with the platform interface
  - Learners view the VW videos for an introduction to the scenario and how to interact with and view objects in the scenario and how to communicate with peers or others in the virtual environment for the scenario
- Action phase
  - Learners enter the VW scenario created for them
  - Learners are given the scenario for the VL experience
  - Learners interact in the environment based on the design of the simulation, which may be acting alone or working in teams and collaborating with others
- Debriefing stage (Billings & Halstead, 2012)
  - A key feature in designing VWs and should be done after each VL experience
  - Educators facilitate the reflection (reflective observation) of learners' experiences during the simulation
  - Meaning (abstract conceptualization) is derived from the experience
  - Further application of the meaning may be initiated

EVIDENCE-BASED SIMULATION PRACTICE 13.1

A study was designed to learn the perceptions and experiences of nursing students using a virtual game (Chia, 2013).

Purpose: To examine the perception and experiences of nursing students using a virtual game prior to the related simulation-based activity in the simulation laboratory.

Design: The game was designed to reinforce knowledge about chronic obstructive pulmonary disease (COPD) and to teach students how to apply this knowledge in the simulated clinical setting.

Method: One hundred sixty-one second-year diploma students participated in the study. Ten students were absent for the virtual game, thereby yielding a response rate of 94.8%. A self-developed questionnaire was used to ask students about their perception and experiences of using the virtual game to collect data. The game was available to the students for 1 week prior to the simulation-based learning (SBL) session. Feedback through a questionnaire was obtained from the participants and included whether or not they felt the virtual game prepared them for the simulated learning experience.

Results: Overall, the participants felt that the game did prepare them for the SBL activity in the laboratory and that it was relevant. A total of 91% of participants felt that their knowledge base on patient management was enhanced in managing the care of patients with COPD.

Conclusions: The results of the study provided useful data to use in phase 2 of the design of the game. The next phase will incorporate constructivist learning theory resulting in more challenging segments in patient assessment and history.

> **EVIDENCE-BASED SIMULATION PRACTICE 13.2**
>
> A study was designed to determine the efficacy of learning clinical reasoning skills by playing 3-D simulation games (Koivisto et al., 2016).
>
> **Purpose:** To investigate nursing students' experiences of learning clinical reasoning by playing a 3-D simulation game.
>
> **Design:** The game consisted of patient scenarios designed around a specific clinical situation requiring clinical reasoning. This was phase 2 of the project.
>
> **Method:** Data were collected during 13 gaming sessions from nursing students in the surgical nursing course. One hundred sixty-six students participated in the sessions. The sessions involved two to five postoperative patient scenarios that lasted 30 to 40 minutes. The game was built around the clinical reasoning process. Participants assumed the role of the nurse and were guided to collect and process information, identify problems and issues, establish goals, take action, and evaluate outcomes related to postoperative patient scenarios. Participants completed an online questionnaire after completing the game.
>
> **Results:** A majority of the students felt they learned the phases of clinical reasoning quite or moderately well. Students felt they learned best how to collect information and to take action, but were less successful in establishing patient goals or in evaluating effectiveness of interventions. There was a moderate to strong positive correlation between the application of nursing knowledge and learning of the clinical reasoning process with the strongest correlation in the area of identification of problems and issues.
>
> **Conclusions:** The results of the study showed that 3-D simulation games can be used for learning of clinical reasoning skills in nursing students. Games allow students to combine theory and practice using a systematic approach. Game mechanics need to be built around the clinical reasoning process and integrate engaging gaming elements.

There are many virtual learning websites with new ones appearing everyday. Some of the more popular sites are listed in Table 13.2.

TABLE 13.2 Virtual Learning Websites

WEBSITE ADDRESS	PURPOSE
Second Life www.secondlife.com	Serious game platform using 3-D technology to create avatars
Voki www.voki.com	Voki is a free collection of customizable speaking avatars for teachers and students that enhances classroom instruction, class engagement, and lesson comprehension.

(continued)

TABLE 13.2
Virtual Learning Websites (*continued*)

WEBSITE ADDRESS	PURPOSE
vSim from Laerdal www.nln.org	News release from the National League for Nursing about Laerdal V simulations
Serious Games and Simulation www.3dseriousgamesandsimulations.com/showcase/healthcare-serious-game	Serious games and simulations use 3-D technology to create healthcare and nursing games and simulations for the trauma unit
SimTab www.simtabs.com/	Develop virtual medical simulations and healthcare serious games
Free Nursing Simulation Scenarios www.healthysimulation.com/1947/more-free-nursing-simulation-scenarios/	Free library of simulation scenarios designed by nursing faculty for nursing and allied health programs
Twinity www.twinity.com	Free virtual 3-D world and 3-D community chats can be created using avatars

3-D, three dimensional.

■ SUMMARY

This chapter discussed VL modalities, including VR, VPs, VRS, MUVEs, and serious games, and has looked at the design of these modalities and their effectiveness in the learning environment. Second Life and mSTREET were two examples of serious game platforms discussed, including factors that need to be considered when designing a game for educational purposes. There are concrete advantages to using VL environments, which include promoting interprofessional collaboration and providing experiences that mimic real-life situations and are easily transferred to the clinical practice setting. Disadvantages of VL include the cost and extensive faculty development required to design the scenario. The learner must also be oriented to the VL platform in order to be successful in maneuvering within the scenario to enhance the learning experience. VL and VRSs can be used in both prelicensure and postlicensure education when there is a great demand for clinical placement and, at the same time, fewer resources available, both time and space, for learning. The uses of VL and their outcomes are in the infancy stages of development and show much promise in enhancing the learning environment.

> **CASE STUDY 13.1**
>
> Students in their last semester of nursing at the local university are enrolled in the community health nursing course. The course has been designed within the context of public health nursing. Disaster preparedness is one of the topics taught in the course. The faculty member has collaborated with faculty in other disciplines, including medical students, physician-assistant students, and emergency management services (EMS) as well as paramedic students, to plan a VR learning experience in the management of disasters. Faculty members are developing the scenario, but are not sure how to design the simulation using Second Life as the VL platform. How should they begin the process to design the simulation so that it is a meaningful learning experience?
>
> **Discussion:** A major factor to consider is the cost of designing the virtual simulation. Does the university support the learning platform, and is it willing to provide funds for the project? An initial action to be considered when designing the virtual serious game is the determination of the purpose of the activity. The scenario should be designed based on the objectives and outcomes of the exercise. That is the key factor in developing a VL situation. It is advisable to base the VW on a sound learning theory, which then influences the activities that are constructed within the activity. Faculty should receive some professional development on how to design the simulation using the Second Life platform. What computer requirements are needed for the learner to interact in the VW? Instructional technology services at the university need to be available to support both faculty and students through the process. Faculty should conduct an assessment of the students' abilities and/or needs to interact with technology and plan orientation based on the data obtained. The value of professional collaboration across disciplines, especially in disaster preparedness, should be emphasized prior to the start of the VL simulation so that learners from all of the disciplines are actively involved in the game.

PRACTICE QUESTIONS

1. The novice simulation educator needs additional understanding when he states virtual reality (VR) platforms:

    A. "Are designed for distance education learners"
    B. "Can be three-dimension (3-D) to enhance immersion"
    C. "Are a mechanism to teach teamwork"
    D. "Provide an opportunity for students to manipulate equipment"

2. Virtual worlds (VW) provide the learner with all the following elements except:

    A. Dynamic feedback
    B. Increased attentiveness
    C. Creativity
    D. Decreased anxiety

3. The main objective of using a virtual patient (VP) in virtual worlds is to:

    A. Entertain while learning
    B. Practice clinical decision making
    C. Practice skills
    D. Encourage creatively

4. Serious gaming is a method of learning delivery that is associated with which educational theory?

   A. Behaviorism
   B. Realism
   C. Emancipatory
   D. Constructivism

5. A novice simulation educator is designing a virtual world, which of the following concepts should not be included:

   A. There should be a sense of immersion for the participant.
   B. Real-world scenarios should be replicated.
   C. No opportunities for social networking are provided so as to keep students on track.
   D. Learners should be allowed to experiment in the scenario.

6. The primary purpose of a serious game is to:

   A. Allow entertainment to lower stress.
   B. Design the learning experience so only one response is correct.
   C. Meet educational and professional goals.
   D. Create the game using a one-dimensional approach.

7. The professor wants to design a scenario on the proper method to use for intubation. Which platform is the best choice for this learning experience?

   A. Second Life
   B. Task trainer
   C. Voki
   D. SimTab

8. The design of a simulation or serious game based on Vygotsky's theory would include:

   A. An opportunity for social interaction between learners
   B. Recall of previously learned information
   C. Development of an avatar by the instructor
   D. Application of Maslow's hierarchy of needs

9. When developing a serious game, the first action the teacher must perform is which of the following?

   A. Determine the platform to use to design the game.
   B. Require students to have taken a computer course on using the technology.
   C. Conduct a debriefing about the experience.
   D. Develop objectives for the activity.

10. During the action phase of the multi-user virtual environment (MUVE), the learner does which of the following?

    A. Creates her or his avatar.
    B. Watches videos to familiarize him- or herself with the requirements for the activity.
    C. Interacts in the environment created in the simulation.
    D. Discusses what he or she has learned during the game or simulation.

REFERENCES

Anderson, J. K., Page, A. M., & Wendorf, D. M. (2013). Avatar-assisted case studies. *Nurse Educator, 38*(3), 106–109. doi:10.1097/NNE.0b013e31828dc260

Bai, X., Duncan, R. O., Horowitz, B. P., Graffeo, J. M., Glodstein, S. L., & Lavin, J. (2012). The added value of 3D simulations in healthcare education. *International Journal of Nursing Education, 4*(2), 67–72.

Billings, D. M. (2009). Teaching and learning in virtual worlds. *Journal of Continuing Education in Nursing, 40*, 489–490. doi:10.3928/00220124-20091023-04

Billings, D. M., & Halstead, J. M. (2012). *Teaching in nursing* (4th ed.). St. Louis, MO: Elsevier.

Charsky, D. (2010). From entertainment to serious games: A change in the use of game characteristics. *Games and Cultures, 5*, 177–198. doi:10.1177/1555412009354727

Chia, P. (2013). Using a virtual game to enhance simulation based learning in nursing education. *Singapore Nursing Journal, 40*(3), 21–26.

Cook, M. J. (2012). Design and initial evaluation of a virtual pediatric primary care clinic in Second Life. *Journal of the American Academy of Nurse Practitioners, 24*, 521–527. doi:10.1111/j.1745-7599.2012.00729.x

dit Dariel, O. J., Raby, T., Ravaut, F., & Rothan-Tondeur, M. (2013). Developing the serious games potential in nursing education. *Nurse Education Today, 12*, 1569–1575. doi:10.1016/j.nedt.2012.12.014

Farra, S. L., & Miller, E. T. (2013). Integrative review: Virtual disaster training. *Journal of Nursing Education and Practice, 3*, 93–101. doi:10.5430/jnep.v3n3p93

Farra, S. L., Miller, E. T., & Hodgson, E. (2015). Virtual reality disaster training: Translation to practice. *Nurse Eduction in Practice, 15*(1), 53–57 doi:10.1016/j.nepr.2013.08.017

Green, J., Wyllie, A., & Jackson, D. (2014). Virtual worlds: A new frontier for nurse education? *Collegian, 21*, 135–141.

Guise, V., Chambers, M., & Valimaki, M. (2012). What can virtual patient simulation offer mental health nursing education? *Journal of Psychiatric and Mental Health Nursing, 19*, 410–418. doi:10.1111/j.1365-2850.2011.01797.x

Herold, D. K. (2012). Second Life and academia—Reframing the debate between supporters and critics. *Journal of Virtual Worlds Research, 5*, 1–22. doi:10.4101/jvwr.v5i1.6156

Hogan, M., Kapralos, B., Cristancho, S., Finney, K., & Dubrowski, A. (2011). Bringing community health nursing education to life with Serious Games. *International Journal of Nursing Education Scholarship, 8*, 1–13. doi:10.2202/1548-923X.2072

Johnsen, H. M., Fossum, M., Vivekananda-Schmidt, P., Fruhling, A., & Slettebo, A. (2016). Teaching clinical reasoning and decision-making skills to nursing students: Design, development, and usability evaluation of a serious game. *International Journal of Medical Informatics, 94*, 39–48. doi:10.1016/j.ijmedinf.2016.06.014

Kaplan, B. G., Holmes, L., Mott, M., & Atallah, H. (2011). Design and implementation of an interdisciplinary pediatric mock code for undergraduate and graduate nursing students. *CIN: Computers, Informatics, Nursing, 29*(9), 531–538. doi:10.1097/NCN.0b013e31821a166e

Keating, S. B. (2011). *Curriculum development and evaluation in nursing* (2nd ed.). New York, NY: Springer Publishing.

Kilmon, C. A., Brown, L., Ghosh, S., & Mikitiuk, A. (2010). Immersive virtual reality simulations in nursing education. *Nursing Education Perspectives, 31*, 314–317.

Knowles, M. S. (1978). *The adult learner: A neglected species* (2nd ed.). Houston, TX: Gulf.

Koivisto, J., Multisilta, J., Niemi, H., Katajisto, J., & Eriksson, E. (2016). Learning by playing: A cross-sectional descriptive study of nursing students' experiences of learning clinical reasoning. *Nurse Education Today, 45*, 22–28. doi:10.1016/j.nedt.2016.06.009

Kolb, D. A. (1984). *Experiential learning: Experience as the source of learning and development.* Englewood Cliffs, NJ: Prentice Hall.

Patel, V., Aggarwal, R., Cohen, D., Taylor, D., & Darzi, A. (2013). Implementation of an interactive virtual-world simulation for structured surgeon assessment of clinical scenarios. *Journal of the American College of Surgeons, 217*, 270–279. doi:10.1016/j.jamcollsurg.2013.03.023

Ricciardi, F., & DePaolis, L. T. (2014). A comprehensive review of serious games in health professions. *International Journal of Computer Games Technology, 2014,* 1-11. doi:10.1155/2014/787968

Rogers, L. (2011). Developing simulations in multi-user virtual environments to enhance healthcare education. *British Journal of Educational Technology, 42,* 608–615. doi:10.1111/j.1467-8535.2010.01057.x

Second Life. (n.d.). *Second Life.* Retrieved from http://secondlife.com

Nurse Training: Trauma Unit. Retrieved from http://www.3dseriousgamesandsimulations.com/showcase/healthcare-serious-game

Society for Simulation in Healthcare. (2018). *Certified Healthcare Simulation Educator Examination Blueprint, 2018 Version.* Retrieved from http://www.ssih.org/Portals/48/Certification/CHSE_Docs/CHSE_Examination_Blueprint.pdf

SimTab. (n.d.). Leading developer of virtual medical simulations and healthcare serious games. Retrieved from http://www.simtabs.com

Tiffany, J., & Hoglund, B. A. (2014). Teaching/learning in second life: Perspectives of future nurse-educators. *Clinical Simulation in Nursing, 10,* e19–e24. doi: 10.1016/j.ecns.2013.06.006

Voki. (2018). Voki classroom. Retrieved from http://www.voki.com

Vygotsky, L. S. (1978). *Mind in society: The development of higher psychological processes.* Cambridge, MA: Harvard University Press.

Walsh, M., & van Soeren, M. (2012). Interprofessional learning and virtual communities: An opportunity for the future. *Journal of Interprofessional Care, 26,* 43–48. doi:10.3109/13561820.2011.620187

Woolfolk, A. (2010). *Educational psychology* (11th ed.). Upper Saddle River, NJ: Merrill.

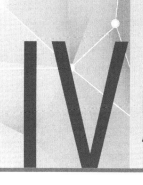

Domain III: Educational Principles Applied to Simulation

14 Educational Theories, Learning Theories, and Special Concepts

RUTH A. WITTMANN-PRICE AND SAMUEL W. PRICE

> *The teacher who is indeed wise does not bid you to enter the house of his wisdom but rather leads you to the threshold of your mind.*
> —Khalil Gibran

This chapter addresses Domain III: Educational Principles Applied to Simulation (Society for Simulation in Healthcare, 2018).

[LEARNING OUTCOMES]

- Discuss educational philosophies and theories in relation to simulation education.
- Discuss learning and motivational theories.
- Discuss concepts related to simulation education.

Understanding educational and learning theories increases awareness of what, why, and how educators teach and how learners assimilate knowledge presented. A simulation environment is an excellent milieu in which to synthesize cognitive, psychomotor, and affective learning. Development of competence in all three learning realms is necessary for healthcare providers. The goal of simulation learning experiences for teaching and assessment is to promote patient safety and provide healthcare learners with the best possible safe learning environment (Bastin, Cook, & Flannery, 2017).

Educational theories are contextual and spurn learning theories or how students grasp, understand, and apply knowledge. This chapter provides an overview of educational theories, including those educational concepts applied specifically to simulation learning and evaluation.

EDUCATIONAL PHILOSOPHIES AND THEORIES

To facilitate learning in a simulation environment, a simulation educator must build experiences on sound theoretical foundations that include understanding the essence of educational philosophies, which:

- Date back to ancient times, are never stagnant, and change as the larger social system matures
- Provide the foundations on which learning theories and educational pedagogies are built
- Consider the branch of philosophy that addresses why we teach, how we teach, and what the goals of education are for learners and society (Walton & Hill, 2016)

Traditional educational theories were teacher centered and based on what the educator could provide to the student. Postmodern theories more often take into account the social meaning of learning, the relationship of knowledge and power, and are more likely to consider multiple and innovative ways of learning (Turner, 2017).

Worldviews about education categorize how an educational philosophy relates to the social context. Learning theories have more defined concepts that are more applicable to teaching situations. Teaching is the act of facilitating learning through instruction, guidance, and coaching. In today's social context, teaching is student centered (McInerney & Green-Thompson, 2017).

Learning is how people understand information and how they store, connect, discover, and retrieve skills and information has been well studied and formalized into many theoretical frameworks. These frameworks explain how knowledge is built and what paradigms are used to advance healthcare research. Figure 14.1 shows the frameworks used in developing research knowledge for healthcare professionals (Win, 2016).

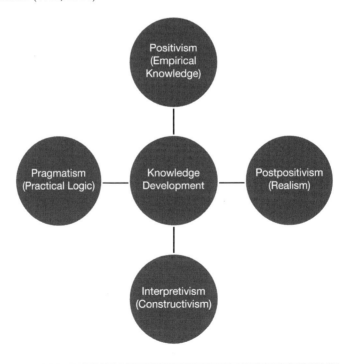

FIGURE 14.1 Knowledge development philosophies.

The two main learning theories discussed and used currently in education are mainly *behaviorism* and *constructivism*. Behaviorism is an ingrained theory in education and structures teaching plans. Constructivism is an ideal theory to encapsulate, ground, and expand what is done in the simulation laboratory because its major tenets promote active learning.

Behaviorism

Behaviorism is a learning theory that was developed in the 1940s. Some of the major tenets of behaviorism are:

- Learning is observable through behavior.
- Learning is reinforced by response.
- Behavior modification leads to control.
- Token economies may be used for classroom management.
- Instructional objectives guide learning (Tyler, 1949).
- Learning is shaped by others.
- Learning is teacher centered.
- Behaviorists include Watson, Skinner, Pavlov, and Bandura.

> **SIMULATION TEACHING TIP 14.1**
>
> Interprofessional education (IPE) using simulation can increase confidence in students, promote communication, and increase positive interactions (Anderson, Hughes, Patterson, & Costa, 2017).

Behaviorism posed a couple of difficult issues for education, including the following:

- Behaviorism does not explain the intrinsic motivation of the learner.
- All learning is not displayed in behavior.
- By predetermining objectives or outcomes, the depth and breadth of the learners' experiences may be squelched (Bevis & Watson, 1989; Diekelmann, 1997, 2005).

It is difficult, at best, to package the human intellect into a modifiable mold for convenience of grouping, evaluating, and justifying what is being taught or presented and what a learner carries forth from an experience. Behaviorism was made popular by Tyler's landmark book *Basic Principles of Curriculum and Instruction* (1949) in relation to writing instructional objectives or what the teacher expected the learner to learn by the end of a teaching session or course.

Constructivism

Currently, constructivism is the theoretical paradigm that best fits educational processes and the social context of today. Constructivists view learning as an active process that builds new knowledge on knowledge already obtained, thereby connecting what is unknown to what is known. Adaptive behaviors are produced when learners take received stimuli and convert it or construct it into cognitive knowledge that makes sense to them. Constructivism is based in the reality of the learner and is therefore learner focused. The faculty role in constructivism includes coaching and facilitating (Le Coze, 2017). Learning using simulation fits well into the constructivist theoretical framework because it is problem based and individually constructed knowledge though experiential learning (Brown & Watts, 2016).

IV DOMAIN III: EDUCATIONAL PRINCIPLES APPLIED TO SIMULATION

LEARNING THEORIES

Experiential Learning Theory

A learning theory that fits within the constructivist framework is experiential learning. Experiential learning theory (ELT) is widely used in simulation experiences. It is defined as "the process whereby knowledge is created through the transformation of experience. Knowledge results from the combination of grasping and transforming an experience" (Kolb, 1984, p. 41).

There are four major concepts within Kolb's ELT:

1. **Concrete experience** (**CE**), or experiences built from reality
2. **Abstract conceptualization** (**AC**), or thinking about an experience
3. **Reflective observation** (**RO**), or taking in the experience
4. **Active experimentation** (**AE**) using hands-on experiences to learn (Kolb, Boyatzis, & Mainemelis, 1999)

ELT is student centered because the learners are in control of the direction the simulation scenario takes. Although the student learning outcomes (SLOs) are formulated by the certified healthcare educator, the students are in control of their actions and the consequences. As students become more advanced in their healthcare studies, they are able to forsake a more passive role in scenarios and increase their active roles and feelings of being prepared to participate in experiential learning (Bastin et al., 2017). The change from passive to active learning is depicted in Figure 14.2.

Gibbs (1988) also has a model for planning experiential learning, which includes the following:

- Planning for action
- Carrying out the action
- Reflecting on the action
- Relating the action back to the theory

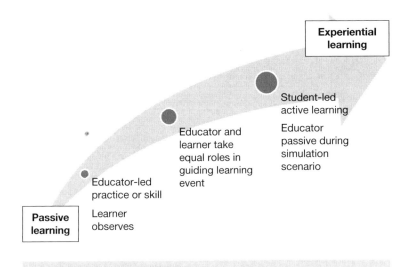

FIGURE 14.2 Change in learning from passive to active.

Grant and Marsden (1992) explain experiential learning as having the following components:

- Providing an experience
- Thinking about the experience
- Identifying improvements
- Planning the learning needed
- Putting the learning into practice

Simulation is well suited for experiential learning because it is a practiced experience in a controlled environment that allows for reflection (thinking) and ultimately changes in practice (doing) by adult professionals (Griffith, Steelman, Wildman, LeNoble, & Zhou, 2017).

Scaffolding Learning Theory

Congruent with ELT is cognitive scaffolding. This theory was introduced by Vygotsky (1978) to explain how a novice learns to be an expert. Just as a scaffold supports a building under construction, the novice learner needs resources and support from experts or mentors to increase cognitive knowledge in a subject and build it progressively. The scaffolding sets the framework for learning and is intentionally established as a "stretch" for the learner. In order for the learner to reach higher levels of knowledge or understanding about a situation or process, supports must be in place, such as:

- Constructive feedback
- Explanations
- Reflection
- Revision of knowledge building

Scaffolding learning has been noted to promote deeper learning and student confidence (Lauerer, Edlund, Williams, Donato, & Smith, 2017; Figure 14.3).

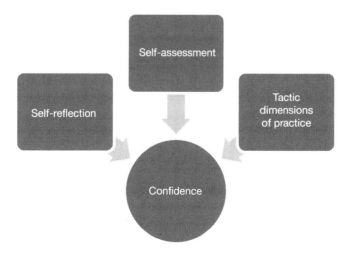

FIGURE 14.3 Outcomes of scaffolding learning.

Social Learning (Cognitive) Theory

Social learning theory is also a proponent of reinforcement and modeling new behavior as learners observe it from certified healthcare educators. Behavior is determined by social determinants, such as demographics and economics, behavioral influences such as those characteristics innate to a person, and environmental elements such as resources (Sriramatr, Silalertdetkul, & Wachirathanin, 2016).

Another popular concept that was attributed to social learning theory is self-efficacy coined by Bandura (1997). Self-efficacy is often measured in healthcare learners, and progressive or ongoing simulation experiences are an ideal environment for its measurement. Self-efficacy is the perception of confidence in one's self in a given situation. Self-efficacy is based on four principles:

1. **Mastering experiences**—The learner's own history of success
2. **Vicarious experiences**—The observed behaviors of a role model being successful at a task
3. **Verbal persuasion**—Telling individuals they will be successful
4. **Physiological states**—The person's "gut feeling" that success can be achieved

PEDAGOGY VERSUS ANDRAGOGY AS EDUCATIONAL CONCEPTS

Pedagogy is generally defined as the art and science of teaching. It refers to the manner in which educators instruct. Its development was intended for children, but all curricula development incorporates pedagogy to some extent and developing effective pedagogy assists students in the learning process (Cadieux et al., 2017). *Andragogy* is the art and science of teaching adults and was coined by Malcolm Knowles in 1980 (Table 14.1).

Adult learners display a variety of learning characteristics.

- The most common reason an adult enters any learning experience is to create change in the following:
  - Skills
  - Behavior
  - Knowledge level
  - Attitudes about things

Adult learners sometimes experience unique barriers to learning, which include the following:

- Lack of time
- Lack of confidence
- Lack of information about opportunities to learn
- Scheduling problems
- Red tape (Carpenter-Aeby & Aeby, 2013)

It is important to incorporate adult learning principles into simulated learning experiences to maximize learning potential for this population. Adult learner characteristics include the following:

- Developed self-concept
- Rich in experiences

TABLE 14.1
Andragogy and Pedagogy

EDUCATIONAL CONSIDERATIONS	ANDRAGOGY	PEDAGOGY
Demands of learning	Learners have life demands besides school.	Learners can devote more time to the demands of learning because responsibilities are minimal.
Role of instructor	Learners are autonomous and self-directed. Educators facilitate the learning, but do not supply all the facts.	Teacher centered because the educator directs the learning. Often uses surface learning.
Life experiences	Learners have a tremendous amount of life experience. Learners connect the learning to their knowledge base. Learners must recognize the value of learning.	Learners do not have the knowledge base to make the connections of new knowledge to life experiences without facilitation.
Purpose of learning	Learners have a goal in sight for their learning.	Learners cannot always see the long-term necessity of information.
Permanence of learning	Learning is self-initiated and tends to last a long time.	Learning is compulsory and tends to disappear shortly after instruction.

- Ready to learn
- Application of knowledge is preferred
- Enjoy problem-based learning (PBL) (Carpenter-Aeby & Aeby, 2013)

SIMULATION LEARNING FRAMEWORKS

Several simulation learning frameworks describe how simulation specifically affects learning.

Kneebone

Kneebone (2005) describes simulation learning using the following elements. Simulation should

1. Allow for deliberate practice (DP) in a safe environment.
2. Provide expert tutors to be available to the learners.
3. Include experiences similar to real life.
4. Be student centered.

Kirkpatrick

Kirkpatrick (1998) discusses four levels of learning with simulation as depicted in Figure 14.4.

> **SIMULATION TEACHING TIP 14.2**
>
> Simulation principles and stages have been effective for teaching surgical technical and nontechnical skills (Sadideen, Goutos, & Kneebone, 2017).

Doerr and Murray

Doerr and Murray (2008) describe the teaching–learning process of simulation by using the model of a four-step plan, which includes the following:

1. The plan
    a. Developing learning outcomes
    b. Description of the scenario and certified healthcare educator responses to the learners
    c. Scripts for standardized (simulated) patients (SPs)
2. The situation
3. Debriefing
4. Transference

Meller

Meller (1997) described the elements of activity in relation to simulation.

- **Passive elements**—Those things that try to stage the realism of the simulation experience, such as moulage (refer to Chapter 9)
- **Active elements**—Those things that are programmed into the simulation experience that cause the learner to respond
- **Interactive elements**—Those changes that the certified healthcare educator makes in reaction to the actions of the learner

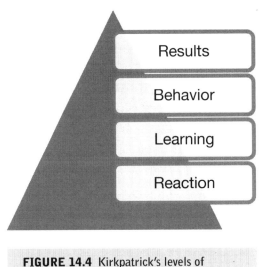

FIGURE 14.4 Kirkpatrick's levels of simulation learning.

REALISM IN SIMULATION

Although realism is a traditional worldview of education, it takes on a slightly different interpretation when applied to simulation. A certain amount of realism must be present during a scenario to meet SLOs. Some points about simulation scenario realism are as follows:

- The goal is to acquire experience in a safe environment.
- The scenario must be real enough to suspend disbelief.
- The scenario must mimic as closely as possible a real clinical scenario.
- SPs, along with mannequins, increase the realism.
- The environmental setup is also important in producing a realistic scenario.
- SPs provide a transition from role-playing to real patients for healthcare professionals.
- SPs can provide learners with "authentic" assessment.

Patient-focused simulation (PFS) includes using a hybrid method of simulations either with a part-task trainer or a mannequin along with an SP. PFS promotes realism because it combines the art of caring with learning clinical skills (Dunbar-Reid, Sinclair, & Hudson, 2015).

Realism is sometimes referred to as the fidelity of the simulation experience. Issenberg, McGaghie, Issenberg, Petrusa, and Scalese (2010) describe fidelity as the exactness of duplication and remind us that simulation is never isomorphic with real life. The higher fidelity may be equated with increased realism. The goal of a simulated environment is to replicate a realistic situation. Fidelity in simulation includes the following:

- **Physical fidelity**: How real does the mannequin appear?
- **Psychological fidelity**: How mentally prepared are the learners?
- **Equipment fidelity**: What can the mannequin, task trainer, or virtual reality platform do?
- **Environmental fidelity**: How do the surroundings look (Dieckmann, Gaba, & Rall, 2007)?

Dieckmann et al. (2007) warn that high fidelity does not necessarily equate with better learning outcomes. Laucken (2003) describes reality as three ways of thinking that are interactive with one another to create reality for the individual person in the experience. Figure 14.5 demonstrates the interconnectiveness of Laucken's theory of how reality is conceptualized.

Suspending Disbelief

Suspending disbelief or engaging in a fiction contract in a simulation experience encompasses the appropriate use of the "as-if" concept (Vaihinger, 1927). Certified healthcare educators running a scenario must integrate information that is believable and within the framework of the scenario, and learners must be open to changing information and understand that the scenario represents actual patient care. There have been elements that lead students to be able to suspend belief. Some elements, according to Muckler (2017), include: "fidelity, psychological safety, emotional buy-in, the fiction contract, and how learners assign meaning" (p. 3).

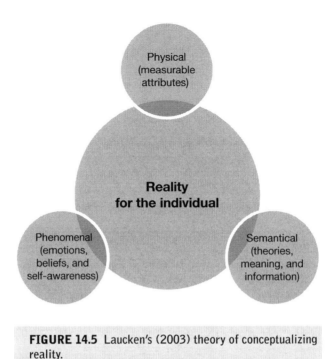

FIGURE 14.5 Laucken's (2003) theory of conceptualizing reality.

Factors that prevent students from just pretending to actually suspending disbelief should be identified by research (Muckler, 2017).

Deliberate Practice

One of the founding teaching principles of simulation is DP. Ericsson, Krampe, and Tesch-Römer (1993) discussed DP as a method of teaching and reinforcing skills for healthcare providers; it is a forerunner to simulation. Ericsson and colleagues understood the implications of translating practice on nonhuman materials to the clinical area as a means to promote expertise and safety.

DP can help ensure competence, retention of skills, and mastery of learning (Gonzalez & Kardong-Edgren, 2017).

Team-Based Learning

Team-based learning (TBL) encourages cooperation in small groups and is appropriate for healthcare students. TBL has three main components:

1. A preparation phase that the student completes individually prior to the group activity
2. Affirming the content is understood

> **SIMULATION TEACHING TIP 14.3**
>
> DP is effective for influencing medical team performance when coupled with a similar model of the situation (shared situation model). DP may assist in reducing barriers in medical teams and enhance cooperation (Harris, Eccles, & Shatzer, 2017).

3. Group activity. The first element requires students (Zachry, Nash, & Nolen, 2017). Simulation encourages TBL through open communication in a safe space that protects the discussion while leveling the playing field. The safe-space concept of learning through simulation contains the following features.

> **EVIDENCE-BASED SIMULATION PRACTICE 14.1**
>
> Levinson et al. (2017) used small-group PBL and simulation with students and found that students perceived the instruction as relevant. It increased understanding of patient safety and patient assessment. Students stated that the small groups contributed to theory and practice integration, clinical reasoning, and communication skills.

LEARNING DOMAINS

Learning is discussed as a process that takes place in three domains: cognitive, affective, and psychomotor, or as stated by the Quality and Safety Education for Nurses (QSEN) program (2005), knowledge, skills, and attitudes (KSAs; Case Western Reserve University, 2014). Learners in healthcare programs are evaluated for growth in all three domains due to the nature of the service work that they will provide to humanity. Bloom's taxonomy (1956; Table 14.2) identifies learning mainly in the cognitive (knowledge) domain. Psychomotor (skills) domains are evident in the application of knowledge, such as demonstrations, and are not difficult to evaluate because they produce observable behavior. Psychomotor learning is often related to procedures, skills, and interventions, all of which can be evaluated in the simulation laboratory. The affective (attitudes) domain of learning is more difficult to assess because it is related to judgment and values such as changes in feelings, interests, and values (caring). Affective learning also includes metacognition or learning how to learn (Burwash & Snover, 2016).

Wong and Driscoll (2008) describe the learning development of the affective domain in five stages:

1. **Receiving**: Learners attend, listen, watch, and recognize.
2. **Responding**: Learners answer, discuss, respond, reply, and actively participate.
3. **Valuing**: Learners accept, adopt, initiate, or demonstrate a preference.
4. **Organizing**: Learners formulate, integrate, modify, and systematize.
5. **Internalizing**: Learners commit, exemplify, and incorporate professionalism into practice.

Simulation can evaluate students' knowledge acquisition in all three domains (Drasovean, 2017). Simulation learning can evaluate students in an environment that contains standard conditions. Evaluation of simulation experiences is thoroughly addressed in Chapter 19.

TABLE 14.2
Bloom's Taxonomy

LEVEL	CONCEPT	VERBS USED WHEN WRITING LEARNING OUTCOMES
Evaluating (formerly called *evaluation*)	Judgment, selection	Appraise, argue, assess, attach, choose, compare, defend, estimate, judge, predict, rate, select, support, value, evaluate
Creating (formerly called *synthesis*; this step formerly occurred before evaluating)	Productive thinking, novelty	Arrange, assemble, collect, compose, construct, create, design, develop, formulate, manage, organize, plan, prepare, propose, set up
Analyzing (formerly called *analysis*)	Induction, deduction, logical order	Analyze, appraise, calculate, categorize, compare, contrast, criticize, differentiate, discriminate, distinguish, examine, experiment, question, test
Applying (formerly called *application*)	Solution, application	Apply, choose, demonstrate, dramatize, employ, illustrate, interpret, operate, practice, schedule, sketch, solve, use, write
Understanding (formerly called *comprehension*)	Explanation, comparison, illustration	Classify, describe, discuss, explain, express, identify, indicate, locate, recognize, report, restate, review, select, translate
Remembering (formerly called *knowledge*)	Memory, repetition, description	Arrange, define, duplicate, label, list, memorize, name, order, recognize, relate, recall, repeat, reproduce, state

Source: Adapted from Bloom, B., Englehart, M., Furst, E., Hill, W., & Drathwohl, D. (Eds.). (1956). *Taxonomy of educational objectives.* New York, NY: Longmans, Green.

MODES OF THINKING

Laucken (2003) describes three modes of *realistic* learner thinking during a simulation experience.

1. **Physical mode** of thinking includes the actual equipment and the fidelity of the equipment. Although mannequins simulate humans, there are many unrealistic attributes, and the same is true for other laboratory equipment.
2. **Semantical mode** of thinking includes the situation created in humans containing information that represents an event. For example, the situation of a patient having a myocardial infarction would include ECG and vital sign changes that would indicate to a learner that this was the event taking place.
3. **Phenomenal mode** of thinking includes the learners' perceptions, emotions, and thinking process during the simulation experience, as well as the participants'

understanding of the relationship of the simulated experience to actual clinical practice.

Specifically in simulation experiences, the right fidelity in the experience needs to be used to emphasize the goal of the experience. The experience needs to be constructed with the goal in mind and framed within the learning outcomes. In addition, the fidelity being used should match the educational level of the student (Lubbers & Rossman, 2017).

CRITICAL THINKING AND METACOGNITION

Critical thinking as an educational concept can be traced back to 1941, when Glaser defined composites of knowledge (Glaser, 1941). Other historical developments in the concept of critical thinking are as follows:

- Miller and Malcolm (1990) adapted Glaser's definition into a model for critical thinking and advised educators to pay closer attention to learners' mental processes.
- In the early days of concept development, educators were concerned with finding an appropriate definition for critical thinking in order to evaluate learners.
- A multitude of definitions arose, and some of the more prominent ones are listed in Table 14.3.

Educators can *role-model critical thinking* and *create opportunities for learners to develop their own critical thinking skills* by asking higher level questions and "thinking out loud," or dialoguing, about a simulation scenario from different perspectives in order to synthesize a solution. The authors of the *ISNA Bulletin* (2014) define attributes or characteristics that enhance and deter critical thinking; these are listed in Table 14.4.

TABLE 14.3
Descriptions of Critical Thinking

AUTHOR	DESCRIPTION OF CRITICAL THINKING
Facione, Facione, and Sanchez (1994)	Critical thinking is the process of purposeful, self-regulating judgment.
Paul and Elder (2007)	Attitudes are central, rather than peripheral, to critical thinking as is independence, confidence, and responsibility, which are needed to arrive at one's own judgment.
Bandman and Bandman (1995)	Critical thinking is the rational examination of ideas, inferences, assumptions, principles, arguments, conclusions, issues, statements, beliefs, and actions. It covers scientific reasoning, decision making, and reasoning in controversial issues. It also includes deductive, inductive, informal, and practical reasoning.

TABLE 14.4

Attributes or Characteristics That Enhance and Deter Critical Thinking

CHARACTERISTICS OF CRITICAL THINKING	CHARACTERISTICS THAT DETER CRITICAL THINKING

• Universal intellectual standards are upheld and include:
  ▪ Clarity
  ▪ Accuracy
  ▪ Precision
  ▪ Relevance
  ▪ Depth
  ▪ Breath
  ▪ Logic
• Intellectual humility as opposed to intellectual arrogance
• Intellectual courage as opposed to intellectual cowardness
• Intellectual empathy as opposed to intellectual narrow-mindedness
• Intellectual autonomy as opposed to intellectual conformity
• Intellectual integrity as opposed to intellectual hypocrisy
• Intellectual perseverance as opposed to intellectual laziness
• Confidence in reason as opposed to distrust of reason and evidence
• Fair-mindedness as opposed to intellectual unfairness
• Reasoning
• Divergent thinking
• Creativity
• Clarification
	• Egocentrism fallacy
	  ▪ It's true because I believe it
	  ▪ It's true because we believe it
	  ▪ It's true because I want to believe it
	  ▪ It's true because I have always believed it
	  ▪ It's true because it is in my selfish interest to believe it
	• Omniscience fallacy
	• Omnipotence fallacy
	• Invulnerability fallacy
	• The halo effect

Source: ISNA Bulletin. (2014). Developing a nursing IQ-Part 1 Characteristics of critical thinking: What critical thinkers do, what critical thinkers do not do. *ISNA Bulletin, 41*(1), 6–14.

Ritchie and Smith (2015) propose that critical thinking is the seventh "C" needed in community health nursing along with:

1. Care
2. Compassion
3. Competence
4. Communication
5. Courage
6. Commitment
7. Critical thinking

> **EVIDENCE-BASED SIMULATION PRACTICE 14.2**
>
> Shin, Ma, Park, Ji, and Kim (2015) studied the relationship of pediatric simulation learning experiences with the development of critical thinking skills in undergraduate nursing students ($N = 237$). The results of using the simulation software on three university sites were measured with Yoon's Critical Thinking (CT) Disposition tool (2004), which was used to measure students' CT abilities. Results demonstrated that it took three exposures to the simulation software to show critical thinking gain in the prudence, systematicity, healthy skepticism, and intellectual eagerness subcategories.

Assessment of learners' critical thinking skills has been completed by use of several different tools. Two of the most widely used tools are listed here.

- The California Critical Thinking Disposition Inventory. This tool evaluates seven "habits of the mind," which are:
  1. Truth seeking
  2. Open-mindedness
  3. Analyticity
  4. Systematicity
  5. Self-confidence
  6. Inquisitiveness
  7. Cognitive maturity

- The Watson–Glaser Critical Thinking Appraisal (WGCTA) (Watson & Glaser, 1964) is available in three different formats; the newest version has 16 scenarios and 40 items. There are five subcategories:
  1. Inference
  2. Recognition of assumptions
  3. Deduction
  4. Interpretation
  5. Evaluation

Mindfulness

A related term to critical thinking is *mindfulness*. The *ISNA Bulletin* (2014) defines *mindfulness* as: "You are engaged with a certain activity, focused, and actively thinking about whatever it is you are undertaking at the moment" (p. 6).

Metacognition

Metacognition is a different concept from critical thinking. "Metacognition is an active process of knowing, or being acutely aware of one's cognitive state with the ability to complete a given task" (Hsu & Hsieh, 2014, p. 234). Metacognition is the process of evaluating your own learning and ideas and being able to change them to understand and promote your own learning success.

> **EVIDENCE-BASED SIMULATION PRACTICE 14.3**
>
> Hsu and Hsieh (2014) completed a study to examine the influence of demographic learning involvement and learning performance variables on metacognition of RN to BSN nursing students ($N = 99$). The correlational study using analysis of online dialogues, the Case Analysis Self Evaluation Scale, and the Blended Learning Satisfaction Scale found that they were all significant independent predictors of metacognition and accounted for over 50% of the variance in metacognition.

EVIDENCE-BASED SIMULATION PRACTICE

The foundations of evidence-based simulation practice (EBSP) are analogous to evidence-based practice (EBP). Healthcare educators use the same method of synthesizing and appraising evidence in the simulation environments in order to draw a conclusion or develop an opinion that is grounded and derived from logical, common ideas in the literature (Leibold, 2017).

Overall, more research needs to be completed in order to produce evidence to support specific learning activities. Pearson, Wiechula, Court, and Lockwood (2007) opined that faculty members should use the acronym FAME when planning to make a change based on evidence:

F = Feasibility
A = Appropriateness
M = Meaningfulness
E = Effectiveness

> **EVIDENCE-BASED SIMULATION PRACTICE 14.4**
>
> Gallagher et al. (2016) used a five-stage simulation exercise to demonstrate to stakeholders the family members' perceptions of adverse healthcare events. The HealthPact Patient and Family Advisory Council (PFAC) sponsored the half-day exercise and then synthesized the planning notes, attendee evaluations ($N = 194$), and exercise discussion notes. Findings demonstrated that response to adverse events are complex, siloed, and uncoordinated and leave a great amount of potential for improvement.

GOFFMAN'S THEORY OF FRAME ANALYSIS

In order to make sense out of a situation, such as a simulated experience, Goffman (1974), who developed a theory about experience interpretation, discusses human perception in frames.

- **Primary frames** describe how the learner's mind or cognition makes sense out of a situation.
- **Natural primary frames** are those that include natural law (physics, anatomy, and physiology).
- **Social primary frames** include human factors such as decision making and communication.

- **Modulations** are learners' understanding that they are in a "what-if" situation that is predefined by the situation in the primary frame. Modulations should hold to learning rules, such as
  - Be within the primary frame and not be a surprise or deception
  - Have a time frame that is appropriate
  - Know the rules and roles within the modulation (Muckler, 2017)

THEORIES OF KNOWING

Healthcare education also draws on theories about how learners come to understand concepts. There are two classic models that have been significant in healthcare education for the past several decades and are widely used as the theoretical foundations for many studie and curricula, as well as learning activity development. They are Barbara Carper's (1978) Ways of Knowing and Patricia Benner's (1982) novice-to-expert theory.

Carper (1978) described four ways that healthcare professionals understand practice situations:

1. **Empirical knowledge,** or scientific knowledge (this includes EBSP)
2. **Personal knowledge,** or understanding how you would feel in the patient's position
3. **Ethical knowledge,** or attitudes and understanding of moral decisions
4. **Esthetic knowledge,** or understanding the situation of the patient at the moment

> **SIMULATION TEACHING TIP 14.4**
>
> Using the new ISBARR (originally, S is for *situation*, B is for *background*, A is for *assessment*, and R is for *recommendation*) communication tool during simulation, as in practice, may mitigate some of the study results that were identified, because the "I" is for *introduction* and the second "R" is for *repeating the orders or results*.

Munhall (1993) added a fifth way of knowing: *unknowing,* or understanding that one cannot know everything about the patient and that one must place oneself in a position of willingness to learn from the patient's perspective.

DEEP, SURFACE, AND STRATEGIC LEARNING

Deep learning is a term first described by Marton and Saljo (1976) to refer to a learning approach and type of knowledge acquisition. The approach a learner takes to information presented in the classroom can be classified into three types of learning styles: deep, surface, and strategic.

1. A deep learning approach is accomplished when a learner addresses material with the intent to understand both the concepts and meaning of the information.
   - The learner relates new ideas to existing experiences and formulates links in long-term memory.
   - The motivation for a deep learning approach is primarily intrinsic, created from the learner's interest and desire to understand the relevance of the information to applied practice

2. A surface learning, or atomistic, approach facilitates learning by:
   - Memorization of facts and details. Surface learning is similar to rote learning in that the learner assimilates information presented at face value.
   - Motivation for surface learning, which is primarily extrinsic, is driven by either the learner's fear of failing or the desire to complete the course successfully.
3. When using a strategic learning approach, the learner does what is needed to complete a course. Strategic learning uses a mixture of both deep and surface learning techniques.
   - All three approaches to learning can be measured by the Approaches and Study Skills Inventory for Students (ASSIST) (Entwistle, 1999; Ramsden & Entwistle, 1981).

> **EVIDENCE-BASED SIMULATION PRACTICE 14.5**
>
> Heid (2015) developed an online clinical postconference pilot study to evaluate the development of deep learning through the use of scenarios and guided discussion. Senior nursing students were provided with online clinical postconference activities for 30 minutes each week. Evaluations of students' satisfaction, integration of nursing concepts, and application from practice to theory were positive.

MOTIVATIONAL THEORIES

Not only do simulation educators need to know how students acquire information, they also need to know why they learn. What are their motivating factors? Motivation has been linked to student retention and success. Many variables effect motivation; motivation can be influenced by the need for achievement or curiosity, or it can be a function of the situation at hand or a person's ability. A learner's *locus of control* can be *extrinsically or intrinsically motivated*. Motivation includes a student's goals, beliefs, perceptions, and expectations (Hanifi, Parvizy, & Joolaee, 2013).

- Extrinsic motivations are those based on external variables, such as grades or earning money, and in today's environment there are many social pressures for students to become nurses.
- Intrinsic motivation has to do with the feeling of accomplishment, of learning for the sake of learning, or the feeling that being a nurse is something the learner always wanted to do. Hanifi et al. (2013) identified internal motivators as spirituality, selflessness, and serving people and that these assist students to remain in school (Nesje, 2015). Intrinsic motivation is correlated with *self-determination theory* developed by Deci and Ryan (Deci, Eghrari, Patrick, & Leone, 1994). According to this theory, humans have three types of needs:
  - To feel competent
  - To feel related
  - To feel autonomous

Following are some traditional models to better explain student motivation:

ARCS Model

Keller (1987) talks about the factors educators can implement to motivate learners in the ARCS model.

    A: Attention—Keep the learner's attention through stimulus changes in the environment

    R: Relevance—Make the information relevant to the learner's goals

    C: Confidence—Make expectations clear so the learner will engage in learning

    S: Satisfaction—Have appropriate consequences for the learner's new skills

Brophy Model

Brophy (1986) listed the following methods by which motivation is formed:

- Modeling
- Communication of expectations
- Direct instruction
- Socialization by parents and educators

Vroom's Expectancy Model

Vroom's expectancy model (VEM; Vroom, 1964) describes what people want and whether they are positioned to obtain it. The Vroom model describes three concepts, which are:

1. **Force (F)**: The amount of effort a person will place into reaching a goal
2. **Valence (V)**: How attractive the goal is to the person
3. **Expectancy (E)**: The possibility of the goal being achieved

The equation for the VEM model is $F = V \times E$ (Vroom, 1964).

DeYoung's Motivational Model

DeYoung (2009) lists 10 principles to motivate learners; they are applicable to a laboratory and virtual learning environment as well as to a traditional setting.

1. Use several senses.
2. Actively involve the learner.
3. Assess readiness.
4. Determine whether the learner thinks the information is relevant.
5. Repeat information.
6. Generalize information.
7. Make learning pleasant.
8. Begin with what is known.
9. Present information at an appropriate rate.
10. Provide a learning-friendly environment.

LEARNER SOCIALIZATION IN THE VIRTUAL, SIMULATION, AND SKILLS ENVIRONMENT

Simulation experiences are a social practice (Underman, 2015) because they encompass a goal-oriented situation that calls for participant interaction in a setting (module) that influences behavior. The simulation setting includes the following:

- Introduction
- Simulator briefing
- Scenario
- Debriefing, which can be done during the simulation or after the learning experience (Karkowsky et al., 2016)
- Session ending (Dieckmann et al., 2007)

The social practice goal of simulation is to enhance positive learner socialization and extend it to healthcare practice. Socialization is the process of internalizing the norms, beliefs, and values of a professional culture to which one hopes to gain admission (Peddle, Bearman, & Nestel, 2016).

- New healthcare students are instructed in ways and attitudes of the organization and gradually adopt the attitudes, values, and unspoken messages within the organization (Rudd, 2014).
- It is important to note that a lack of socialization has been associated with negative job satisfaction, which results in high turnover rates (Yanchus, Periard, & Osatuke, 2017).

The transition of a healthcare learner to the professional environment is challenging. Simulation environments are being used to decrease reality shock and familiarize learners using both social practice and social aspects within the social practice. Social aspects include interdisciplinary communication, teamwork, and role identification (Dieckmann et al., 2007).

Kramer (1974) describes *reality shock* as what takes place when a neophyte realizes that what was learned in school does not match that which is experienced in actual clinical practice.

Kramer's four phases of reality shock are:

1. Honeymoon
2. Shock or rejection
3. Recovery
4. Resolution

Designed Experiences Through "Serious Gaming"

Another topic in simulation related to socialization is the use of serious gaming. Serious gaming uses the video game simulation platform to build educational programs that enhance learning by *being* or becoming the character in the game and by *doing* to create and organize for a functional epistemology. Using an epistemology in which one learns through doing and through performance is a new frontier in education, but this mode of simulation also lacks research. Some of the concepts associated with serious gaming include:

- **Interactivity**: Serious games can be played alone or as part of a community.
- **Agency**: The simulated world grants the player the right to create.
- **Parameters**: These are built-in barriers by the game designers (Squire, 2007).

Additional information about Second Life and gaming is provided in Chapter 13.

THE ART OF TEACHING SIMULATION

LeFlore and Anderson (2009) explain that most simulation scenarios begin with a "stem," or some information about the case, and then teaching during simulation experiences can take on one of three levels of facilitation by certified healthcare educators:

1. **Self-directed**: This approach allows experienced learners to proceed through scenarios without assistance from the certified healthcare educator.
2. **Cueing students**: In this approach, the certified healthcare educator provides hints or cues to the learners to ensure they progress through the scenario.
3. **Expert or instructor model**: This is an approach in which the certified healthcare educator instructs during the scenario as the learners are experiencing the situation.

LEARNING OUTCOMES VERSUS LEARNING OBJECTIVES

Historically, healthcare education has used objectives for learning since Tyler's landmark book, *Basic Principles of Curriculum and Instruction* (1949), encouraged educators to develop behavioral objectives to organize their teaching. Therefore, objectives are part of the behavioral paradigm. To standardize the format of objectives, educators have incorporated the action verbs outlined in Bloom's taxonomy (1956), which has since been revised.

Bloom's Taxonomy

Bloom's *Taxonomy of Educational Objectives* (1956) describes an end behavior (see Table 14.2). The taxonomy uses "behavioral terms" to divide learning into leveled achievement, from knowledge acquisition to the synthesis of new ideas (Novotny & Griffin, 2006).

Most teaching sessions begin with objectives or learning outcomes to frame the content or experience. *Objectives* and *learning outcomes* are the two terms used often in healthcare education and some professions will also use the term *goals*. All the terms are trying to depict what the student will have acquired by the end of the class, session, or scenario. The most common method of developing a measurable objective or learning outcome is depicted in Table 14.5.

Depending on the length of the simulation scenario and the level of the practitioners, educators usually have several objectives in mind. The number of learning objectives/outcomes should be reasonable and related to the intent of the learning session and the time allotted to the scenario. Objectives and learning outcomes

TABLE 14.5

Learning Outcomes

ANTECEDENT	LEARNER	VERB DESCRIBING BEHAVIOR	CONTENT	CONTEXT	CRITERIA
"By the end of this session"	"The learner will"	"Demonstrate"	Sterile gloving	In clinical settings	100% of the time
"By the end of this session"	"The learner will"	"Compare"	Different cultures	Related to childbearing experiences	By Interviewing two culturally differed patients

are reflected in the evaluation of the learning session. Most lists of objectives or learning outcomes are prefaced with the statement, "By the end of this scenario the student will be able to..." Evaluating learning that takes place in simulation is addressed in Chapter 19. Simulation as an evaluation tool has become widespread because it occurs in a controlled environment where all learners can be presented with testing in similar conditions using a leveled playing field. Traditional clinical experiences were not able to provide that, because educational opportunities may differ from day to day (Drasovean, 2017).

EVALUATING SIMULATION LEARNING EXPERIENCES

Simulation learning experiences are used for either formative and summative learner assessment or evaluation. Evaluation practices themselves need to be assessed so that healthcare professionals are more confident they are preparing competent practitioners for the future (Logue, 2017). Simulation-based evaluation is one method used to evaluate learning and the goals of the students' learning can be short term such as the following:

1. Has the student met the learning objectives/outcomes?
2. Did the scenario improve patient care and safety?

An important consideration when using simulation-based evaluation is validity. Is the simulation experience measuring what it is intended to measure? Kane (2006) discusses the evaluation process of testing by breaking it down into four key areas:

1. **Scoring**: Was the test provided to learners under fair and consistent conditions?
2. **Generalization**: Are the results reliable and consistent when the evaluation technique is used with different groups?
3. **Extrapolation**: Is the assessment measuring the construct it is supposed to measure and not extraneous variables?
4. **Decision/interpretation**: Are the scores being used for their intended purpose and without manipulation?

Current literature discusses developing instruments to evaluate students' learning through the use of simulation. Hung, Liu, Lin, and Lee (2016) developed a 37-item Simulation-Based Learning Evaluation Scale (SBLES) that is based on competencies and is valid and reliable. Some tools are specific, whereasothers can be used in a variety of simulation learning experiences. The Team Performance Observation Tool was developed to assess interprofessional simulation experiences (Zhang, Miller, Volkman, Meza, & Jones, 2015). Chapter 21 will discuss in detail the current research being completed in relation to simulation learning and evaluation.

GAGNE'S CONDITIONS OF LEARNING

Gagne's (1970) steps for instruction are a classic list of tasks that is still referenced today and suited for learning in a simulated environment. Gagne's (1970) nine events of instruction are shown in Table 14.6.

TABLE 14.6
Gagne's Conditions of Learning

INSTRUCTIONAL EVENT	ACTIVITIES OF TEACHING–LEARNING
1. Gains attention of the learner	Stimuli activates receptors
2. Informs learners of objectives	Sets expectations for the learner
3. Stimulates recall of prior learning	Activates short-term memory and the retrieval of information by asking questions
4. Presents the content	Presents content with features that can be remembered
5. Provides "learning guidance"	Assists the learner to organize the information for long-term memory
6. Elicits performance (practice)	Asks learners to perform to enhance encoding and verification
7. Provides appropriate feedback (feedback about simulation experiences is covered in Chapter 18)	Encourages performance
8. Assesses performance	Evaluates performance
9. Enhances retention and transfer	Review periodically to decrease memory loss of information

LEARNING ACTIVITIES USED IN SIMULATION ENVIRONMENTS

Interprofessional Learning

Interprofessional learning is needed to prepare students for the future of healthcare (Brown & Miller, 2016). Team-based education is needed for quality patient care and is the focus of many healthcare education and simulation initiatives. The goal of interprofessional learning is to have all health professional learners "deliberately working together" as stated by the Interprofessional Educational Collaboration (IPEC), which is made up of six professional organizations (American Association of Colleges of Nursing, American Association of Colleges of Osteopathic Medicine, American Association of Colleges of Pharmacy, American Dental Education Association, Association of American Medical Colleges, and Association of Schools of Public Health, 2011). The IPEC outlined four core competencies needed for healthcare professionals to function effectively in interprofessional teams. The domains of the four major competencies and related criteria are fully explained in Chapter 6.

Problem-Based Learning

Problem-based learning (PBL) is a teaching strategy that was developed in the 1970s as a student-centered approach. It uses patient problems of increasing complexity to assist students to understand clinical decision making individually and in a group format (MacVane, Fiona, Whitney, Meddings, & Evans, 2015). Lee, Nam, and Kim (2017) studied PBL and simulation and it has positive effects on team efficacy and learning attitudes in healthcare students.

Self-Directed Learning

Self-directed learning (*SDL*) is another term often heard in healthcare education and refers to a collection of learning activities that are truly learner focused. It originated with Knowles (1980) and is a process in which the learner decides his or her own learning needs. The learner formulates the goals, develops the networking and resources, does the learning, and evaluates the learning. Learners must be ready to take on the task of SDL and they need to have the confidence, maturity, and tenacity to engage in SDL (Ha, 2016). SDL activities can include virtual learning modules. To assess whether learners are ready for this type of knowledge acquisition, the Self-Directed Learning Readiness Scale (SDLRS) is used.

Reflection

Reflection is a method used to develop critical thinking and is used extensively in simulation experiences through debriefing (Chapter 17) and feedback (Chapter 18). Please refer to these chapters to better understand the essence of reflection, which is a critical component of simulation learning.

Environmental Management

The underpinning of positive learning environment management is respect for the learners. Once an atmosphere of trust and respect is established, there should be very few management issues. Chickering and Gamson's (1987) seven principles of good teaching practice are applicable to simulation learning environments and are listed here:

1. Encourage contact between learners and educators.
2. Develop reciprocity and cooperation among learners.
3. Encourage active learning.
4. Give prompt feedback.
5. Emphasize time on task.
6. Communicate high expectations.
7. Respect diverse talents and ways of learning.

According to Mulligan (2007), there are four pillars of classroom management; these are discussed here because they also fit the simulation learning environment very well.

1. Pillar 1: Educators should use instructional strategies (active learning strategies) that motivate and keep learners interested and engaged.
2. Pillar 2: Educators need to use instructional time wisely and take a proactive approach to teaching by charging the learners to be accountable for their learning.
3. Pillar 3: Social behaviors that need attention and correcting should be dealt with immediately, face to face, and privately.
4. Pillar 4: Educators need to create a flexible environment in order to adjust to the learners' needs.

SUMMARY

Simulation as a learning tool has a history of success in healthcare education. The theoretical foundations of experiential learning and realism are well represented in simulation. Successful simulation for healthcare education contains the following best practice attributes as identified in a mega-analysis completed by McGaghie et al. (2010).

- Feedback: Formative or summative (discussed in Chapters 17 and 18)
- DP: Encompasses nine educational goals:
  1. Occurs with motivated learners
  2. Defines the learning outcomes
  3. Keep the experience at the appropriate level for the learner
  4. Repeat the exercise or skill to gain proficiency
  5. Promote rigor in skill to ensure best practice
  6. Provide learner with feedback
  7. Promote self-regulation in learners
  8. Evaluate to reach a mastery standard
  9. Start process again with another task (McGaghie, Siddall, Mazmanian, & Myers, 2009)
- Curriculum integration
- Outcome measurement

- Simulation fidelity
- Skill acquisition and maintenance
- Mastery learning
- Transfer to practice
- Team training
- High-stake testing
- Instructor training
- Educational and professional context

> **CASE STUDY 14.1**
>
> Joseph is a new faculty member at a small baccalaureate school with premed, nursing, and prepharmaceutical programs. He is full time, tenure track, and working on his doctoral degree. Joseph is assigned a mentor and a 12-credit/semester teaching load, which is normal for many institutions. He meets with his mentor, who goes over his syllabus with him. The mentor asks Joseph why he has so many assignments for the learners to do after they have completed their hybrid simulation experience. Joseph states that he believes that the learners' writing skills are lacking, and they need writing assignments and he has them expand on the simulation day by describing the illness process of the simulated patient scenario in depth. If you were the mentor and saw a novice place 50% of the clinical course grade on writing assignments related to simulation, how would you handle it?

■ PRACTICE QUESTIONS

1. A healthcare simulation educator is developing a scenario for a student to learn newborn care and would like to use the constructivist theory as the foundation. The best method would be:

   A. Have the student repeat a newborn assessment several times to get procedures correct.
   B. Use a newborn mannequin that simulates an active newborn and have the student approach the assessment without interfering and discuss later.
   C. Develop a scenario that changes the newborn's status if an assessment is performed wrong.
   D. Change the newborn's status to mimic a healthy newborn if the assessment is done correctly.

2. The student needs additional understanding when he states, "A constructivist approach to this scenario includes..." the following:

   A. "Using the material we learned yesterday and applying it today."
   B. "Starting with what we know about this situation and then assessing the patient."
   C. "Approaching the patient as if we have no information."
   D. "Relating what is similar in this case to other cases we have worked through."

3. During a team-based simulation scenario, one student takes the lead and approaches the patient first and takes blood pressure when the mannequin tells

the group that she feels lightheaded. This student who takes the blood pressure is displaying which of Kolb's learning styles?

A. Concrete experience (CE)
B. Abstract conceptualization (AC)
C. Reflective observation (RO)
D. Active experimentation (AE)

4. The simulation healthcare educator has developed a simulation scenario based on the scaffolding learning theory and presents it to a group of students. The students are provided with an explanation of the case that becomes increasingly difficult. The group was unable to formulate a cohesive plan for the patient. One of the learning elements missing may have been:

A. Instructor presence
B. Realism
C. Constructive feedback
D. Knowledge

5. Guided by social learning theory, the healthcare simulation educator demonstrates to a student who has low self-efficacy how to insert chest tubes correctly. The principle that the healthcare simulation educator is using is:

A. Mastering experience learning
B. Vicarious experience learning
C. Verbal persuasion
D. Modulating psychological state

6. One of the healthcare students was previously an emergency medical technician (EMT) and during a simulation prebriefing she states that she would like to advance her splinting skills. The student is demonstrating which type of educational concept?

A. Pedagogy
B. Realism
C. Behavioralism
D. Andragogy

7. The new healthcare simulation educator needs additional information when she lists Kneebone's (2005) simulation learning principles as (p. 63):

A. It should occur in a safe environment.
B. Tutors should be available to learners.
C. Principles are teacher centered.
D. They should mimic real life.

8. Kirkpatrick's (1998) simulation learning principles are orderly and once learning is achieved, the healthcare simulation educator should expect the students to:

A. Display a reaction
B. Describe results
C. Continue to learn
D. Demonstrate the behavior

9. The last step of Doerr and Murray's (2008) simulation teaching–learning process is:

    A. Debriefing
    B. Transference
    C. Developing learning outcomes
    D. Creating the situation

10. A simulation educator is developing student objectives/learning outcomes and would like to assess students at the application level. Which objective/learning outcome would best fit the application level?

    A. Observe the hybrid simulation procedure.
    B. Discuss the clinical decision for starting cardiopulmonary resuscitation.
    C. Decide on the priority intervention.
    D. Evaluate the intervention's effect.

REFERENCES

Anderson, G., Hughes, C., Patterson, D., & Costa, J. (2017). Enhancing inter-professional education through low-fidelity simulation. *British Journal of Midwifery*, 25(1), 52–58. doi:10.12968/bjom.2017.25.1.52

Bandman, E. L., & Bandman, B. (1995). *Critical thinking in nursing* (2nd ed.). Norwalk, CT: Appleton & Lange.

Bandura, A. (1997). *Self-efficacy: The exercise of control*. New York, NY: W. H. Freeman.

Bastin, M. L., Cook, A. M., & Flannery, A. H. (2017). Use of simulation training to prepare pharmacy residents for medical emergencies. *American Journal of Health-System Pharmacy*, 74(6), 424–429. doi:10.2146/ajhp160129

Benner, P. (1982). From novice to expert. *American Journal of Nursing*, 82(3), 402–407.

Bevis, E., & Watson, J. (1989). *Toward a caring curriculum: A new pedagogy for nursing*. New York, NY: National League for Nursing.

Bloom, B., Englehart, M., Furst, E., Hill, W., & Drathwohl, D. (Eds.). (1956). *Taxonomy of educational objectives*. New York, NY: Longmans, Green.

Brophy, J. (1986). *On motivating students. Occasional Paper No. 101*. East Lansing, MI: Institute for Research on Teaching, Michigan State University.

Brown, M. R., & Miller, B. (2016). Incorporating clinical laboratory science students into interprofessional simulation. *Clinical Laboratory Science*, 29(4), 247–251.

Brown, M. R., & Watts, P. (2016). Primer on interprofessional simulation for clinical laboratory science programs: A practical guide to structure and terminology. *Clinical Laboratory Science*, 29(4), 241–246. doi:10.29074/ascls.29.4.241

Burwash, S. C., & Snover, R. (2016). Up Bloom's pyramid with slices of Fink's pie: Mapping an occupational therapy curriculum. *Open Journal of Occupational Therapy*, 4(4), 1–8. doi:10.15453/2168-6408.1235

Cadieux, D. C., Lingard, L., Kwiatkowski, D., Van Deven, T., Bryant, M., & Tithecott, G. (2017). Challenges in translation: Lessons from using business pedagogy to teach leadership in undergraduate medicine. *Teaching & Learning in Medicine*, 29(2), 207–215. doi:10.1080/10401334.2016.1237361

Carpenter-Aeby, T., & Aeby, V. G. (2013). Application of andragogy to instruction in an MSW practice class. *Journal of Instructional Psychology*, 40(1–4), 3–13.

Carper, B. A. (1978). Fundamental patterns of knowing in nursing. *Advances in Nursing Science*, 1(1), 13–24. doi:10.1097/ANS.0b013e3181c9d5eb

Case Western Reserve University. (2014). QSEN Institute. Retrieved from http://qsen.org/about-qsen

Chickering, A. W., & Gamson, Z. F. (1987). Seven principles for good practice in undergraduate education. *Wingspread Journal*, 9(2). Retrieved from https://files.eric.ed.gov/full-text/ED282491.pdf

Deci, E., Eghrari, H., Patrick, B. C., & Leone, D. R. (1994). Facilitating internalization: The self-determination theory perspective. *Journal of Personality*, 62(1), 119–142. doi:10.1111/j.1467-6494.1994.tb00797.x

DeYoung, S. (2009). *Teaching strategies for nurse educator* (2nd ed.). Upper Saddle River, NJ: Prentice Hall.

Dieckmann, P., Gaba, D., & Rall, M. (2007). Deepening the theoretical foundations of patient simulation as social practice. *Simulation in Healthcare*, 2, 183–193. doi:10.1097/SIH.0b013e3180f637f5

Diekelmann, N. L. (1997). Creating a new pedagogy for nursing. *Journal of Nursing Education*, 36(4), 147–148. doi:10.3928/0148-4834-19970401-03

Diekelmann, N. L. (2005). Engaging the students and the teacher: Co-creating substantive form with narrative pedagogy. *Journal of nursing Education*, 44(6), 249–252.

Doerr, H., & Murray, W. B. (2008). How to build a successful simulation scenario = obstacle-course + treasure hunt. In R. R. Kyle & W. B. Murray (Eds.), *Clinical simulation: Operations, engineering and management* (pp. 745–749). London, UK: Elsevier/Academic Press.

Drasovean, Y. (2017). Optimizing learner assessment in a respiratory therapy clinical simulation course. *Canadian Journal of Respiratory Therapy*, 53(1), 17–22.

Dunbar-Reid, K., Sinclair, P. M., & Hudson, D. (2015). Advancing renal education: Hybrid simulation, using simulated patients to enhance realism in haemodialysis education. *Journal of Renal Care*, 41(2), 134–139. doi:10.1111/jorc.12112

Entwistle, N. J. (1999). Approaches to studying and levels of understanding: The influences of teaching and assessment. In J. C. Smart (Ed.), *Higher education: Handbook of theory and research* (p. xv). New York, NY: Agathon Press.

Ericsson, K. A., Krampe, R. T., & Tesch-Römer, C. (1993). The role of deliberate practice in the acquisition of expert performance. *Psychology Review*, 100(3), 363–406. doi:10.1037/0033-295X.100.3.363

Facione, N. C., Facione, P. A., & Sanchez, C. A. (1994). Critical thinking disposition as a measure of competent judgment: The development of the California Critical Disposition Inventory. *Journal of Nursing Education*, 33, 345–350. doi:10.3928/0148-4834-19941001-05

Gagne, R. (1970). *The conditions of learning* (2nd ed.). New York, NY: Holt, Rinehart and Winston.

Gallagher, T. H., Etchegaray, J. M., Bergstedt, B., Chappelle, A. M., Ottosen, M. J., Sedlock, E. W., & Thomas, E. J. (2016). Improving communication and resolution following adverse events using a patient-created simulation exercise. *Health Services Research*, 51, 2537–2549. doi:10.1111/1475-6773.12601

Gibbs, G. (1988). *Learning by doing: A guide to teaching and learning methods*. London, UK: Fell.

Glaser, E. M. (1941). *An experiment in the development of critical thinking*. New York, NY: Teacher's College, Columbia University.

Goffman, E. (1974). *Frame analysis. An essay on the organization of experience*. Boston, MA: Northeastern University Press.

Gonzalez, L., & Kardong-Edgren, S. (2017). Deliberate practice for mastery learning in nursing. *Clinical Simulation in Nursing*, 13(1), 10–14. doi:10.1016/j.ecns.2016.10.005

Grant, J., & Marsden, P. (1992). *Training senior house officers by service based training*. London, UK: Joint Conference for Education in Medicine.

Griffith, R. L., Steelman, L. A., Wildman, J. L., LeNoble, C. A., & Zhou, Z. E. (2017). Guided mindfulness: A self-regulatory approach to experiential learning of complex skills. *Theoretical Issues in Ergonomics Science*, 18(2), 147–166. doi:10.1080/1463922X.2016.1166404

Ha, E. (2016). Undergraduate nursing students' subjective attitudes to curriculum for simulation-based objective structured clinical examination, 36, 11–17. doi:10.1016/j.nedt.2015.05.018

Hanifi, N., Parvizy, S., &; Joolaee, S. (2013). Motivational journey of Iranian bachelor of nursing students during clinical education: A grounded theory study. *Nursing & Health Sciences, 15*(3), 340–345. doi:10.1111/nhs.12041

Harris, K., Eccles, D., & Shatzer, J. (2017). Team deliberate practice in medicine and related domains: A consideration of the issues. *Advances in Health Sciences Education, 22*(1), 209–220. doi:10.1007/s10459-016-9696-3

Heid, C. L. (2015). Fostering deep learning: An on-line clinical postconference pilot study. *Teaching & Learning in Nursing, 10*(3), 124–127. doi:10.1016/j.teln.2015.02.002

Hsu, L., & Hsieh, S. (2014). Factors affecting metacognition of undergraduate nursing students in a blended learning environment. *International Journal of Nursing Practice, 20*(3), 233–241. doi:10.1111/ijn.12131

Hung, C., Liu, H., Lin, C., & Lee, B. (2016). Development and validation of the simulation-based learning evaluation scale. *Nurse Education Today, 40,* 72–77. doi:10.1016/j.nedt.2016.02.016

Indian State Nurses Foundation & Indian State Nurses Association. (2014). Developing a nursing IQ Part 1 Characteristics of critical thinking: What critical thinkers do, what critical thinkers do not do. *ISNA Bulletin, 41*(1), 6–14.

Issenberg, S. B., McGaghie, W. C., Issenberg, E. R., Petrusa, D. L., & Scalese, R. J. (2010). Features and uses of high-fidelity medical simulations that lead to effective learning: A BEME systematic review. *Medical Teacher, 27*(1), 10–28. doi:10.1080/01421590500046924

Kane, M. (2006). Validation. In R. L. Brennan (Ed.), *Educational measurement* (4th ed., pp. 17–64).Westport, CT: American Council on Education/Praeger.

Karkowsky, C. E., Landsberger, E. J., Bernstein, P. S., Dayal, A., Goffman, D., Madden, R. C., & Chazotte C. (2016). Breaking bad news in obstetrics: A randomized trial of simulation followed by debriefing or lecture. *Journal of Maternal–Fetal & Neonatal Medicine, 29*(22), 3717–3723. doi:10.3109/14767058.2016.1141888

Keller, J. M. (1987). Development and use of the ARCS model of motivational design. *Journal of Instructional Development, 10*(3), 2–10.

Kirkpatrick, D. L. (1998). *Evaluating training programs: The four levels* (2nd ed.). San Francisco, CA: Berrett-Koehler.

Kneebone, R. (2005). Evaluating clinical simulations for learning procedural skills: A theory-based approach. *Academic Medicine, 80*(6), 549–553. doi:10.1097/00001888-200506000-00006

Knowles, M. (1980). *The modern practice of adult education.* Chicago, IL: Follett.

Kolb, D. A. (1984). *Experiential learning: Experience as the source of learning and development.* Upper Saddle River, NJ: Prentice Hall.

Kolb, D. A., Boyatzis, R. E., & Mainemelis, C. (1999). *Experiential learning theory: Previous research and new directions.* Department of Organizational Behavior, Weatherhead School of Management, Case Western Reserve University. Hillsdale, NJ: Lawrence Erlbaum. Retrieved from http://www.d.umn.edu/~kgilbert/educ5165-731/Readings/experiential-learning-theory.pdf

Kramer, M. (1974). *Reality shock: Why nurses leave nursing.* St. Louis, MO: Mosby.

Laucken, U. (2003). *Theoretical psychology.* Oldenburg, Germany: Biblioteks und Information system der Univeritat.

Lauerer, J., Edlund, B. J., Williams, A., Donato, A., & Smith, G. (2017). Scaffolding behavioral health concepts from more simple to complex builds NP students' competence. *Nurse Education Today, 51,* 124–126. doi:10.1016/j.nedt.2016.08.016

Le Coze, J. (2017). Reflecting on Jens Rasmussen's legacy (2) behind and beyond, a "constructivist turn." *Applied Ergonomics, 59*(Part B), 558–569. doi:10.1016/j.apergo.2015.07.013

Lee, M., Nam, K., & Kim, H. (2017). Effects of simulation with problem-based learning program on metacognition, team efficacy, and learning attitude in nursing students. *CIN: Computers, Informatics, Nursing, 35*(3), 145–151. doi:10.1097/CIN.0000000000000308

LeFlore, J. L., & Anderson, M. (2009). Alternative educational models for interdisciplinary student teams. *Simulation in Healthcare, 4,* 135–142. doi:10.1097/SIH.0b013e318196f839

Leibold, N. (2017). Virtual simulations: A creative, evidence-based approach to develop and educate nurses. *Creative Nursing*, 23(1), 29–34. doi:10.1891/1078-4535.23.1.29

Levinson, M., Kelly, D., Zahariou, K., Johnson, M., Jackman, C., & Mackenzie, S. (2017). Description and student self-evaluation of a pilot integrated small group learning and simulation programme for medical students in the first clinical year. *Internal Medicine Journal*, 47(2),211–216. doi:10.1111/imj.13332

Logue, N. C. (2017). Evaluating practice-based learning. *Journal of Nursing Education*, 56(3), 131–138. doi:10.3928/01484834-20170222-03

Lubbers, J., & Rossman, C. (2017). Satisfaction and self-confidence with nursing clinical simulation: Novice learners, medium-fidelity, and community settings. *Nurse Education Today*, 48, 140–144. doi:10.1016/j.nedt.2016.10.010

MacVane, P., Fiona, E., Whitney, E., Meddings, F., & Evans, M. (2015). Embedding the 6 Cs: Problem-based learning the Bradford way. *British Journal of Midwifery*, 23(5), 330–335. doi:10.12968/bjom.2015.23.5.330

Marton, F., & Saljo, R. (1976). On qualitative differences in learning: I—Outcome and process. *British Journal of Educational Psychology*, 46(1), 4–11. doi:10.1111/j.2044-8279.1976.tb02980.x

McGaghie, W. C., Issenberg, S. B., Petrusa, E. R., & Scalese, R. J. (2010). A critical review of simulation-based medical education research: 2003–2009. *Medical Education*, 44, 50–63. doi:10.1111/j.1365-2923.2009.03547.x

McGaghie, W. C., Siddall, V. J., Mazmanian, P. E., & Myers, J. (2009). Lessons for continuing medical education from simulation research in undergraduate and graduate medical education: Effectiveness of continuing medical education: American College of Chest Physicians evidence-based educational guidelines. *Chest*, 135(Suppl. 3), 62–68. doi:10.1378/chest.08-2521

McInerney, P. A., & Green-Thompson, L. P.(2017). Teaching and learning theories, and teaching methods used in postgraduate education in the health sciences: a systematic review protocol. *JBI Database of Systematic Reviews & Implementation Reports*, 15(4), 899–904. doi: 10.11124/JBISRIR-2016-003110

Meller, G. (1997). A typology of simulators for medical education. *Journal of Digital Imaging*, 10(3, Suppl. 1), 194–196. doi:10.1007/BF03168699

Miller, M. A., & Malcolm, N. S. (1990). Critical thinking in the nursing curriculum. *Nursing & Healthcare*, 11(2), 66–73.

Muckler, V. C. (2017). Exploring suspension of disbelief during simulation-based learning. *Clinical Simulation in Nursing*, 13(1), 3–9. doi:10.1016/j.ecns.2016.09.004

Mulligan, R. (2007). Management strategies in the educational setting. In B. Moyer & R. A. Wittmann-Price (Eds.), *Teaching nursing: Foundations of practice excellence* (pp. 109–125). Philadelphia, PA: F. A. Davis.

Munhall, P. L. (1993). Unknowing: Toward another pattern of knowing in nursing. *Nursing Outlook*, 41(3), 125–128.

Nesje, K. (2015). Nursing students' prosocial motivation: Does it predict professional commitment and involvement in the job? *Journal of Advanced Nursing*, 71(1), 115–125. doi:10.1111/jan.12456

Novotny, J., & Griffin, M., T. (2006). *A nuts-and-bolts approach to teaching nursing*. New York, NY: Springer Publishing.

Paul, R., & Elder, L. (2007). Critical thinking: The nature of critical and creative thought. *Journal of Developmental Education*, 32(2), 34–35.

Pearson, A., Wiechula, R., Court, A., & Lockwood, C. (2007). A reconsideration of what constitutes "evidence" in the healthcare professions. *Nursing Science Quarterly*, 20, 85–88. doi:10.1177/0894318406296306

Peddle, M., Bearman, M., & Nestel, D. (2016). Virtual patients and nontechnical skills in undergraduate health professional education: An integrative review. *Clinical Simulation in Nursing*, 12(9), 400–410. doi:10.1016/j.ecns.2016.04.004

Ramsden, P., & Entwistle, N. J. (1981). Effects of academic departments on students' approaches to studying. *British Journal of Educational Psychology*, 51, 368–383. doi:10.1111/j.2044-8279.1981.tb02493.x

Ritchie, G., & Smith, C. (2015). Critical thinking in community nursing: Is this the 7th C? *British Journal of Community Health, 20*(12), 578–579. doi:10.12968/bjcn.2015.20.12.578

Rudd, A. (2014). *Examining professional stereotypes in an interprofessional education simulation experience* (Doctoral dissertation). University of Alabama, Tuscaloosa.

Sadideen, H., Goutos, I., & Kneebone, R. (2017). Burns education: The emerging role of simulation for training healthcare professionals. *Burns, 43*(1), 34–40. doi:10.1016/j.burns.2016.07.012

Shin, H., Ma, H., Park, J., Ji, E. S., & Kim, B. H. (2015). The effect of simulation courseware on critical thinking in undergraduate nursing students: Multi-site pre–post study. *Nurse Education Today, 35*(4), 537–542. doi:10.1016/j.nedt.2014.12.004

Society for Simulation in Healthcare. (2018). *Certified Healthcare Simulation Educator Examination Blueprint, 2018 Version*. Retrieved from http://www.ssih.org/Portals/48/Certification/CHSE_Docs/CHSE_Examination_Blueprint.pdf

Squire, K. D. (2007). Games learning, and society: Building a field. Educational Technology, p. 51-54. Retrieved from https://website.education.wisc.edu/~kdsquire/manuscripts/gls.pdf

Sriramatr, S., Silalertdetkul, S., & Wachirathanin, P. (2016). Social cognitive theory associated with physical activity in undergraduate students: A cross-sectional study. *Pacific Rim International Journal of Nursing Research, 20*(2), 95–105.

Turner, S. (2017). Using high-fidelity simulation scenarios in the classroom to engage learners. *Creative Nursing, 23*(1), 35–41. doi:10.1891/1078-4535.23.1.35

Tyler, R. W. (1949). *Basic principles of curriculum and instruction*. Chicago, IL: University of Chicago Press.

Underman, K. (2015). Playing doctor: Simulation in medical school as affective practice. *Social Science & Medicine, 136,* 180–188. doi:10.1016/j.socscimed.2015.05.028

Vaihinger, H. (1927). *The philosophy of the as-if system of the theoretical, pragmatic, and religious fictions of mankind based on an idealistic positivism*. Aalen, Germany: Scientia.

Vroom, V. (1964). *Work and motivation*. New York, NY: Wiley.

Vygotsky, L. S. (1978). *Mind in society: The development of higher mental processes*. Belmont, CA: Wadsworth.

Walton, I. J., & Hill, L. J. (2016). Integrating services and education in primary care. International *Journal of Integrated Care, 16*(6), 1–2. doi:10.5334/ijic.2943

Watson, G., & Glaser, E. M. (1964). *Critical thinking appraisal*. Orlando, FL: Harcourt, Brace & Jovanovich.

Win, W. (2016). Research philosophy in pharmacy practice: Necessity and relevance. *International Journal of Pharmacy Practice, 24*(6), 428–436. doi:10.1111/ijpp.12281

Wong, C. K., & Driscoll, M. (2008). A modified Jigsaw method: An active learning strategy to develop the cognitive and affective domains through curricular review. *Journal of Physical Therapy Education, 21*(3), 15–23. doi:10.1097/00001416-200801000-00004

Yanchus, N. J., Periard, D., & Osatuke, K. (2017). Further examination of predictors of turnover intention among mental health professionals. *Journal of Psychiatric & Mental Health Nursing, 24*(1), 41–56. doi:10.1111/jpm.12354

Zachry, A. H., Nash, B. H., & Nolen, A. (2017). Traditional lectures and team-based learning in an occupational therapy program: A survey of student perceptions. *Open Journal of Occupational Therapy, 5*(2), 1–10. doi:10.15453/2168-6408.1313

Zhang, C., Miller, C., Volkman, K., Meza, J., & Jones, K. (2015). Evaluation of the team performance observation tool with targeted behavioral markers in simulation-based interprofessional education. *Journal of Interprofessional Care, 29*(3), 202–208. doi:10.3109/13561820.2014.982789

15 Implementing Simulation in the Curriculum

NINA MULTAK

Learn from yesterday, live for today, hope for tomorrow.
The important thing is not to stop questioning.

—Albert Einstein

his chapter addresses Domain III: Educational Principles Applied to Simulation (Society for Simulation in Healthcare, 2018).

[LEARNING OUTCOMES]

- Describe the principles of integrating simulation into a curriculum.
- Identify the learning domains to which simulation-based learning can be applied.
- Discuss effective utilization of resources.

Simulation can be used to help learners acquire new knowledge and to better understand concepts needed for safe and effective patient care. By implementing simulation into healthcare curricula, educators will be able to more adeptly assess applied knowledge and skills. Issenberg, McGaghie, Petrusa, Gordon, and Scalese (2005) describe the best practices of simulation in their critical review of simulation-based healthcare education. Curricular integration rated highly among the dozen best practices and was noted as being essential for the effective use of simulation. It is widely accepted that simulation-based learning is most effective when integrated with other learning events and focused on specific learning outcomes. In addition, simulation-based healthcare education is identified as being complementary to clinical education.

Healthcare educators should understand the principles of integrating simulation into a curriculum and identify the curricular areas in which simulation can be effectively implemented. Resources should be used effectively and efficiently. Simulation-based healthcare education and evaluation need to be planned, scheduled, and carried out with consideration given to the entire curriculum

(Scalese & Issenberg, 2008). Simulation should involve all educational stakeholders and garner the necessary administrative support, including funding and materials (Issenberg et al., 2005).

DEVELOPMENT OF A CURRICULUM

Healthcare educators seeking to implement simulation into the curriculum should consider the needs of the learners throughout their training. Educators should consider learners to be at the novice level, progressing in the curriculum to an expert level and utilizing a vertical approach to curricular integration. Consideration should also be given to integrating simulation with inclusion of learners from other professions and disciplines.

It is important to keep measurable objectives in mind, as the design of the simulation activity is critical to its success. Effective simulation is designed using sound methods and principles with the goal that students gain competence in or observe and assess the outlined learning objectives within a safe, learning-conducive environment. Simulation activities are commonly developed in the areas of education (conceptual knowledge, skills), assessment, system integration, and for research purposes (Palaganas, Maxworthy, Epps, and Mancini, 2015).

The initial steps of curriculum development, according to Kern and colleagues, can be effectively applied to simulation.

- The first step in the model of Kern and colleagues is problem identification with a subsequent needs assessment. Effective simulation activities begin with a needs assessment that identifies the learners, the knowledge of the learners, and the skills that will be taught. The needs assessment helps educators to develop measurable learning objectives. This should include an evaluation of the problem, identifying both the current educational approach and the ideal educational approach. Following structured needs assessment will help to develop more educationally sound and meaningful simulation programs.

The next step includes a focused assessment of the learners and the most ideal learning environment. For simulation-based healthcare education, the educator should decide in which of the following environments the information would best be learned: a simulation lab, a classroom, or in situ. It is important to identify the participants in the simulation curriculum. The knowledge and skills that novices need to learn is not the same as the knowledge needed by advanced students, and so it is important to develop learning objectives that provide the appropriate balance of guidance and autonomy for students' levels of sophistication and to identify whether students will be evaluated individually or as part of a team.

The Certified Healthcare Simulation Educator™ (CHSE™) should analyze the current educational approach along with practitioners and the healthcare educational system to address the students' current educational needs. The difference between the ideal approach and current approach represents a gap and identifies a general needs assessment. A targeted needs assessment should include an assessment of the following:

- The needs of a specific learner group
- The healthcare institution and specific learning environment, which may differ from the needs of the specific student population (Kern, Thomas, & Hughes, 2009)

Setting goals and objectives serves as a basis for assessment, and specific measurable learning objectives should be considered. This includes:

- Cognitive (knowledge) domain
- Affective (attitudinal) domain
- Psychomotor domain (skill and behavioral) (Kern et al., 2009)

Educational strategies considered should be specific to learners and content of the curriculum.

Healthcare faculty are often challenged to identify educational strategies that depart from structured learning and reactive thinking to reflective and proactive thinking. Experiential learning strategies using active learning approaches in which students become engaged with educational materials as active learners is replacing some of the classroom-based instruction (Jeffries & Clochesy, 2012). Simulation-based education bridges the classroom and clinical arena and engages learners with broad perspectives to reflect and reframe their understanding of concepts important for clinical practice. Educators use simulation as a way to provide rich learning experiences that can imitate clinical experiences and integrate simulation into the curriculum with clear connections toward achievement of student learning outcomes.

Implementation of simulation in a curriculum requires consideration of many specific issues.

Considerations for implementation include the following:

- Obtain political support.
- Identify and procure resources.
- Identify and address barriers to implementation.
- Introduce the curriculum (piloting or phasing-in).
- Administer the curriculum and refine the curriculum over successive cycles.

The final step in the model of Kern and colleagues includes evaluation and feedback. This can be used to drive ongoing support, justify additional resources, and answer research questions about the effectiveness of specific curriculum elements. Table 15.1 outlines the model's steps and acknowledges the actual work needed to complete the steps.

A needs assessment for a curriculum can be accomplished by many methods, including the following:

- Informal discussions
- Questionnaires
- Surveys
- Interviews
- Focus groups
- Observations
- Tests
- Literature review
- Available published documents

TABLE 15.1
Steps to Curriculum Development According to the Model of Kern and Colleagues

STEPS	WORK NEEDED TO COMPLETE THE STEPS
Step 1: Problem identification and general needs assessment • Identify the problem or educational gap • Identify the current approach (who is doing what, when, and how; resource limitations) • Identify the ideal approach • Ideal approach − current approach = general assessment	Work for Steps 1 and 2 • Systematic review of literature • Needs assessment report • Assessment tool
Step 2: Needs analysis of targeted learners • Identify the learners, level of training, previous experience, current performance, learning styles, and preferences • Identify barriers or enabling factors • Identify the available resources for this group (simulation, faculty, and clinical experiences) • Identify multiple ways to obtain information/needs assessment (Kern et al., 2009)	
Step 3: Goals and objectives • Review types and levels of objectives • Learning domains: cognitive, psychomotor, and affective • Review Bloom's taxonomy of educational objectives • Write specific, measurable, achievable, relevant, and timely objectives	Work for Steps 3 and 4 • Identification of a new educational tool or method • Development of simulation scenarios • Research on the merits of educational processes or tools

Step 4: Educational strategies
• Use multiple educational methods and match methods to objectives
• Review/discuss pros and cons of different methods
• Choose methods that are feasible in terms of resources
• Consider different simulation options
  ▪ Computer-based virtual patients
  ▪ Role-playing
  ▪ Standardized (simulated) patients
  ▪ Task trainers or models
  ▪ Virtual reality simulators
  ▪ Mannequin simulators
  ▪ Hybrid simulation
  ▪ Group learning projects
  ▪ Supplemental interactive activities	

(continued)

TABLE 15.1
Steps to Curriculum Development According to the Model of Kern and Colleagues (*continued*)

STEPS	WORK NEEDED TO COMPLETE THE STEPS
Step 5: Implementation • Consider resources: Personnel, time, facilities, and funding/costs • Administration and operations • Piloting, phasing-in, full implementation	Work for Steps 5 and 6 • Descriptive study of curriculum implementation • Cost-effective analysis report • Assessment tool
Step 6: Evaluation and feedback • Identify users and use (formative, summative), resources for evaluation, questions to ask, evaluation design • Select measurement method • Assess ethical issues • Data collection and analysis • Identification of results	

Source: Adapted from Kern, D. E., Thomas, P. A., and Hughes, M. T. (2009). *Curriculum development for medical education: A six step approach* (2nd ed.). Baltimore, MD: Johns Hopkins University Press.

DELIBERATE PRACTICE

Research on expert performance has transformed the way healthcare educators approach how clinicians acquire clinical competence and how expertise is defined (Ericsson, 2004, 2008).

Deliberate practice is the path to acquiring expertise and the goal of deliberate practice is to improve performance. Repeated behaviors become automatic habits. Students who master the art of deliberate practice are committed to being lifelong learners—always exploring and experimenting and refining. This requires sustained effort and concentration. The concept of deliberate practice, in which education is focused on improving particular tasks, has been essential to the development of the simulation-based experiential learning paradigm and has been implemented by healthcare educators across many disciplines (Ericsson, 2008).

LEARNING DOMAINS

Simulation can measure outcomes in the cognitive, affective, and psychomotor domains. Cognitive domain learning may include the acquisition and recall of facts and figures, concepts, and principles. Cognitive learning outcomes have been identified as a basic strategy for the assessment of student learning. A traditional lecture followed by a multiple-choice or short-answer exam is an example of cognitive evaluation. Healthcare simulation offers an opportunity for teaching and evaluation of higher level cognitive functions, such as the application, synthesis, and evaluation of healthcare knowledge (Kardong-Edgren, Adamson, & Fitzgerald, 2010).

Learning in the affective domain includes the values, attitudes, and beliefs that are essential for a healthcare provider. Assessment of the affective domain requires educators to identify and verify that healthcare learners have absorbed the values, attitudes, and beliefs essential for a healthcare provider and that these are reflected in their professional practice. Mannequin simulation allows opportunities for learners to reveal their competency in the affective domain through participation in simulation scenarios.

Technical skill performance is an example of the assessment of psychomotor learning. Using task trainers, virtual reality simulators, and mannequin simulators, the CHSE can assess the acquisition of technical skills (Jeffries & Norton, 2005). Using a case scenario to evaluate technical skills allows CHSEs to teach and evaluate psychomotor skills in a setting that is more realistic than a traditional skills station (such as suturing on a task trainer or starting an intravenous [IV] line using a simulated IV arm) and much safer than an actual patient care setting, such as a live patient in an emergency department. Evaluation instruments that measure preestablished outcomes may be used for a comprehensive evaluation of learning (Kardong-Edgren et al., 2010).

■ INTEGRATING SIMULATION

Simulation training can be implemented in various components of a curriculum.

- Basic science courses can effectively use simulation modalities. Pharmacologic effects can be simulated on a mannequin for usual dosage ingestion or overdose. Medication effects can also be taught in code or Advanced Cardiac Life Support scenarios.
- Simulators can be used to teach vital-sign assessment as well as evaluation of cardiac and pulmonary conditions to healthcare learners.
- Crisis management training can be implemented with consideration of complex details of realistic case scenarios.

Effectively directing simulation resources can result in an educator's ability to implement simulation successfully in the educational curriculum. These resources are shown in Figure 15.1.

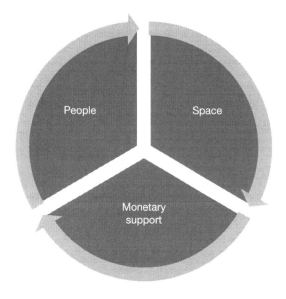

FIGURE 15.1 Resources needed to include simulation in a curriculum.

Organizational barriers can hinder the implementation of simulation-based education in the curriculum. Scheduling trainees to attend simulation activities can be a challenge. It is suggested that leaders in the institution support simulation programming by encouraging faculty to become involved and avoid learner scheduling and space issues (Exhibit 15.1). Faculty and financial resources can also be supported by administrative personnel (McGaghie, Issenberg, Petrusa, & Scalese, 2010).

> **EVIDENCE-BASED SIMULATION PRACTICE 15.1**
>
> Bennett, Rodgers, Fitzgerald, and Gibson (2017) completed a literature search about using simulation in occupational therapy curricula. The researchers found most articles discussed the use of simulation in foundational courses and for preparation for fieldwork, and to address competencies necessary for newly graduating therapists. Most studies were descriptive of students' perception about simulation, indicating further outcomes research is needed.

EXHIBIT 15.1

Considerations for Simulation Implementation

The Type of Knowledge, Skill, Attitudes, or Behavior Addressed in Simulation Include:

Conceptual knowledge	Technical skills	Decision-making skills	Attitudes and behavior

Purpose

Education	Assessment	Clinical training	Research

Experience Level of Participants

Preprofessional training	Initial professional education	Clinical training/ Residency	Continuing education

Source: Gaba, D. M. (2004). The future vision of simulation in health care. *Quality & Safety in Health Care, 13,* i2–i10. doi:10.1136/qshc.2004.009878

■ SIMULATION CONCEPTS

It is important to imbed simulation throughout a curriculum, instead of implementing simulation exercises as independent curricular elements (Burns, O'Donnell, & Artman, 2010). It is also vital to consider a vertical as well as horizontal approach to implementing simulation in the curriculum. Simulations should be developed for novice, experienced, and expert clinicians. An interprofessional or multidisciplinary approach to simulation programming should also be implemented in order to give learners experience developing their skills in a team-based setting. Establishing the best approach to integrating simulation in a curriculum can be determined by the institution as well as by the discipline and can address the potential effect of combining simulation-based healthcare education with other educational strategies (McGaghie et al., 2010).

Prior to curricular implementation, educators should consider the following simulation-based considerations:

- **Realism:** Educational goals should match simulation type. Task trainers should be used for procedural skills, whereas complex events should involve a high-fidelity mannequin simulator (McGaghie et al., 2010).
- **Reliability (e.g., assessment tools, implementation process):** The development of effective evaluation tools should follow an organized process with a clearly defined endpoint (Kardong-Edgren et al., 2010).
- **Validity (e.g., content, construct):** Ideally, simulation evaluation instruments validly measure each of the three domains of student performance: cognitive, psychomotor, and affective. Several types of validity need to be considered when using tools for evaluation, including the following:
  - Content validity—Refers to the appropriateness of each item and comprehensiveness of the measurement.
  - Construct validity—Refers to the process of establishing that an action accurately represents the concept being evaluated (Kardong-Edgren et al., 2010).
  - Face validity—Does the evaluation tool appear to be measuring the concept it is supposed to measure?
  - Predictive ability—Is there a correlation between the responses and an expectation (Zheng & Agresti, 2000)?
- **Feasibility (e.g., efficient, effective, achievable):** There should be possibilities for replication of some or nearly all of the essential aspects of a clinical situation so that the situation can be readily understood and managed when it occurs in actual clinical practice (Cant & Cooper, 2010).
- **Learner-centered education:** Students can use deliberate practice in a focused manner to master skills at their own pace (Ericsson, 2004).
- **Interprofessional education:** Interprofessional education (IPE) has been recognized by various international professional societies (e.g., World Health Organization, Institute of Medicine) and accreditation organizations as foundational to achieving safe, high-quality, accessible, patient-centered care.
- **Teamwork:** Critical teamwork competencies should be identified and used as a focus for training content; teamwork simulations need to be designed to improve team processes (Salas, Diaz-Granados, Weaver, & King, 2008).
- **Human factors:** Engaging learners in repetitive practice is suggested as a primary factor in studies showing skill transference to real patients. With increased

> **SIMULATION TEACHING TIP 15.1**
>
> Simulation program development should occur in conjunction with other curriculum programming. Simulation can be used for both formative and summative assessments and therefore is most valuable when integrated throughout the training curriculum. Involving faculty in the development of assessment tools enables more faculty involvement in simulation programming.

simulator availability, learning curves are shortened, which leads to faster skill automaticity. Simulators must be made available at a convenient location that accommodates learners' schedules (Issenberg et al., 2005).

- **Patient safety:** Simulation is an important educational technique for improving clinical training and patient safety (Groves et al., 2017).

SUMMARY

Simulation-based educators should highlight evidence-based information, which supports the best practices of simulation (McGaghie et al., 2010). Implementing simulation in the curriculum is among the top objectives in the best practice list according to research. Other best practices noted in this research include feedback, deliberate practice, outcome measurement, appropriate fidelity, attention to skill acquisition and maintenance, mastery in learning, transference to practice, team training, high-stakes training, instructor training, and appropriate educational and professional context.

> **CASE STUDY 15.1**
>
> Schools of Health Sciences are being developed all over the country in academic institutions to accommodate the market demand for healthcare practitioners. If you were the founding dean of a health sciences program that included the disciplines of nursing, physician assistant studies, physical therapy, and occupational therapy, how would you develop the interprofessional simulation program in order to integrate simulation throughout all curricula?

PRACTICE QUESTIONS

1. The expert simulation educator understands that integrating simulation throughout the curriculum involves:

    A. Resources
    B. A new building
    C. High-fidelity equipment
    D. Staff approval

2. The first step in integrating simulation throughout a curriculum should be to:

    A. Acquire equipment.
    B. Develop student learning outcomes.
    C. Discuss the best learning environment.
    D. Perform a needs assessment.

3. The novice simulation educator needs better understanding when she states that learning goals need to be established in the following domain:

    A. Psychomotor
    B. Cognitive
    C. Empathetic
    D. Affective

4. The final step of developing an integrative simulation curriculum is:

   A. Evaluation
   B. Teaching methods
   C. Developing student learning outcomes
   D. Discussing the mission

5. The novice simulation educator understands deliberate practice when she states:

   A. "It has the goal of developing perfect skills."
   B. "It is a method to evaluate and grade students."
   C. "It is a method to ensure appropriate formative evaluation."
   D. "It is a method to use to practice skills to become better at doing them."

6. A student who is practicing insertion of central lines on a task-trainer is learning mainly in which domain?

   A. Affective
   B. Psychomotor
   C. Cognitive
   D. Psychosocial

7. A scenario in which a student is telling family members "bad news" about a patient is developing skill in which domain?

   A. Affective
   B. Psychomotor
   C. Cognitive
   D. Psychosocial

8. A student who is calculating the correct morphine dosage in a simulation to complete a patient-controlled analgesic (PCA) pump setup is developing skill in which domain?

   A. Affective
   B. Psychomotor
   C. Cognitive
   D. Psychosocial

9. A simulation principle that is followed by educators is:

   A. Educational goals should match the simulation type.
   B. Always use the lowest simulation type to accomplish a task.
   C. The more real the environment, the better the learning outcome will be.
   D. All students should be exposed to all simulation types.

10. A summation educator has used an evaluation tool for three different groups and the scores are inconsistent. The simulation educator concludes the tool lacks:

    A. Content validity
    B. Face value
    C. Construct validity
    D. Relatability

REFERENCES

Bennett, S., Rodgers, S., Fitzgerald, C., & Gibson, L. (2017). Simulation in occupational therapy curricula: A literature review. *Australian Occupational Therapy Journal, 64*(4), 314–327. doi:10.1111/1440-1630.12372

Burns, H. K., O'Donell, J., & Artman, J. (2010). High-fidelity simulation in teaching problem solving to 1st-year nursing students. *Clinical Simulation in Nursing, 6*(3), e87–e95. doi:10.1016/j.ecns.2009.07.005

Cant, R., & Cooper, S. (2010). Simulation-based learning in nurse education: Systematic review. *Journal of Advanced Nursing, 66*(1), 3–15. doi:10.1111/j.1365-2648.2009.05240.x

Deutsch, E., & Palaganas, J. (2015). SSH accreditation standards. In J. Palaganas, J. Maxworthy, C. Epps & M. Mancini (Eds.), *Developing excellence in simulation programs* (pp. 2–16). Baltimore, MD: Lippincott Williams & Wilkins.

Ericsson, K. A. (2004). Deliberate practice and the acquisition and maintenance of expert performance in medicine and related domains. *Academic Medicine, 79*(10), S70–S81. doi:10.1097/00001888-200410001-00022

Ericsson, K. A. (2008). Deliberate practice and acquisition of expert performance: A general overview. *Academic Emergency Medicine, 15*(11), 988–994. doi:10.1111/j.1553-2712.2008.00227.x

Gaba, D. M. (2004). The future vision of simulation in health care. *Quality & Safety in Health Care, 13*, i2–i10. doi:10.1136/qshc.2004.009878

Groves, P. S., Bunch, J. L., Cram, E., Farag, A., Manges, K., Perkhounkova, Y., & Scott-Cawiezell, J. (2017). Priming patient safety through nursing handoff communication: A simulation pilot study. *Western Journal of Nursing Research, 39*(11), 1394–1411. doi:10.1177/0193945916673358

Issenberg, S. B., McGaghie, W. C., Petrusa, E. R., Gordon, D. L., & Scalese, R. J. (2005). Features and uses of high-fidelity medical simulations that lead to effective learning: A BEME systematic review. *Medical Teacher, 27*, 10–28. doi:10.1080/01421590500046924

Jeffries, P. R., & Clochesy, J. M. (2012). Clinical simulations: An experiential, student-centered pedagogical approach. In D. M. Billings & J. A. Halstead (Eds.), *Teaching in nursing: A guide for faculty* (4th ed., 352–368). St. Louis, MO: Elsevier Health Sciences.

Jeffries, P. R., & Norton, B. (2005). Selecting learning experiences to achieve curriculum outcomes. In D. M. Billings & J. A. Halstead (Eds.), *Teaching in nursing: A guide for faculty* (2nd ed., pp. 187–212). St. Louis, MO: Elsevier.

Kardong-Edgren, S., Adamson, K. A., & Fitzgerald, C. (2010). A review of currently published evaluation instruments for human patient simulation. *Clinical Simulation in Nursing, 6*, e25–e35. doi:10.1016/j.ecns.2009.08.004

Kern, D. E., Thomas, P. A., & Hughes, M. T. (2009). *Curriculum development for medical education: A six step approach* (2nd ed.). Baltimore, MD: Johns Hopkins University Press.

McGaghie, W., Issenberg, S. B., Petrusa, E. R., & Scalese, R. J. (2010). A critical review of simulation-based medical education research: 2003–2009. *Medical Education, 44*, 50–63. doi:10.1111/j.1365-2923.2009.03547.x

Palaganas, J. C., Maxworthy, J. C., Epps, C. A., & Mancini, M. (2015). Defining excellence in simulation. Washington, DC: Society for Simulation in Healthcare.

Salas, E., Diaz-Granados, D., Weaver, S. J., & King, H. (2008). Does team training work? Principles for health care. *Academic Emergency Medicine, 11*, 1002–1009. doi:10.1111/j.1553-2712.2008.00254.x

Scalese, R. J., & Issenberg, S. B. (2008). Simulation-based assessment. In E. S. Holmboe & R. E. Hawkins (Eds.), *Practical guide to the evaluation of clinical competence* (pp. 179–200). Philadelphia, PA: Mosby Elsevier.

Society for Simulation in Healthcare. (2018). *Certified Healthcare Simulation Educator Examination Blueprint, 2018 Version*. Retrieved from http://www.ssih.org/Portals/48/Certification/CHSE_Docs/CHSE_Examination_Blueprint.pdf

Zheng, B., & Agresti, A. (2000). Summarizing the predictive power of a generalized linear model. *Statistics in Medicine, 19*, 1771–1781. doi:10.1002/1097-0258(20000715)19:13<1771::AID-SIM485>3.0.CO;2-P

16
Planning Simulation Activities
KAREN K. GITTINGS

It takes as much energy to wish as it does to plan.
—Eleanor Roosevelt

This chapter addresses Domain III: Educational Principles Applied to Simulation (Society for Simulation in Healthcare, 2018).

[LEARNING OUTCOMES]

- Discuss the importance of developing goals and objectives for simulation activities that are relevant to student learning outcomes.
- Describe formative and summative methods that can be used to evaluate learning outcomes for simulation activities.
- Design a simulation day or simulation activities to promote learning.

Simulation activities are a valuable adjunct for student learning and evaluation if linked appropriately to student learning outcomes. Planning ahead is vitally important for the overall success and effectiveness of simulation activities. The process begins with an assessment of learner needs, after which goals for the simulation activities and measurable learning objectives must be identified. The educator must then decide on whether the evaluation should be formative or summative and what methods of evaluation would be most appropriate. After these initial steps are completed, the simulation activities are designed with consideration to resources needed and those that are available. A well-planned simulation activity will minimize problems in the implementation phase. The focus of this chapter is to discuss the planning process for simulation activities; a sample simulation day is reviewed to illustrate each step in the process.

NEEDS ASSESSMENT

The first step in the planning process for simulation activities is to identify the needs of the learners. This can be accomplished through several methods. In some instances, it may be helpful to administer a formal needs assessment at the onset of the planning process; this allows learners to self-identify their educational needs. The needs assessment can also be done informally by the educator who is responsible for the simulation activities and has the most knowledge of the context in which the simulation is being used and how it links to student learning outcomes. Both methods will serve to provide a starting point for the planning process and further guide the development of goals and objectives.

> **CASE STUDY 16.1**
>
> Karen, a nurse educator, is planning a simulation day for her learners. To begin the process, she reviews the student learning outcomes of her Adult Health II course. The learners are first-semester seniors (third-semester nursing students) in a baccalaureate nursing program. Karen identifies areas of new content and skills that will be introduced to learners this semester, and from those, determines what knowledge and skills would be best taught through simulation activities. It is decided that learners will be taught intravenous (IV) insertion and principles of IV therapy during the simulation day.
>
> In further assessing her learners' needs, Karen recognizes that they gain little clinical experience in working with
>
> - Nasogastric (NG) tubes
> - Small-bore feeding tubes
> - Tube feeding
> - Administration of medications through enteral feeding tubes
>
> Even though learners are introduced to these skills in the fundamentals of nursing course, they may not have the opportunity to use them again because of their clinical placement. It was therefore decided to include these skills as part of the simulation day for review and reeducation.
>
> With an understanding of learner needs, Karen is able to develop goals for the simulation day. It is important to keep student learning outcomes for the course in mind to ensure that the goals are relevant and support learning within the course. Goals include the following:
>
> 1. The simulation day will enable learners to develop an understanding of IV insertion and principles of IV therapy.
> 2. The simulation day will enable learners to review knowledge and skills related to feeding-tube insertion, tube feedings, and enteral medication administration.
>
> After setting her goals for the simulation day, Karen develops measurable objectives that will be used to evaluate the effectiveness of the simulation activities. Objectives include the following:
>
> At the completion of the simulation day, learners will
>
> 1. Demonstrate correct technique in IV insertion using the IV simulator.
> 2. Demonstrate the correct steps for hanging a secondary IV and programming the smart pump.

CASE STUDY 16.1 (*continued*)

3. Assess and perform nursing interventions for a simulated patient having abdominal pain.
4. Demonstrate the correct technique for NG insertion and enteral administration of medications.

In deciding whether to use formative or summative evaluation, Karen considers her goals for the day. Because the simulation day is designed to introduce new skills related to IV therapy and reinforce knowledge related to NG tubes and enteral medication administration, Karen decides to use this day as a teaching opportunity with formative evaluation to assess learners' progress. At each learning station, students will be required to return demonstrate their new skills. Faculty members are responsible for facilitating the learning of new skills and correction of identified learning deficits.

As learners will only attend one simulation day associated with the Adult Health II course, a summative evaluation will be completed by learners and faculty. This evaluation will be used to determine whether the learning activities were effective in meeting the planned goals and objectives.

> **SIMULATION TEACHING TIP 16.1**
>
> Let learners know up front that they will be evaluated the day and provide them with the criteria so that, as they move through the day, they have an idea of what aspects they should be paying particular attention to in order to complete the appraisal.

For the purposes of formative evaluation, Karen elects to use debriefing, observation, and feedback. Debriefing will follow the high-fidelity simulation of the patient with abdominal pain. Each simulation will run 15 to 20 minutes followed by a 30-minute debriefing. The simulation coordinator will lead the debriefing because of her expertise and advanced training in this skill.

Faculty members will use observation and feedback at the three other low-fidelity simulation stations. Skills' checklists or other tools will be used to objectively document learner performance. Learners will be provided feedback during their performance to assist with process improvement.

Learners and faculty will be asked to complete a brief survey at the conclusion of the simulation day. This tool will be developed with the assistance of the simulation coordinator. Information will be collected anonymously and used to determine whether learning objectives were met. Suggestions for further improvement will also be solicited.

Because the simulation day is designed to provide opportunities for learners to acquire new knowledge and skills, Karen elects to use skills' checklists at the IV therapy and NG tube stations to evaluate learner performance. At the conclusion of the day, learners will be asked to complete a survey that is a self-report of their satisfaction with the simulation day activities, and their confidence in meeting the learning objectives. In the future, when simulation activities are used to document competency, a more valid and reliable evaluation tool will need to be used.

In the nursing department where Karen teaches, course coordinators are given the opportunity to schedule a week for simulation activities for their courses. Karen elects to schedule her simulation week early in the semester so

(*continued*)

CASE STUDY 16.1 (continued)

learners will have the opportunity to learn new skills (IV therapy) and review old skills (NG tubes) prior to starting back to clinical in the hospital setting. She further decides to have four simulation stations that will support the identified learning objectives. The first station will be an IV station where learners will learn proper technique for IV insertion. The second station will be an IV station where learners will learn principles of IV therapy, including hanging a secondary medication and programming the smart pump. At the third station, learners will be required to assess and intervene in a simulated patient having abdominal pain. Last, learners will review procedures for inserting NG tubes and administering enteral medications. These simulation activities will be scheduled over a period of 7.5 hours. In order to keep the number of learners low, only two clinical groups (16 learners) will be scheduled per day. Learners will be divided into four groups of four. For a class of 50 learners, 3 to 4 days will be necessary to rotate all learners in the Adult Health II course through the simulation activities. A sample schedule for the simulation day is noted in Table 16.1.

TABLE 16.1
Sample Schedule for Simulation Day

TIMES	STATION 1 IV SIM	STATION 2 IV PUMP	STATION 3 SIMULATOR	STATION 4 NG/MEDS
8:30–9:45 a.m.	Orientation	Orientation	Orientation	Orientation
9:50–10:40 a.m.	Blue Team	Green Team	Purple Team	Red Team
10:45–11:35 a.m.	Red Team	Blue Team	Green Team	Purple Team
11:35–12:35 p.m.	Lunch	Lunch	Lunch	Lunch
12:40–1:30 p.m.	Purple Team	Red Team	Blue Team	Green Team
1:45–2:35 p.m.	Green Team	Purple Team	Red Team	Blue Team
2:40–3:00 p.m.	Evaluations	Evaluations	Evaluations	Evaluations
3:00–4:00 p.m.	Math Work	Math Work	Math Work	Math Work

IV, intravenous; MED, medication; NG, nasogastric; SIM, simulator.

CASE STUDY 16.1 (continued)

Karen continues planning for the simulation day by identifying the simulation modalities that will be used at each station. In the first station, learners will work with the screen-based IV computer simulator to learn correct technique for IV insertion; because this program provides feedback at the conclusion of each scenario, learners will be provided with an objective evaluation of their technique.

At the second station, learners will have the opportunity to work with IV equipment and practice priming IV lines, hanging secondary IVs, and programming the smart pump. This simulation activity involves the use of a task trainer (smart pump) in which learners have the opportunity to practice IV therapy skills.

Learners will work with a high-fidelity mannequin at the third station, where they will be required to assess and intervene with a patient having abdominal pain. Learners will be observed during the simulation activity and feedback will be provided as part of the debriefing process.

The fourth and final station will use low-fidelity simulation to allow learners to practice the technique of NG tube insertion and administration of enteral medications. A task trainer that is a model of a human's head and upper torso will be used to practice NG tube insertion. Enteral medication administration can be practiced with a very simple setup of an NG tube inserted into an empty jug. Evaluation will be through observation and feedback.

In order to plan for simulation and schedule laboratory space each semester, the simulation coordinator requests that course coordinators sign up for their simulation week at the end of the preceding semester. A master schedule is then generated so that all faculty are aware of their simulation week, as well as other courses using the laboratory. Prior to her assigned week, Karen notifies the simulation coordinator of her planned learning activities and space needs so that rooms/space in the laboratory can be designated in advance.

After carefully considering each simulation activity, Karen identifies potential personnel for each station. At the IV simulator station, a full-time faculty or trained adjunct faculty will need to run and demonstrate the IV simulator. The second station with IV therapy can be led by an adjunct clinical faculty member. As the third station involves the high-fidelity mannequin, the simulation coordinator will lead the simulation and debriefing because of her advanced knowledge and skill in this area. The NG tube and enteral medication administration station has previously been designated as a self-directed station, but feedback from previous learners has led to this station also being directed by a content expert. This is a simulation activity that could be led by an adjunct clinical faculty or graduate learner.

In order to have enough content experts to lead each simulation station, Karen needs to recruit at least four additional members to the simulation team. The simulation coordinator is the first person recruited to run the high-fidelity simulation. Three clinical faculty will also be used.

1. The first is an adjunct clinical faculty member who has worked in this adult health course for several years and participated in multiple simulation exercises; as her expertise is IV therapy, she has been asked to lead this station.
2. The second clinical faculty is actually a full-time faculty member with experience on the IV simulator, so she was asked to lead this particular station.
3. The final clinical faculty member is new to this adult health course and simulation. Because her clinical experience is in acute care surgical nursing, she is very comfortable with NG tubes and has agreed to lead this station.

(continued)

CASE STUDY 16.1 (continued)

As the course coordinator, Karen is also in the simulation laboratory with her learners to troubleshoot any problems that may occur.

In order to orient her team members to the simulation activities, Karen sends out, in advance, an agenda with the day's schedule of activities. Learning objectives are shared, and the simulation activities at each station are listed in detail. The goal of the simulation experience and the course coordinator's expectations for the day are made clear to all members. To accommodate everyone's schedule, training is held 1 hour prior to the learners' arrival. As three of the team members have participated in this simulation day previously, only a brief review is necessary. More time is spent with the new adjunct clinical faculty to familiarize her with the equipment and learning objectives for the station she is assigned. Because she is an experienced nurse, she has no difficulty grasping the activities of this station.

Using the university's online learning platform, Karen created a folder within her course's site with information pertaining to simulation day activities. Learners were also encouraged to visit the simulation site to meet their simulated patient and review his past medical–surgical history. This provides learners with additional information about the high-fidelity simulation activity in an attempt to reduce anxiety and fear of the unknown.

As the simulation laboratory is in use at least 3 days a week, Karen and the simulation coordinator prepare the simulation rooms the Friday before simulation activities are scheduled to begin for her adult health course. Handouts are prepared and copied for use at some stations. All equipment and supplies are laid out and organized; computerized simulators are calibrated as necessary. A final walk-through of the stations is conducted early Monday morning before the learners arrive. Because these four simulation activities have been used previously with success, no prior run-through was needed.

GOAL DEFINITION

Once learner needs have been assessed, it is important to set achievable goals for the day. The words *goals* and *objectives* are often erroneously used interchangeably. Goals are usually statements that serve as a long-term target; they describe the expected outcome at the end of the teaching–learning process. Goals can be used to broadly identify the purpose and final outcomes of the day and lead to the development of more specific objectives (Bastable, 2014).

LEARNING OBJECTIVES

Learning objectives are specific actions that are measurable, tangible, and designed to support attainment of the goals. Written to be short term, objectives are a statement about a single behavior that is to be accomplished after a teaching session or within a short period of time. Objectives are often used to describe a behavior or performance that the learner must accomplish before being considered competent (Bastable, 2014).

The number of learning objectives depends on the number of simulation activities and time involved, but generally vary from one to four. In addition to being relevant, the learning objectives should also be at the appropriate level for the learner; for example, the learning objectives for a simulation activity should be different if the learner is a student nurse compared to an experienced practitioner. When running the simulation activities, it is important to always keep the learning objectives in mind. Objectives are the starting point for designing the simulation and will further guide the development of the scenario pertaining to content and complexity (Bailey, 2017).

TYPES OF EVALUATION

Evaluation of simulation activities can be formative or summative. Formative evaluation is done during the learning activity, allowing the educator to assess learners' progress toward achieving learning objectives. In this manner, the learning activity is used to facilitate learning and identify student learning deficits; the activity can also be evaluated and improved upon (Billings & Halstead, 2012).

Summative evaluation is completed at the conclusion of a learning activity, course, or program. The focus is generally on evaluating the extent to which objectives or outcomes were met, leading to a grade assignment. Because summative evaluation occurs at the end, the biggest disadvantage is that nothing can be done to alter the results (Billings & Halstead, 2012).

EVALUATION METHODS

After determining the type of evaluation to be used, different methods of evaluation must be considered. Debriefing is considered an integral part of the teaching–learning process that occurs with high-fidelity simulation. This follow-up discussion provides learners the opportunity to process what they have learned. Learners are able to assess their own performance and, through feedback from faculty and peers, confirm their knowledge and identify areas needing improvement. It is the debriefing process that leads to the long-term acquisition of knowledge (Abelsson & Bisholt, 2017).

When other low-fidelity simulations are used, observation and feedback may be a more appropriate means of evaluation. *Observation* is the direct visualization of learner performance of a task or behavior. This is a useful method for evaluating skills competence. Faculty members observing learner performance are able to provide immediate feedback; in addition, learners have the opportunity to remediate and improve on skills. Using an objective tool with observation is important to avoid bias and accurately record information (Billings & Halstead, 2012).

Feedback is an important evaluative mechanism, but, in order for it to be effective, there must be a clear understanding of what constitutes good performance of the expected standards (Allen & Molloy, 2017). In order to provide appropriate feedback, observation must have occurred. The person providing feedback must also know the standard against which the learner is being compared; for this reason, it is important that the person providing feedback has expertise in the content area.

To evaluate the effectiveness of the simulation day, a survey with a rating scale can be used to elicit learners' and faculty's feedback on the extent to which the day's objectives were met. Objectivity of the evaluation process is increased by using a rating scale (Billings & Halstead, 2012). Information from the survey can identify issues with the learning activities and lead to improvement for future simulation-day activities.

> **EVIDENCE-BASED SIMULATION PRACTICE 16.1**
>
> McDermott, Sarasnick, and Timcheck (2017) discuss the International Nursing Association for Clinical Simulation and Learning (INACSL) newly released Standards of Best Practice™. The Simulation Design Standard (SDS) was used to create a pilot study with sophomore nursing students ($N = 143$) to prepare students for fundamental respiratory concepts. The student perceptions (80%) believed that simulation assisted critical thinking.

EVALUATION TOOLS

Measurements of learner performance can range from self-reporting surveys to external reviewers using validated assessment tools. Many educators use self-reports of satisfaction and confidence to evaluate learning objectives and outcomes. For those educators unskilled in tool development, self-reporting provides a means of evaluation that is easily obtained, although not necessarily a valid measure of simulation effectiveness. Although it was a widely held belief that high-fidelity simulation was effective for student learning, the initial evidence was inconsistent and lacked reporting of validity and reliability (Chen, Huang, Liao, & Liu, 2015). The objective structured clinical examinations (OSCEs) are well known as valid assessment tools used in medical schools for evaluation, but they can also be used to objectively evaluate clinical nursing skills (Zhu et al., 2017). Several evaluation tools that use checklists or evaluation scales are documented in the literature, but many have not been evaluated for reliability or validity. Within the past 5 years, several new instruments have been developed that demonstrate appropriate psychometric properties (Chen et al., 2015).

DESIGNING THE SIMULATION ACTIVITY

Planning and organizing the simulation activities are vital to a successful simulation day. Decisions must be made about the time frame allotted for the learning activities. For example, will the simulations be run during class or clinical time? If simulation activities occur on a clinical day, what will the learners do if simulation activities are completed in less time than their designated clinical hours?

Simulation activities must be planned that are consistent with student learning outcomes for the course. What simulation activities would reinforce student learning and promote achievement of student learning outcomes? How many simulation activities would be appropriate?

Consideration must also be given to the number of learners enrolled in the course. Simulation activities are most effective when learners are placed in small groups. Even when using low-fidelity simulations, fewer learners allow for more time for interaction with faculty members and hands-on practice. This leads to questions about how to schedule the learners in smaller numbers and still fit into the simulation laboratory schedule.

SELECTING THE SIMULATION MODALITY

After designing the simulation day and activities, careful consideration must be given to selection of the modalities that will best support learning objectives. Simulation modalities are referred to as *high fidelity* and *low fidelity*, but with continued technological advances, even the simplest trainers are becoming more realistic. *High fidelity* generally refers to the use of software-controlled, full-body mannequins, whereas *low fidelity* refers to the traditional task trainers that are used for procedural training. Mannequins that partially produce physiologic changes are referred to as *medium fidelity* (Jeffries, Dreifuerst, Aschenbrenner, Adamson, & Schram, 2015).

■ RESOURCE IDENTIFICATION

Once the simulation day has been planned, it is important to identify the resources that will be needed, as well as those that are available. First to consider is the location. Although many nursing/medical schools have simulation laboratories, the size and room availability may be limited. Scheduling and reserving space are an early priority.

Equipment needs should also be identified. This should include a detailed list of everything that is needed at each simulation station. In addition to equipment needs, when planning for the simulation it is also important to consider whether props or moulage are needed to achieve the desired look for the mannequin. A medical record may also be necessary for the scenario to proceed. It is important to carefully plan the details in advance so that the simulation is realistic and complete (Jeffries et al., 2015).

It is also important to identify the content experts/educators and their availability for the simulation activities. Although some low-fidelity simulation activities can be designated as self-directed, generally, a monitor is needed at each station to orient learners to the activity and keep them on target. For simulation done in nursing/medical schools, learners who are at a higher class level could be used to monitor some of the low-fidelity stations. For activities that involve high fidelity or more complex learning activities, an adjunct clinical instructor or a graduate-level learner would be able to function as the content expert in instructing and assisting learners to meet learning objectives. Some schools have dedicated laboratory personnel or technicians whose responsibilities include simulation and management of laboratory activities.

Simulation activities that are carried out in healthcare organizations are usually developed and organized by the staff of the education department. The educators have the primary responsibility of providing and managing the simulation activities, but other resources are often available. Nurses and medical personnel within the organization have unique knowledge and skills that make them valuable resources in assisting with simulation activities. In addition, healthcare organizations that have collaborative relationships with nursing/medical schools can invite faculty to participate in simulation activities.

■ SIMULATION TEAM

Once the resources have been identified, it is important to organize the simulation team. Educators/content experts must be recruited to participate in simulation day activities. In the academic setting, if other faculty are to be used, consideration must be given to their workload and responsibilities. If the simulation activities are to be conducted on the learners' clinical days, the adjunct clinical instructors can be requested to assist with leading the simulation activities on the day their learners are in the laboratory setting. Adjunct clinical instructors may be recruited to assist with other days, but it must be clear whether additional pay is expected and whether departmental or laboratory budgets can support this. Graduate learners can also be recruited, as an example, from the nurse educator students; simulation hours may be used to fulfill hour requirements in a practicum course.

In the healthcare organizational setting, educators who are recruiting assistance from other agency personnel must often request release of the employees from their primary department. Arrangements need to be made as early as possible to prevent scheduling conflicts. This is also true when collaborating with faculty from nursing/medical schools.

If standardized (simulated) patients are used, actors must also be recruited. In collaboration with the drama department in academic settings, drama learners may portray patients as part of an assignment. Other educators or faculty may also be used. Volunteers may be recruited as well. Professional actors skilled in playing standardized (simulated) patients are also available for hire, although costs can be prohibitive.

Once the members of the simulation team have been recruited and confirmed, arrangements must be made to orient and train them for their roles. It can be challenging to schedule extra time for team members to train, especially when they have other jobs and responsibilities. This becomes less of an issue when the same content experts, whether clinical professionals, educators, or adjunct clinical instructors, are used frequently and simulation activities are done repetitively. Standardized (simulated) patients may require a more in-depth orientation and training depending on the role to be played.

PREPARATIONS

Prior to the simulation day, multiple tasks must be accomplished in preparation for the learners and simulation team. A week in advance, learners and team members should be sent an agenda with a schedule of the day's activities. Learners should additionally be provided information about

- Dress requirements
- Equipment required (e.g., stethoscope)
- Any preplanning work/assignment (Exhibit 16.1)

EXHIBIT 16.1

Learner Instructions for Simulation Day

Please bring the following items on your simulation day.

1. Clinical uniform
2. Stethoscope
3. Simulation-day agenda
4. Class notes on nasogastric tubes
5. Medical–surgical nursing textbook
6. Nursing skills book
7. Medications reference

The laboratory must also be prepared with all equipment set up and ready for use. If the laboratory is heavily used, it may not be possible to set up until late in the preceding week. The laboratory setting should be fully prepared and functional so that simulation can be started and kept on schedule. When learners are required to stand around and wait because of lack of planning on the part of the coordinator, it reflects poorly on the simulation day overall. Learners appreciate well-run, organized learning activities.

It may be advisable to pilot a new simulation before conducting it with learners. This can be done in the form of a run-through or field test and can be as simple as the course coordinator and simulation coordinator running the simulation scenario through with various unfolding events or endings. This process assists in identifying potential issues and problems that may occur during the simulation; in addition, this is an opportunity to ensure nothing has been forgotten, all necessary resources are available, and every simulation activity is running seamlessly. Prebriefing may also be used prior to the simulation in order to answer questions. This also provides the opportunity for faculty to ensure that any required preparatory work has been completed by the students (Leighton, 2017).

SUMMARY

Simulation days are very valuable to learners and can provide clinical skill practice that will be needed in the clinical area. Being true to the goals and objectives of the experience is of utmost importance. Deciding on the logistics of how stations will be set up and what type of evaluation of skills will be accomplished is needed. It is also important to organize the day beforehand by setting up the laboratory, notifying people, and providing the learners with expectations.

PRACTICE QUESTIONS

1. A new educator is planning to include simulation in his medical–surgical course. To begin the planning process, the educator should first:

    A. Write a simulation scenario on a topic of interest.
    B. Assess the needs of the learners in the course.
    C. Determine the methods of evaluation to be used.
    D. Develop a schedule for the simulation activities.

2. In planning the simulation, the educator should give priority to including:

    A. Skills that students have requested
    B. Scenarios that are difficult and challenging
    C. Topic areas recommended by clinical faculty
    D. Activities that will help meet student learning outcomes

3. A simulation educator is developing goals for the simulation activities to be included in her course. The best example of a goal is:

    A. "Learners will demonstrate the correct technique for inserting a nasogastric tube."
    B. "Learners will demonstrate the correct technique for administering enteral medications."

C. "Simulation activities will enable learners to demonstrate their knowledge and skills with nasogastric tubes."
D. "Learners will demonstrate the correct technique for checking tube-feeding residuals."

4. In developing objectives for a simulation exercise planned for her course, the simulation educator should write objectives that are:

   A. Measurable and relevant
   B. Broadly written and long term
   C. Complex and difficult to achieve
   D. Vague and intangible

5. A simulation educator elects to use formative evaluation to evaluate student learning following simulation activities. The best example of a method of formative evaluation is to:

   A. Administer a survey at the end of the simulation.
   B. Include questions on the next exam that address the simulation objectives.
   C. Encourage learners to give return demonstrations following skill demonstrations.
   D. Include simulation skills as part of the end-of-semester evaluation tool.

6. When planning an evaluation method that will provide the learner with constructive critique for improvement and the opportunity for self-reflection, the simulation educator should select:

   A. Observation
   B. Surveys
   C. Skills checklists
   D. Debriefing

7. When using simulation to document competencies, the experienced simulation educator would choose an evaluation tool which is valid and reliable such as:

   A. Objective structured clinical exams (OSCEs)
   B. Self-reporting surveys
   C. Skills checklists
   D. Debriefing

8. What statement by the simulation educator would indicate that she has a good understanding of designing simulation activities?

   A. "I will have students arrive at 8:30 a.m., and we will see how long the simulation takes."
   B. "I will schedule small groups of learners for each simulation activity."
   C. "I will have the adjunct clinical faculty develop objectives for the day."
   D. "I will bring a large group of students in to get them all done at one time."

9. When discussing plans for a simulation day with his mentor, the new simulation educator demonstrates evidence of his knowledge of simulation modalities by stating:

   A. "Intravenous (IV) arms are a great use of high-fidelity simulation."
   B. "High-fidelity mannequins have limited use with new nursing students."

C. "A task trainer can be effective in teaching new skills."
D. "Debriefing is an effective method for evaluating skill acquisition with task trainers."

10. Which statement by the novice simulation educator would need to be corrected by the simulation coordinator?
    A. "A skill station designed for a review can be self-directed."
    B. "A basic skill station could be monitored by a senior level or graduate student."
    C. "An adjunct clinical instructor can teach a skill within their expertise."
    D. "The lab technician will serve as content expert for the high-fidelity simulation."

REFERENCES

Abelsson, A., & Bisholt, B. (2017). Nurse students learn acute care by simulation—Focus on observation and debriefing. *Nurse Education in Practice, 24,* 6–13. doi:10.1016/j.nepr.2017.03.001

Allen, L., & Molloy, E. (2017). The influence of a preceptor-student "Daily Feedback Tool" on clinical feedback practices in nursing education: A qualitative study. *Nurse Education Today, 49*), 57–62. doi:10.1016/j.nedt.2016.11.009

Bailey, C. (2017). Human patient simulation. In M. J. Bradshaw & B. L. Hultquist (Eds.), *Innovative teaching strategies in nursing and related health professions* (pp. 245–267). Burlington, MA: Jones & Bartlett Learning.

Bastable, S. B. (2014). *Nurse as educator: Principles of teaching and learning for nursing practice* (4th ed.). Burlington, MA: Jones & Bartlett Learning.

Billings, D. M., & Halstead, J. A. (2012). *Teaching in nursing: A guide for faculty* (4th ed.). St. Louis, MO: Saunders.

Chen, S. L., Huang, T. W., Liao, I. C., & Liu, C. (2015). Development and validation of the simulation learning effectiveness inventory. *Journal of Advanced Nursing, 71*(10), 2444–2453. doi:10.1016/j.nedt.2016.11.009

Jeffries, P. R., Dreifuerst, K. T., Aschenbrenner, D. S., Adamson, K. A., & Schram, A. P. (2015). Clinical simulations in nursing education: Overview, essentials, and the evidence. In M. H. Oermann (Ed.), *Teaching in nursing and role of the educator* (pp. 83–101). New York, NY: Springer Publishing.

Leighton, K. (2017). Innovations in facilitating learning using patient simulation. In M. J. Bradshaw & B. L. Hultquist (Eds.), *Innovative teaching strategies in nursing and related health professions* (pp. 269–295). Burlington, MA: Jones & Bartlett Learning.

McDermott, D. S., Sarasnick, J., & Timcheck, P. (2017). Using the INACSL Simulation™ design standard for novice learners. *Clinical Simulation in Nursing, 13*(6), 249–253. doi:10.1016/j.ecns.2017.03.003

Society for Simulation in Healthcare. (2018). *Certified Healthcare Simulation Educator Examination Blueprint, 2018 Version.* Retrieved from http://www.ssih.org/Portals/48/Certification/CHSE_Docs/CHSE_Examination_Blueprint.pdf

Zhu, X., Yang, L., Lin, P., Lu, G., Xiao, N., Yang, S., & Sui, S. (2017). Assessing nursing students' clinical competencies using a problem-focused objective structured clinical examination. *Western Journal of Nursing Research, 39*(3), 388–399. doi:10.1177/0193945916667727

17

Debriefing

LINDA WILSON, JOHN T. CORNELE, AND RUTH A. WITTMANN-PRICE

> *I think the big thing is don't be afraid to fail. It's a part of building character and growing.*
>
> —Nick Foles

This chapter addresses Domain III: Educational Principles Applied to Simulation (Society for Simulation in Healthcare, 2018).

[LEARNING OUTCOMES]

- Discuss the importance of simulation debriefing in the learning process.
- Discuss the principles of simulation debriefing.
- Describe a variety of simulation debriefing methodologies.

When using simulation as a learning tool, debriefing is an essential component of the learning process (Cantrell, 2008). Most simulation experts concur that the debriefing process of learners, which takes place after the simulation experience, is in effect the most important element of the learners' experience. Cant and Cooper (2009) describe debriefing as one of the "core components" of simulation learning. Alinier (2011) describes debriefing by stating, "Experiential learning experience must then be reinforced and analyzed with the participants through a debriefing process that is as, if not more, important than the experience itself as it helps them to reflect about what happened and understand and assimilate the learning objectives" (p. 14). The ultimate goal of the learning process that takes place during debriefing is to foster clinical decision making (Dreifuerst, 2009).

Dewey (1933, p. 9) suggests that reflection is a process and requires a process; he describes reflection as "active, persistent, and careful consideration"; furthermore, Dewey believed that reflection could be caused by "a state of doubt, hesitation, [or] perplexity" (p. 12). This active approach to reflection requires that the learner recognizes actions or events and enters a state of questioning of held beliefs and learned behaviors to identify issues and begin to problem solve.

BACKGROUND

Debriefing was originally used in the military in order for personnel to describe what happened during a mission. Debriefing accomplished two objectives for the military. First, it assisted with operational understanding and strategic planning and, second, it helped to reduce the psychological impact of a traumatic event on the participant. Reconstructing the event through narrative was therapeutic for the participant. By conducting debriefing in groups, participants received several different perspectives (Fanning & Gaba, 2007).

THE DEBRIEFING PROCESS

Learning is facilitated during the debriefing process of simulation (Dieckmann, Lippert, Glavin, & Rall, 2010). Debriefing is a process that commonly involves face-to-face discussion between a group of learners and an educator after a simulation scenario has taken place. Debriefing is often distinguished as a separate process from feedback, which can occur using different modalities (face to face, written, or electronic), and normally occurs between one learner and an educator after a simulation experience (Archer, 2010). When standardized (simulated) patients (SPs) are used in simulation experiences, they are often included in the feedback process to provide insights to the learner, but they are not usually participants in debriefing processes (Barrows, 1993).

The debriefing process is normally facilitated retrospectively with the simulation participants as soon as possible after the experience is completed (Cantrell, 2008), and it includes all the learners actively involved in the entire experience (Alinier, 2011). Timing of the debriefing process is important, and it is beneficial to provide debriefing as close to the simulation experience as possible (Cantrell, 2008).

Some simulation experts refer to the process of debriefing as *team debriefing*, which highlights the aspect that it is a group activity (Alinier, 2011). Debriefing should be facilitated by a certified educator who has observed the entire simulation learning experience and has taken physical or mental notes about the details of the experience (Alinier, 2011). Recording of the simulation experience is important to the debriefing process and can also effectively include videotaping of the experience. Videotaping may assist learners to analyze their performance and provide structure to the debriefing process. At times, depending on the complexity of a scenario, learning is facilitated by having a second certified educator observing the simulation scenario and participating in the debriefing process in order to note all the details of a simulation experience (Alinier, 2011).

Debriefing sessions are often approximately 20 to 30 minutes in length, and researchers have noted that 10-minute debriefing sessions are inadequate to facilitate the learning process (Cantrell, 2008). Therefore, as a critical component of simulation learning, adequate time must be assigned to the debriefing process.

Another type of debriefing is called *in-simulation* debriefing. This debriefing technique is done by suspending the scenario to discuss a specific incident or aspect of learning (Van Heukelom, Begaz, & Treat, 2010).

> **EVIDENCE-BASED SIMULATION PRACTICE 17.1**
>
> Matthews and Viens (1998) found that videotaping a simulation experience and having learners critically critique the experience during debriefing decreased learner anxiety.

Lederman (1984) describes the essential, structural elements of debriefing as having the following seven components.

1. Debriefer, or simulation educator
2. Participants, or learners to debrief
3. A simulation experience
4. The impact of the simulation experience
5. Recollection of the simulation experience
6. Report about the simulation experience
7. Time required for debriefing (Lederman, 1984)

DEBRIEFING AND THE LEARNING PROCESS

Using simulation experiences provides learners an opportunity to practice and acquire knowledge and clinical skills in a safe environment (McGaghie, Issenberg, Petrusa, & Scalese, 2010). Much of the knowledge acquisition is facilitated during the debriefing process because it is a teaching strategy (Cantrell, 2008).

Debriefing as a teaching strategy supports a constructivist theory of education, which is fully explained in Chapters 13 and 14. Some of the learning processes that take place during debriefing include the following:

- Promoting communication skills
- Appropriately integrating emotions into the learning process
- Reinforcing skill acquisition (Cantrell, 2008)

Debriefing is a learning process that ties in all three domains of learning:

1. Psychomotor—during debriefing, skills are analyzed
2. Affective—feelings and emotions are discussed
3. Cognitive—learning takes place by having events deconstructed (Cantrell, 2008)

Warrick, Hunsaker, Cook, and Altman (1979) defined the objectives of debriefing as

1. Identification of the different perceptions and attitudes that have occurred
2. Linking the exercise to specific theory or content and skill-building techniques
3. Development of a common set of experiences for further thought
4. Opportunity to receive feedback on the nature of one's involvement, behavior, and decision making
5. Reestablishment of the desired classroom climate, such as regaining trust, comfort, and purposefulness

DEFINING ATTRIBUTES OF DEBRIEFING

Dreifuerst (2009) describes the following defining attributes of debriefing in a concept analysis:

- Reflection
- Emotion
- Reception
- Integration
- Assimilation

Each attribute is described in the following text.

Reflection

An important aspect of the debriefing process as pointed out by Dieckmann, Gaba, and Marcus (2007) is that no one has the "correct view." Debriefing comprises perceptions of educator(s) and learners of what took place in the simulation experience. Different views assist learners with understanding different elements of the scenario, and in that way, it mimics clinical situations. Debriefing discussions should begin with asking participants about their view of the situation just experienced and initiate the reflective learning process (Dieckmann et al., 2007).

Fanning and Gaba (2007) call reflection "the cornerstone" of both experiential learning and lifelong learning. The following text lists different ways to conceptualize reflection and some important points about using reflection as a learning activity.

- In 1983, Schön published his landmark book, *The Reflective Practitioner: How Professionals Think in Action*, and called on educators to develop themselves as reflective practitioners in order to gain competence in their individual practices.
- Boud, Keogh, and Walker (1985) defined *reflection* as "an important human activity in which people recapture their experience, think about it, mull it over, and evaluate it" (p. 19).
- Reflection is a technique that encourages critical thought, either with oneself (self-dialogue) or another individual or group (dialogue) (Shor, 1992).
- Reflection is a thoughtful and self-regulating process (Kaakinen & Arwood, 2009).

Reflection can be facilitated in different ways.

- Many certified healthcare educators use the technique after an experience in a free-flow attempt to assist learners to uncover what affective behaviors they can identify as assets and to highlight those behaviors that may be deficits.

> **SIMULATION TEACHING TIP 17.1**
>
> Several issues must be considered when asking learners to reflect.
>
> - Reflection is a self-disclosing process that can elicit sensitive information.
> - What one does with information revealed during reflective sessions may become an ethical issue.

- Others pose reflective questions to learners, such as "What was the one thing (incident or patient) that affected you most?" or "What was the best thing that happened to you during the experience?"
- Usually, questions like these are followed up with questions such as, "What one thing would you do differently if you were in that situation again?"

Having learners reflect facilitates finding deeper meanings and thinking critically about experiences, especially critical incidents (Montagna, Benaglio, & Zannini, 2010).

Scanlon and Chernomas (1997) identified three stages of reflection.

1. Awareness
2. Critical analysis
3. New perspective

Riley-Doucet and Wilson (1997) describe a three-step process for reflection:

1. *Critical appraisal* is done by a learner in free form to drill down to the meaning of the experience.
2. *Peer group discussions* share questions that the learners might have become aware of during the experience.
3. *Self-awareness* or *self-evaluation* is the last step and relates the learning outcomes for evaluative purposes.

Montagna et al. (2010) also recommend that educator feedback to learners be done with care and that certain resources are available if needed.

Emotions

Debriefing provides the learner the opportunity to reexamine the experience and deal with emotions, thereby providing an emotional release as well as a thinking process (Dreifuerst, 2009).

Reception

Reception has to do with how "open" the learner is to accepting the information provided or revealed during debriefing. The simulation educator needs to establish an environment that facilitates positive reception by

- Presenting learners' strengths and challenges in a nonthreatening manner
- Maintaining learner–facilitator respect at all times
- Providing confidentiality as appropriate (Dreifuerst, 2009)

Integration

Using a conceptual framework that is familiar to the learners in their discipline and integrating the context of the simulation scenario fosters learning. Integration links knowledge gained from the simulation experience to knowledge already familiar from the learning. By facilitating integration, the simulation educator is promoting deep learning (Dreifuerst, 2009). Refer to Chapter 14 for an explanation of deep, surface, and strategic learning.

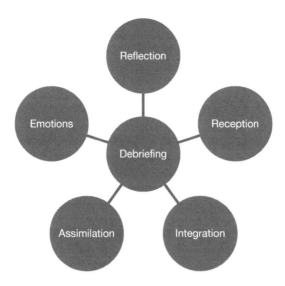

FIGURE 17.1 Attributes of learning in debriefing as defined by Dreifurest (2009).

Assimilation

Assimilation has to do with the ultimate goal of simulation, which is the transfer of knowledge from the experience to actual clinical practice. Further assimilation studies are needed, but assimilation may be encouraged by techniques used by the facilitator, such as the Socratic dialogue. Dreifurest (2009) reminds simulation educators that all attributes defined as elements of debriefing work together to promote learning as shown in Figure 17.1.

ORAL (SOCRATIC) QUESTIONING

Oral questioning, or Socratic dialogue, can promote the learners' critical thinking and prompt them to reflect. Questions that involve synthesizing concepts rather than questions that can be answered with a "yes" or "no" or regurgitating facts are the most beneficial (Exhibit 17.1). Promoting thinking through questioning can be accomplished by using "what-if" questions and changing the situation to encourage learners to think beyond the experience (Dreifuerst, 2009).

EXHIBIT 17.1

Benefits of Questioning

- Increases motivation and participation.
- Helps monitor the learners' acquisition of knowledge and understanding.
- Promotes higher cognition.
- Assesses learners' progress.
- Facilitates environmental management.
- Encourages learners to ask and to answer questions.
- Promotes dialogue/interaction/debate between and among educators and learners (Ralph, 2000).

DEBRIEFING AS AN ASSESSMENT PROCESS

Debriefing, which usually involves a group of learners, is most often used as a formative evaluative mechanism. Summative evaluations of learner performance are most commonly done on an individual basis using feedback (McGaghie et al., 2010). A method of using debriefing as an evaluation has been outlined by Rudolph, Simon, Raemer, and Eppich (2008); it is a four-step process, which is shown diagrammatically in Figure 17.2.

FACILITATOR ROLE IN THE DEBRIEFING PROCESS

Fanning and Gaba (2007) describe facilitator involvement in debriefing as high to low. Table 17.1 demonstrates the differences in involvement.

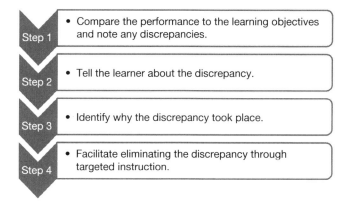

FIGURE 17.2 Four-step evaluation process of Rudolph, Simon, Raemer, and Eppich.

Source: Adapted from Rudolph, J. W., Simon, R., Raemer, D. B., & Eppich, W. J. (2008). Debriefing as formative assessment: Closing performance gaps in medical education. *Academic Emergency Medicine, 15*, 1010–1016.

TABLE 17.1

Involvement of Facilitator in Debriefing

High-level facilitation	The facilitator outlines the debriefing process. Facilitator guides the discussion when necessary. Facilitator has low-level involvement. Learners are highly involved.
Low-level facilitation	Facilitation takes on an involved role. Learners are less involved and have less initiative. Facilitators use a direct debriefing process. Simulation educator may overinstruct.

Source: Fanning, R. M., & Gaba, D. M. (2007). The role of debriefing in simulation-based learning. *Simulation in Healthcare, 2*(2), 115–125. doi:10.1097/SIH.0b013e3180315539

TYPES OF DEBRIEFING METHODS

Structured Debriefing

Debriefing sessions often begin with establishing group rules in order to focus the learners on the meaning of the scenario rather than have them focus on the fidelity of the scenario (Dieckmann et al., 2007). Cantrell (2008) used a structured debriefing process in her study with nursing learners and used guiding questions that were developed by Ham and O'Rouke (2004):

- What were the patient's goals for this episode of care?
- Were these goals met by your nursing behaviors?
- How did you prioritize the patient's needs?
- What would you do differently if actually caring for him or her and the family in an acute care setting?

Structured debriefing provides guidance in the learning process, facilitates the collection of data, and provides insight into the learners' thinking processes.

> **EVIDENCE-BASED SIMULATION PRACTICE 17.2**
>
> Birch et al. (2007) used debriefing in the simulation education of learners using a scenario about postpartum hemorrhage. The study found that those learners who participated in the simulation experience and were debriefed had increased knowledge immediately after the scenario and at 3 months after the scenario.

Case Study Analysis Debriefing

One of the most common methods of debriefing is review of a case study. One method to accomplish this has been outlined in 12 steps by Salas et al. (2008) and includes the following:

1. Use debriefing to diagnose the case.
2. Provide a supportive environment.
3. Always note teamwork, which is critical to patient safety.
4. Team leaders should be educated in debriefing.
5. Members should not be threatened during a debriefing session.
6. Focus on critical incidents during the scenario.
7. Describe the interactions of the team.
8. Use objective data when possible.
9. Provide process feedback before outcome feedback.
10. Provide both individual and team feedback appropriately.
11. Provide feedback as soon as possible.
12. Record outcomes of the debriefing to use in the future.

Debriefing With Good Judgment

A nonjudgmental approach to debriefing uses the simulation educator as a patient advocate by asking questions using "I" and referring to the patient (advocacy). The simulation educator then requests the learner to describe the thought process used, and this is the inquiry process (Rudolph, Simon, Rivard, Dufresne, & Raemer, 2007). There are three phases in this method of debriefing: (a) reactions phase, (b) understanding phase, and the (c) summary phase (Rudolph et al., 2007). An example is provided in Exhibit 17.2.

Debriefing for Meaningful Learning

This method for debriefing focuses on the following: (a) foster student reflective thinking and learning; (b) socratic questioning; (c) principles of active learning; and (d) E5 Model: Engage, Explore, Explain, Evaluate, Extend (or Elaborate) (Dreifuerst, 2015).

Promoting Excellence and Reflective Learning in Simulation

Promoting Excellence and Reflective Learning in Simulation (PEARLS) is a blended approach to debriefing that includes: (a) learner self-assessment, (b) facilitating focused discussion, and (c) providing information via directive feedback and/or teaching. This method of debriefing has four phases: (a) reactions phase, (b) description phase, (c) analysis phase, and the (d) summary phase (Eppich & Cheng, 2015).

3-D Model of Debriefing

This method of debriefing begins with a prebrief. Then the debriefing focuses on the aspects of defusing, discovering, and deepening where the learners will: (a) reflect on the experience, (b) identify mental models that led to specific behavior or cognitive process, and (c) build or enhance new mental models. The debriefing will end with a summary (Zigmont, Kappus, & Sudikoff, 2011).

EXHIBIT 17.2

An Example of an Advocacy–Inquiry Question

Dirty Question (A question that—when asked—puts the learner on the defense): Why did you not verify the patient identification (ID) prior to giving that med?

A-I Question: I noticed that you did not check the patient ID prior to giving the medication. That concerns me because verifying the correct patient is an important part of medication administration. Can you tell me what you were thinking at that time?

By using the advocacy–inquiry technique for questions there is no "guess what I am thinking." We need to understand the thinking behind actions in order to change them.

Source: Adapted from Rudolph, J. W., Simon, R., Rivard, P., Dufresne, R. L., & Raemer, D. B. (2007). Debriefing with good judgment: Combining rigorous feedback with genuine inquiry. *Anesthesiology Clinics, 25,* 361–376. doi:10.1016/j.anclin.2007.03.007

Plus-Delta Debriefing

This method of debriefing focuses on what was accomplished or done well. To facilitate this debriefing the simulation educator will use a two-column tool to have the group identify: (a) what went well, and (b) what can be changed next time (Gardner, 2013). This method of debriefing fosters a method of continuous improvement (Gardner, 2013).

How Do You Choose the Best Method of Debriefing for You?

To decide which method of debriefing is best for you, review all of the debriefing methods and compare them to your educational philosophy. You can also test various debriefing methods over time and evaluate them. Or possibly, your institution has selected a debriefing method that everyone is supposed to use so debriefing is done in a consistent manner.

There are many techniques used during the debriefing process. Table 17.2 describes some of these techniques.

THE DEBRIEFING ENVIRONMENT

The environment in which debriefing is conducted is also important. Besides having an appropriate amount of time set aside for debriefing, there should to be enough room for the members being debriefed. Rooms for debriefing should

TABLE 17.2

Debriefing Techniques

TECHNIQUE	DESCRIPTION OF THE TECHNIQUE
Funneling	Learners are guided during debriefing, but the debriefer does not comment (Fanning & Gaba, 2007).
Framing	A technique used during debriefing to present the simulation experience to the participants in a relevant way (Fanning & Gaba, 2007).
Frontloading	Providing specific questions before the debriefing to guide the direction of the debriefing (Fanning & Gaba, 2007).
Good cop–bad cop	Technique used if there is more than one debriefer. This technique provides opposing sides to an issue (Fanning & Gaba, 2007).
Case review	An organized review of the patient condition starting with diagnosis and then a review of systems.

Source: Adapted from Fanning, R. M., & Gaba, D. M. (2007). The role of debriefing in simulation-based learning. *Simulation in Healthcare, 2*(2), 115–125. doi:10.1097/SIH.0b013e3180315539

be large, private, and comfortable. Large groups of learners pose special challenges to debriefing, and two methods used to overcome group learning that may exclude individuals are the following:

1. Separate groups. Have more than one debriefer and separate the large group into smaller groups.
2. Use the fishbowl method. Have an inner circle of learners and an outer circle. Debrief the learners in the inner circle and then have learners switch to the outer circle and outer-circle learners move in for debriefing (Fanning & Gaba, 2007).

An additional consideration for establishing an environment that feels safe for debriefing includes a space away from where the simulation was conducted, a comfortable and private area (Decker, 2007).

> **SIMULATION TEACHING TIP 17.2**
>
> Dieckmann et al. (2007) discuss the importance of simulation educators paying attention to the semantical sense that learners develop during the analysis of a scenario during debriefing. The use of words and language in descriptions of the scenario can provide insight into how learners phenomenally experienced the scenario.

> **SIMULATION TEACHING TIP 17.3**
>
> Steinwachs (1992) describes using a process of seating that avoids "energy gaps." In order to facilitate this concept, learners must sit next to each other, and there should be no empty spaces. Decker (2007) suggests a circular design for seating that allows spherical movement while questioning the learners as discussion is promoted.

■ DEBRIEFING DIFFICULTIES

Debriefing sessions are goal oriented, but at times difficulties can occur when learners interpret debriefings differently than what was intended in the learning outcomes. In this case, extra time is often needed to explain what was supposed to occur as opposed to what did occur. Many simulation educators then reenact the scenario to accomplish the intended learning outcomes (Dieckmann et al., 2010).

■ PRACTICE QUESTIONS

1. The novice simulation educator who is going to facilitate a debriefing needs further understanding when she:
   A. Observes the entire simulation
   B. Takes notes on observations during the simulation
   C. Has an experienced debriefer with her
   D. Starts debriefing students one at a time

2. A simulation educator is very new to the debriefing process. Which method of debriefing might be easier for the educator to start with?
   A. Debriefing with Good Judgment
   B. Case Study Debriefing
   C. Debriefing for Meaningful Learning
   D. Advocacy Inquiry

3. Ideally, the length of the debriefing time should be:

   A. 5 minutes
   B. Half the time needed to complete the simulation
   C. Equal to the time needed to complete the simulation
   D. Double the time needed to complete the simulation

4. The debriefing method in which the simulation educator facilitates the identification of what went well compared to what can be changed next time is called:

   A. Debriefing with Good Judgment
   B. Case Study Debriefing
   C. Debriefing for Meaningful Learning
   D. Plus Delta

5. The debriefing method in which the simulation educator focuses on defusing, discovering, and deepening is called:

   A. Plus Delta
   B. Debriefing with Good Judgment
   C. 3-D Model of Debriefing
   D. Debriefing for Meaningful Learning

6. The simulation educator wants to learn how to be an effective debriefer. The best method to use to learn debriefing is to:

   A. Read a book about debriefing.
   B. Practice with an experienced debriefer.
   C. Watch a video of a debriefing session.
   D. Attend a lecture on debriefing.

7. How does a simulation educator select the best debriefing method to use?

   A. Review all available methods of debriefing
   B. Compare each debriefing method with your personal educational philosophy
   C. Test out each type of debriefing method
   D. All of the above

8. Which debriefing method includes a technique called *Advocacy Inquiry*?

   A. Plus Delta
   B. Debriefing with Good Judgment
   C. 3-D Model of Debriefing
   D. Debriefing for Meaningful Learning

9. The debriefing environment should be:

   A. Comfortable with seats for everyone
   B. A location away from where the simulation took place
   C. A safe environment
   D. All of the above

10. The simulation educator's role in the debriefing process is that of:
    A. Educator
    B. Researcher
    C. Evaluator
    D. Facilitator

■ REFERENCES

Alinier, G. (2011). Developing high-fidelity health care simulation scenarios: A guide for educators and professionals. *Simulation and Gaming*, 42(1), 9–26. doi:10.1177/1046878109355683

Archer, J. C. (2010). State of the science in health professional education: Effective feedback. *Medical Education*, 44, 101–108. doi:10.1111/j.1365-2923.2009.03546.x

Barrows, H. S. (1993). An overview of the uses of standardized (simulated) patients for teaching and evaluating clinical skills. *Academic Medicine*, 68(6), 443–451. doi:10.1097/00001888-199306000-00002

Birch, L., Jones, N., Doyle, P. M., Green, P., McLaughlin, A., Champney C., ... Taylor, K. (2007). Obstetric skills drills: Evaluation of teaching methods. *Nurse Education Today*, 27(8), 915–922. doi:10.1016/j.nedt.2007.01.006

Boud, D., Keogh, R., & Walker, D. (Eds.). (1985). *Reflection: Turning experience into learning* (pp. 7–8). London, UK: Kogan.

Cant, R. P., & Cooper, S. J. (2009). Simulation-based learning in nursing education: Systematic review. *Journal of Advanced Nursing*, 66(1), 3–15. doi:10.1111/j.1365-2648.2009.05240.x

Cantrell, M. A. (2008). The importance of debriefing in clinical simulation. *Clinical Simulation in Nursing*, 4, e19–e23. doi:10.1016/j.ecns.2008.06.006

Decker, S. (2007). Integrating guided reflection into simulated learning experiences. In P. R. Jeffries (Ed.), *Simulation in nursing education: From conceptualization to evaluation* (pp. 73–85). New York, NY: National League for Nursing.

Dewey, J. (1933). *How we think: A restatement of the relation of reflective thinking to the educative process*. Lexington, KY: D. C. Health.

Dieckmann, P., Gaba, D., & Marcus, R. (2007). Deepening the theoretical foundations of patient simulation as social practice. *Simulation in Healthcare*, 2(3), 183–193. doi:10.1097/sih.0b013e3180f637f5

Dieckmann, P., Lippert, A., Glavin, R., & Rall, M. (2010). When things do not go as expected: Scenario life savers. *Simulation in Healthcare*, 5, 219–225. doi:10.1097/sih.0b013e3181e77f74

Dreifuerst, K. T. (2009). The essentials of debriefing in simulated learning: A concept analysis. *Nursing Education Perspectives*, 30(2), 109–114.

Dreifuerst, K. T. (2015). Getting started with debriefing for meaningful learning. *Clinical Simulation in Nursing*, 11(5), 268–275. doi:10.1016/j.ecns.2015.01.005

Eppich, W., & Cheng, A. (2015). Promoting excellence and reflective learning in simulation (PEARLS). *Simulation in Healthcare*, 10(2), 106–115. doi:10.1097/sih.0000000000000072

Fanning, R. M., & Gaba, D. M. (2007). The role of debriefing in simulation-based learning. *Simulation in Healthcare*, 2(2), 115–125. doi:10.1097/sih.0b013e3180315539

Gardner, R. (2013). Introduction to debriefing. *Seminars in Perinatology*, 37(3), 166–174. doi:10.1053/j.semperi.2013.02.008

Ham, K., & O'Rourke, E. (2004). Clinical strategies. Clinical preparation for beginning nursing students: An experiential learning activity. *Nurse Educator*, 29(4), 139–141.

Kaakinen, J., & Arwood, E. (2009). Systematic review of nursing simulation literature for use of learning theory. *International Journal of Nursing Education Scholarship*, 6(1), 1–20. doi:10.2202/1548-923X.1688

Lederman, L. (1984). Debriefing: A critical reexamination of the post experience analytic process with implications for its effective use. *Simulation Games*, 15, 415–431. doi:10.1177/0037550084154002

Matthews, R., & Viens, D. C. (1988). Evaluating basic nursing skills through group video testing. *Journal of Nursing Education, 27*(1), 44–46.

McGaghie, W. C., Issenberg, S. B., Petrusa, E. R., & Scalese, R. J. (2010). A critical review of simulation-based medical education research: 2003–2009. *Medical Education, 44,* 50–63. doi:10.1111/j.1365-2923.2009.03547.x

Montagna, L., Benaglio, C., & Zannini, L. (2010). Reflective writing in nursing education: Background, experiences and methods. *Assistenza Infermieristica e Ricerca, 29*(3), 140–152.

Ralph, E. (2000). Oral-questioning skills of novice teachers: Any questions? *Journal of Instructional Psychology, 26*(4), 286–296.

Riley-Doucet, C., & Wilson, S. (1997). A three-step method of self-reflection using reflective journal writing. *Journal of Advanced Nursing, 25,* 964–968. doi:10.1046/j.1365-2648.1997.1997025964.x

Rudolph, J. W., Simon, R., Raemer, D. B., & Eppich, W. J. (2008). Debriefing as formative assessment: Closing performance gaps in medical education. *Academic Emergency Medicine, 15,* 1010–1016. doi:10.1111/j.1553-2712.2008.00248.x

Rudolph, J. W., Simon, R., Rivard, P., Dufresne, R. L., & Raemer, D. B. (2007). Debriefing with good judgment: Combining rigorous feedback with genuine inquiry. *Anesthesiology Clinics, 25,* 361–376. doi:10.1016/j.anclin.2007.03.007

Salas, E., Klein, C., King, H., Salisbury, M., Augenstein, J. S., Birnbach, D. J., ... Upshaw, C. (2008). Debriefing medical teams: 12 evidence-based best practices and tips. *Joint Commission Journal on Quality and Patient Safety, 34,* 518–527. doi:10.1016/s1553-7250(08)34066-5

Scanlon, J. M., & Chernomas, W. M. (1997). Developing the reflective teacher. *Journal of Advanced Nursing, 25*(6), 1138–1143. doi:10.1046/j.1365-2648.1997.19970251138.x

Schön, D. A. (1983). *The reflective practitioner: How professionals think in action.* New York, NY: Basic Books.

Shor, I. (1992). *Empowering education: Critical teaching for social change.* Chicago, IL: University of Chicago Press.

Society for Simulation in Healthcare. (2018). *Certified Healthcare Simulation Educator Examination Blueprint, 2018 Version.* Retrieved from http://www.ssih.org/Portals/48/Certification/CHSE_Docs/CHSE_Examination_Blueprint.pdf

Steinwachs, B. (1992). How to facilitate a debrief. *Simulation Gaming, 23,* 186–195. doi:10.1177/1046878192232006

Van Heukelom, J. N., Begaz, T., & Treat, R. (2010). Comparison of postsimulation debriefing versus in-simulation debriefing in medical simulation. *Simulation in Healthcare, 5,* 91–97. doi:10.1097/sih.0b013e3181be0d17

Warrick, D. D., Hunsaker, P. L., Cook, C. W., & Altman, S. (1979). Debriefing experiential learning exercises. *Journal of Experiential Learning and Simulation, 1,* 91–96.

Zigmont, J. J., Kappus, L. J., & Sudikoff, S. N. (2011). The 3D model of debriefing: Defusing, discovering, and deepening. *Seminars in Perinatology, 35*(2), 52–58. doi:10.1053/j.semperi.2011.01.003

18

Standardized Patient Debriefing and Feedback

ANTHONY ERRICHETTI

Thinking is easy, acting is difficult, and to put one's thoughts into action is the most difficult thing in the world.
—Johann Wolfgang von Goethe

This chapter addresses Domain III: Educational Principles Applied to Simulation (Society for Simulation in Healthcare, 2018).

[LEARNING OUTCOMES]

- Discuss debriefing as a self-reflective learning process.
- Describe how debriefing and feedback are necessary components in the patient simulation learning process, requiring learners to reflect on their work.
- Compare the different roles the clinical educators and standardized patients (SPs) have in the debriefing process.
- Discuss SP selection and training for the debriefing–feedback process.

SPs have been used for more than 50 years to teach and assess clinical skills (Barrows, 1993). Originally used to facilitate medical learner training through simulated patient encounters, SPs are now used in high-stakes licensure examinations (Dillon, Boulet, Hawkins, & Swanson, 2004). Their full potential, however, is realized when used in formative assessment exercises where skills assessment and debriefing are part of an educational plan. Selection of appropriate SPs and preparation for the debriefing and feedback process are required. This chapter presents an overview of how SPs can be selected and prepared for debriefing with suggestions for basic to advanced debriefing approaches.

DEBRIEFING FOUNDATIONS

Debriefing, as we know it today, has roots in the military and in adult and experiential learning theories and practices. The military "after-action review" (AAR) is a professional discussion of an event that enables soldiers and units to discover for themselves what happened and develop a strategy for improvement (Bartone & Adler, 1995).

"An AAR is not a critique. No one, regardless of rank, position, or strength of personality, has all of the information or answers. After-action reviews maximize training benefits by allowing soldiers, regardless of rank, to learn from each other" (Department of the Army, 1993, p. 1).

Simulation learning is experiential learning, that is, learning through direct experience (Itin, 1999). American educator John Dewey noted, however, that experience alone does not guarantee learning, but that learning occurs when experience is reflected on or "reconstructed" (Dewey, 1933). Experiential learning therefore requires the learners to reflect on their actions (Kolb, 1984) and, in the context of simulation learning, actions taken during SP and other simulation exercises. It integrates personal experience with academic learning, structures opportunities for reflection, is inquiry based, and facilitates face-to-face communication (Hatcher, 1997).

Debriefing is a process that facilitates learner self-reflection. It is a "rigorous reflection process" (p. 361) that focuses on clinical (e.g., critical thinking and actions) and behavioral (e.g., interpersonal communication) issues raised by a simulation exercise (Rudolph, Simon, Rivard, Dufresne, & Raemer, 2007). Feedback, a tool of debriefing, is information given to the learners about their performance intended to be used to promote positive and desirable development (Archer, 2010). For feedback to be effective, the debriefer must be aware of the needs of the learner and be able to judge whether the learner is ready to accept it.

Adult learners, the focus of simulation education, have life experience, opinions, emotions, and assumptions ("frames"); well-developed personalities; and relationship patterns that drive their behaviors (Rudolph et al., 2007). They expect learning to be goal directed, relevant, and applicable. Simulation learning, the antithesis of teacher-led classroom learning, is learning through experience and interaction with experts who understand adult learners' mind-set. Vygotsky's (1978) "zone of proximal development" (p. 86) describes the stage at which we find many adult learners who are, for example, students of healthcare science, that is, between unsupervised and supervised practice. This transition occurs with expert guidance (Vygotsky, 1978), the type of guidance that could come from a debriefing encounter.

SPs CORE COMPETENCIES

SPs are professionals trained to accurately simulate medical problems and conditions, document and assess skills, and provide feedback (Boulet & Errichetti, 2008). They must continually demonstrate a number of "core competencies" to remain effective. The following is a list of those competencies, from the basic/foundational to the advanced, all of which are directly or indirectly related to mastering the debriefing process (Exhibit 18.1).

Foundational Competencies

Professional Conduct

SPs are required to demonstrate professional behaviors that guide their actions. These include the following:

- **Reliability**: Being on time and carrying out scheduled activities as planned
- **Emotional intelligence**: The ability to be aware of and monitor one's own emotions as well as others' (Mayer & Salovey, 1997)
- **Social intelligence**: The awareness of how one interacts in social situations (Goleman, 2006; Thorndike, 1920)
- **Lifelong learning**: The willingness and ability to learn new things (e.g., medical problems and conditions) in new ways (e.g., through experiential and web-based learning)

Acting/Simulating

SPs have the ability to learn patient roles and credibly simulate or imitate a patient's condition, including physical symptoms, believably enough to convince learners that they are in an authentic clinical encounter. It requires SPs to play a role while simultaneously observing the learner for postencounter assessment and debriefing. Overidentifying with a role (e.g., when portraying an illness one actually has) or getting too deeply into it (e.g., through "method acting") undermines the learner assessment and debriefing. SPs must come out of the character immediately and prepare for postencounter activities.

Professionalism and credible acting may be all that are needed for clinical simulations that do not require the following advanced competencies.

Advanced Competencies

Documentation

When history taking and physical examination skills are used, SPs must be able to memorize the checklist items, observe the learner during the encounter, and then document on the checklists what the learner accomplished.

Communication Assessment

SPs are in the best position to assess the interaction and communication skills of the learner. They are in close proximity to the leaner in the exam room during the encounter and are observing such skills as rapport building, empathic responses, nonverbal communication, eliciting information, active listening, information exchange, and physical examination quality.

Debriefing and Feedback

These are arguably the most difficult skills for SPs to master, requiring SPs to come out of their characters immediately, assess the learner, and quickly formulate a debriefing agenda. SPs, using their social and emotional intelligence, engage the learner for a short, productive review of the encounter. They must be prepared

> **EXHIBIT 18.1**
>
> **Standardized Patient Core Competencies**
>
> FOUNDATIONAL SKILLS
> Professional conduct
> Acting/simulating
>
> ADVANCED SKILLS
> Documenting skills (checklists)
> Assessing communication
> Debriefing–feedback

to work with learners whose responses to the SP exercise can range from apathy to engagement. And most important, SPs must create a climate of psychological safety in which learners disclose and discuss needed areas of improvement (Schön, 1983). Indeed, empathy and compassion for the learner are key debriefing requirements.

■ SELECTING SPs FOR DEBRIEFING—SCREENING PROCESS

Not every SP is appropriate for debriefing and feedback activities. These are tasks requiring maturity, psychological awareness, discernment, and the ability to communicate with and coach learners. Before SPs can be used for this purpose, they must be rigorously screened to determine whether they have the potential to demonstrate the communication assessment and debriefing core competencies. They must be literate, have the ability and willingness to learn, and demonstrate the goodwill toward learners that is critically important to debriefing (Adamo, 2003). A robust screening process will determine whether SP candidates can be trained to engage learners in debriefing. The following are suggested steps to SP selection.

Prescreening SP Candidates

The following suggested activities can evaluate SP capabilities:

- Candidates should submit a curriculum vitae (CV) to evaluate their experience and assess their writing skills.
- Candidates complete an electronic application to determine a candidate's comfort level with technology.
- Provide candidates with an "SP Program Information Sheet," listing job skills, activities, and requirements to review before the first interview.
- A phone or video (e.g., Skype) interview with the SP recruiter to evaluate the motivation, for example, the candidate's attitude toward the medical healthcare field, why she or he wants to do this work, and whether he or she has read and

comprehended the SP Program Information Sheet. The candidate's work history, understanding of SP work, and comfort level with educational technology can also be assessed during this online interview.

> **EVIDENCE-BASED SIMULATION PRACTICE 18.1**
>
> Keiser and Turkelson (2017) studied the development and implementation of SPs using healthcare students and community members in simulation-based learning experiences (SBLEs) and found the total cost for training SPs was $1,500. The outcomes of the program yielded SPs providing 730 hours of SP service in 20 different low-stakes SBLEs for 862 student encounters. A survey of the SPs demonstrated that participants were satisfied and felt confident performing as an SP.

SP Information Meeting

If candidates are appropriate, they are invited to an unpaid "information meeting," an extended group interview and exercise that provides a didactic and experiential overview of the work. The goal of the meeting is to get an impression of the candidates' abilities to demonstrate and master the SP core competencies.

Group Interview and Introduction

- Candidates introduce themselves.
- Group question: "What draws you to this work?"
- SP trainer provides an overview of SP work through, for example, presenting SP–learner encounter videos.
- Candidates are asked to give their opinion about the quality of the work demonstrated by the learners on the videos.
- "Veteran" SPs discuss their experience.

This process allows candidates to present themselves as they might be when functioning as SPs and reveals their potential to provide debriefing. For example, some candidates will demonstrate respect and consideration for other candidates, will listen and respond appropriately, and ask questions. The process may also reveal candidates who lack emotional and social intelligence, for example, by "grandstanding" or making themselves the center of attention. Or candidates may appear to be overly reticent to speak, ask questions, or render an opinion. By reviewing and discussing videos, one can access whether candidates view learners' behaviors in a positive light. A "red flag" would be raised if candidates are overly judgmental in their opinion of a learner (Exhibit 18.2).

Experiential SP Exercise

Candidates learn a short sample SP case in order to assess reading ability and memory. They are then asked to voluntarily play the case as an SP several times and provide feedback to a simulated "learner" played by an SP. Feedback given

> **EXHIBIT 18.2**
>
> **Standardized Patient Selection Process: Steps**
>
> 1. Prescreening
>   - Submit CV and application
>   - Phone/video interview
> 2. SP information meeting
>   - Group interview
>   - SP exercise
>   - Candidate debriefing

CV, curriculum vitae; SP, standardized patient.

could include how the learner communicated and interacted with the SP. This exercise provides candidates the opportunity to "try out" different components of SP work and for the trainer to determine candidate capabilities.

SP Candidate Debriefing

Following this exercise, the candidates are debriefed about the SP information meeting. "What was the meeting like for you?" "What did you learn about SP work? "What did you learn about yourselves?" "Any suggestions about how to improve this process?" It is important that the SP trainer conducting the meeting understands and demonstrates an empathic debriefing approach as a prelude to preparing new SPs for debriefing training, that is, they try to understand how SPs think about the experience, and whether they are able to provide the trainer with useful feedback.

PREPARING SPs FOR DEBRIEFING AND FEEDBACK

After it has been determined whether SPs have the potential ability to provide debriefing and feedback, they are trained for the process. Although there is considerable variability among SP programs regarding how debriefing and feedback are conducted, the following learning points are general guidelines for all programs.

Debriefing Concepts for SPs

- *Understand the difference between debriefing and feedback.* If debriefing is a process used to reflect on work, feedback is a tool of debriefing that clearly articulates "positive feedback" (what was done well) and "constructive feedback" (what could be improved upon with continued practice).
- *Coaching follows debriefing.* The debriefer engages the learner to assist the learner to reflect of his or her work.
- *Debriefing is conducted in an empathic but straightforward way* that models the ideal healthcare encounter SPs expect from learners. It creates a climate of "psychological safety" in which learners can disclose without shame or humiliation.

- *Feedback and inquiry are linked.* The debriefer seeks to understand the learner through *empathic inquiry* (Rudolph et al., 2007).
- *SP debriefing is focused on interpersonal and communication skills.* Because debriefing potentially has a medical/healthcare component (e.g., reviewing how a differential diagnosis was determined, critical thinking and problem solving, and patient management) and an interpersonal and communication component, experienced clinician would address the healthcare issues and the SP would address the interpersonal and communication element.
- *Understand the goals and objectives of the exercise.* SPs are briefed on what the learners are expected to accomplish during a given exercise.
- *Understand the learner's level of training and expertise.* SPs are instructed, for example, to not expect expertise in novice learners and to avoid comparing student learners to the ideal healthcare provider.

Small-Group Debriefing and Feedback Exercises

Moving from concepts to practice, the following small-group training methods help SPs understand how they will follow a debriefing plan:

- *Review and discuss* the debriefing–feedback model used.
- *View videos depicting "gold standard" debriefing examples.* These can come from actual encounters or simulated encounters that illustrate appropriate debriefing and feedback approaches.
- *View SP–learner encounter videos and rate communication* as a group, compare ratings, and discuss: "What positive and constructive feedback would you give this learner?"
- *Role-play and discuss.* SPs greatly benefit from small-group practice and receiving immediate feedback. Role-play option: Pair SPs, one playing the learner, the other playing the SP who will give feedback. The SP as learner can be coached to portray a common learner issue, for example, a nervous learner who has difficulty making eye contact.
- *Use side coaching*: The trainer sits close to the SP and quietly gives instructions or redirects actions during role-play training.
- *Use earbud coaching*: A variation of side coaching, the SP in training wears an earbud during debriefing and receives instructions or redirections from the trainer.

> **SIMULATION TEACHING TIP 18.1**
>
> Watch a prerecorded actual learner–SP encounter, make notes on learner communication issues to be addressed, and then have one SP portray the learner and the other assume the role of the SP who gives feedback.

DEBRIEFING AND FEEDBACK MODELS

Models of debriefing range from the basic (giving positive and constructive feedback) to the reflective/exploratory (encouraging learner self-reflection and exploring learner "frames of reference"). All models require giving specific feedback on observable behavior. Also, the SP debriefer must prepare by reviewing learner communication ratings and/or exercise objectives and identify areas to review.

The following are several examples of feedback and debriefing for SP encounters.

Basic Feedback Approach

The *feedback sandwich* (Chowdhury & Kalu, 2004) softens constructive feedback by *sandwiching* it between two examples of positive performance (Exhibit 18.3).

- Advantages: Easy to teach to SPs and satisfactory to learners who want specific feedback: "Tell me what I did well, and what I could have done better."
- Disadvantages: Prescriptive, formulaic; reinforces passivity on the part of the learner; more a report than a reflection on work done.

Pendleton's Rules

Pendleton's Rules (Exhibit 18.4) structures feedback so that positive feedback is highlighted first, followed by a discussion of "what could have been done differently" (Pendleton, Schofield, Tate, & Havelock, 1984, p. 247).

EXHIBIT 18.3

Feedback Sandwich

Positive feedback: "This is what I thought you did well."
Constructive feedback: "When you did x, I would have preferred y."
Positive feedback: "This is another example of what I thought you did well."

EXHIBIT 18.4

Pendleton's Rules—Steps

Learners
Self-assess performance
List two things done well and two things the learner could improve on with more practice.

SPs
Assess learner
List two things done well and two things the learner could improve on with more practice.

SP and Learner
Compare notes, discussing areas of agreement and disagreement, and actions that could improve performance.

SP, standardized patient.

- Advantages: Learners actively prepare themselves for debriefing by identifying strengths and areas to improve. SPs can address and focus on areas to improve identified by the learner.
- Disadvantages: By rigidly focusing on the positives first, valuable debriefing time may be lost that could have been spent discussing more relevant issues.

Reflective Debriefing Model

Based on the work of Rudolph, Simon, Rivard, Dufresne, and Raemer (2006, 2007), this approach promotes reflection on the work between learner and SP in which the SP encourages self-reflection, provides concrete and specific feedback, and most important attempts to understand the learners' "frame of reference" or assumptions about why she or he did what she or he did (Exhibit 18.5). In this approach, the SP debriefer raises issues of concern (e.g., why the learner did not demonstrate empathy during a "giving bad news" exercise), but tries to understand the learner's point of view. The SP models empathy and the desire to understand the other, a fundamental stance of patient-centered treatment. This, like other feedback and debriefing models, requires the debriefing facilitator to create a climate of psychological safety in which the learner will feel comfortable discussing and critiquing his or her work. The SP is a learner in this process as well because the learner's frame of reference is inferred and not always evident through his or her actions. Therefore, the learners' rationale for his or her actions may either be accepted

---

EXHIBIT 18.5

Standardized Patient Reflective Debriefing Steps

Standardized Patient

- Encourage learner self-reflection by first taking the *emotional pulse* of the learner.
- "How are you? How did you feel during the encounter?" (Focus on the learner's affect)
- Encourage the learner to self-reflect on *positive actions.*
  - "What do you think went well?"
- Encourage the learner to self-reflect on *future actions.*
  - "With enough practice, what do you think could be improved?"
- When done well, the learner's concerns and questions are the primary focus of attention.

When Feedback Is Given

- Positive, specific feedback is given when appropriate.
- Constructive feedback (areas of questions or concerns) is given, but the learner's frame of reference is explored
- "Here is some feedback… help me to understand why you did x."
- Empathically explore the learner's thinking and be prepared to change your mind about your own assumptions or make rational challenges.

("Now I understand, that makes sense") or challenged ("Now I understand what you were doing, but let's explore another option").

- Advantages: Promotes mutual understanding of the learner's frame of reference, models empathy, and promotes true experiential learning.
- Disadvantages: Requires a high level of training, maturity, and psychological sophistication on the part of the SP learner.

Debriefing the Physical Examination

If the physical examination was technically correct but of poor quality, or if done with thoroughness and care but technically incorrect, SPs are encouraged to have the learners retry the exam in question and correct the technique.

STARTING DEBRIEFING

The following are suggested openings appropriate for all types of debriefing and feedback.

Set the Stage

- Debriefing dress: Wear a robe, gym pants, and so on, over the exam gown if wearing one.
- Welcome the learner: Open the door, invite the learner in, and make the individual feel comfortable: "Please come in and have a seat."

Set the Collaborative Agenda

"We have x minutes to discuss your work. We're going to focus on your communication and our patient–clinician relationship. I will not be reviewing your clinical reasoning, the questions you asked, and so forth. This is a dialogue so please ask me any questions. How does this sound?"

ADDITIONAL APPROACHES TO ENSURE DEBRIEFING QUALITY

- To ensure debriefing and feedback quality, SP encounters should be video recorded and those videos reviewed on a regular basis. A debriefing quality-assurance checklist can be used to note SP behaviors. Such a checklist would note, for example, whether the SP began the debriefing appropriately, maintained a positive attitude toward the learner, modeled empathy by attempting to understand the learners' frame of reference, and ended the debriefing encounter on a respectful note.
- Prepare learners for debriefing. If learners are to get the most from the debriefing–feedback process, they can be instructed on how the process works, what they should expect from the SP, how they can participate in the process, and how they should prepare themselves for the debriefing.

SUMMARY

Debriefing and feedback are sophisticated skills, arguably among the most difficult to master. SPs must be screened for appropriateness. Although there are no formal screening exams to determine skill and psychological readiness, the experienced SP trainer can determine, through experiential exercises and communication assessment training, the most appropriate candidates. SPs must have a high degree of emotional and social intelligence, and have the ability to distinguish between low- and high-quality performances appropriate for the level of learner. They must practice, receive feedback, and be debriefed in such a way that closely approximates the model of debriefing used. Indeed, debriefing trainers must model debriefing and feedback's best practices.

CASE STUDY 18.1

You are interviewing three SPs and ask them to role-play a patient with active appendicitis. The first one doubles over and moans continuously while you are trying to examine him. The second SP states that he has a pain level of 3 on a scale of 0 to 10 and is sitting on the table smiling. The third one asks several questions about the condition and asks whether he can "read up" on it first on his electronic device. Assess all three SPs for their appropriateness to provide SP service and feedback to learners.

PRACTICE QUESTIONS

1. Feedback is:
   A. Another term for *debriefing*
   B. A tool of debriefing
   C. Best delivered when something positive is said first
   D. A process of self-reflection

2. Preparing the learner for debriefing:
   A. Helps teach the learner how to debrief
   B. Is optional
   C. Is required
   D. Helps the learner to participate more effectively in the process

3. Debriefing is an advanced standardized patient (SP) core competency because:
   A. Not every SP is capable of providing feedback.
   B. It is more difficult than communication assessment.
   C. It is of more use than just giving feedback.
   D. Debriefing is arguably the most complex activity for SPs to master.

4. The reason standardized patients (SPs) provide feedback on communication is:
   A. They are arguably in the best position to judge, and therefore debrief, the communication quality of the learners.
   B. It is easier to evaluate communication than the physical examination.

C. They are trained to do it.
D. They are trained to assess communication.

5. One of the best ways to debrief the physical examination is:
    A. Telling the learner directly what he or she did incorrectly
    B. Showing the learner how the physical exam should be performed
    C. Asking the candidate to retry the exam and correct as necessary
    D. The standardized patient (SP) should never debrief the physical exam

6. The advantage of using Pendleton's Rules for debriefing is:
    A. It helps both the standardized patient (SP) and the learner prepare for debriefing by listing positive performance as well as what could have been done differently.
    B. It is an easy technique for SPs to remember.
    C. Research shows it is an effective debriefing process.
    D. Learners like to get both positive and negative feedback.

7. To ensure standardized patient (SP) debriefing quality:
    A. Give the SP feedback about the debriefing.
    B. Ask SPs to self-assess their work.
    C. Question the SP about his or her knowledge of debriefing.
    D. Use a debriefing quality-assurance checklist to note SP behaviors.

8. Empathy is important to the debriefing process because:
    A. It helps the standardized patient (SP) understand the learner's frame of reference.
    B. It demonstrates that the SP is a warm and caring person.
    C. It creates psychological safety for the learner.
    D. It is an important adult learning approach.

9. Reflective debriefing models:
    A. Promote positive learning
    B. Are always appropriate
    C. Get the learners to self-assess their work so that in actual practice they can self-correct their performance
    D. Get the standardized patients (SPs) to reflect on the quality of the learner's work

10. One disadvantage of using the sandwich style of feedback is:
    A. It makes learners passive recipients of the debriefer's information.
    B. It does not work well as reflective feedback.
    C. It does not work well with physical examination debriefing.
    D. It puts the debriefer in charge of what to discuss.

REFERENCES

Adamo, G. (2003). Simulated and standardized patients in OSCEs: Achievements and challenges 1992–2003. *Medical Teacher*, 25(3), 262–270. doi:10.1080/0142159031000100300

Archer, J. C. (2010). State of the science in health professional education: Effective feedback. *Medical Education*, 4(1), 101–108. doi:10.1111/j.1365-2923.2009.03546.x

Barrows, H. S. (1993). An overview of the uses of standardized patients for teaching and evaluating clinical skills. *AAMC Academic Medicine*, 68(6), 443–451. doi:10.1097/00001888-199306000-00002

Bartone, P. T., & Adler, A. B. (1995). Event-oriented debriefing following military operations: What every leader should know. *US Army Pamphlet*, 95(2), 1–12. doi:10.21236/ada300953

Boulet, J. R., & Errichetti, A. (2008). Training and assessment with standardized patients. In R. H. Riley (Ed.), *Manual of simulation in healthcare*. New York, NY: Oxford University Press.

Chowdhury, R. R., & Kalu, G. (2004). Learning to give feedback in medical education. *Obstetrician and Gynaecologist*, 6, 242–247. doi:10.1576/toag.6.4.243.27023

Department of the Army. (1993). *A leader's guide to after-action reviews* [Training circular] (pp. 25–20). Washington, DC: Author.

Dewey, J. (1933). *How we think: A restatement of the relation of reflective thinking to the educative process*. Boston, MA: D. C. Heath.

Dillon, G. F., Boulet, J. R., Hawkins, R. E., & Swanson, D. B. (2004). Simulations in the United States Medical Licensing Examination (USMLE). *Quality & Safe Health Care*, 13(Suppl. 1), i41–i45. doi:10.1136/qhc.13.suppl_1.i41

Goleman, D. (2006). *Social intelligence: The new science of human relationships*. New York, NY: Bantam Dell.

Hatcher, J. A. (1997). The moral dimensions of John Dewey's philosophy: Implications for undergraduate education. *Michigan Journal of Community Service Learning*, 4(1), 22–29. Retrieved from http://hdl.handle.net/2027/spo.3239521.0004.103

Itin, C. M. (1999). Reasserting the philosophy of experiential education as a vehicle for change in the 21st century. *Journal of Experiential Education*, 22(2), 91–98. doi:10.1177/105382599902200206

Keiser, M. M., & Turkelson, C. (2017). Using students as standardized patients: Development, implementation, and evaluation of a standardized patient training program. *Clinical Simulation in Nursing*, 13(7), 321–330. doi:10.1016/j.ecns.2017.05.008

Kolb, D. A. (1984). *Experiential leaning theory: Experience as the source of learning and development*. Englewood Cliffs, NJ: Prentice Hall.

Mayer, J. D., & Salovey, P. (1997). What is emotional intelligence? In P. Salovey & D. Sluyter (Eds.), *Emotional development and emotional intelligence: Implications for educators* (pp. 3–31). New York, NY: Basic Books.

Pendleton, D., Schofield, T., Tate, P., & Havelock, P. (1984). *The consultation: An approach to teaching and learning*. Oxford, UK: Oxford University Press.

Rudolph, J. W., Simon, R., Rivard, P., Dufresne, R. L., & Raemer, D. B. (2006). There's no such thing as non-judgmental debriefing: A theory and method of debriefing with good judgment. *Simulation in Healthcare*, 1(1), 49–55. doi:10.1097/01266021-200600110-00006

Rudolph, J. W., Simon, R., Rivard, P., Dufresne, R. L., & Raemer, D. B. (2007). Debriefing with good judgment. *Anesthesiology Clinics*, (15), 361–376. doi:10.1016/j.anclin.2007.03.007

Schön, D. (1983). *The reflective practitioner*. New York, NY: Basic Books.

Society for Simulation in Healthcare. (2018). *Certified Healthcare Simulation Educator Examination Blueprint, 2018 Version*. Retrieved from http://www.ssih.org/Portals/48/Certification/CHSE_Docs/CHSE_Examination_Blueprint.pdf

Thorndike, E. L. (1920). Intelligence and its use. *Harper's Magazine*, 140, 227–235.

Vygotsky, L. (1978). Interaction between learning and development. *Mind in society* (pp. 79–91). Cambridge, MA: Harvard University Press.

19 Evaluation of Simulation Activities

MELANIE LEIGH CASON AND FRANCES WICKHAM LEE

One of the great mistakes is to judge policies and programs by their intentions rather than their results.
—Milton Friedman

This chapter addresses Domain III: Educational Principles Applied to Simulation (Society for Simulation in Healthcare, 2018).

[LEARNING OUTCOMES]

- Discuss the basic components of performance and activity evaluation.
- Discuss the importance of evaluation of simulation activities.
- Identify current practices for individual learner evaluation, team evaluation, and activity evaluation in simulation-based training (SBT).
- Discuss the future of evaluation in SBT.

The healthcare world continues to evolve at an amazing speed with increasing individual and organizational accountability at the forefront. Experts agree that simulation is a valuable tool for healthcare education learning and for determining clinical competency (Cant & Cooper, 2010; Chappell & Koithan, 2012; Wilhaus, Burleson, Palaganas, & Jeffries, 2014). However, the question remains: How does one determine the effectiveness of simulation at the individual, team, organizational, and system levels? Assessing learner outcomes, whether for students or practicing healthcare professionals, individually or in teams, requires valid and reliable tools to ensure that instructional goals are achieved (Boulet et al., 2011). Although a variety of SBT and simulation-based team training (SBTT) evaluation tools exist, there continues to be a need for establishing the validity and reliability of both the simulator and the tools (Adamson & Kardong-Edgren, 2012; Eppich,

Howard, Vozenilek, & Curran, 2011; Rosen, Salas, Silvestri, Wu, & Lazzara, 2008; Schaefer et al., 2011). In addition to accurately evaluating learners, outcome data are needed to determine the overall effectiveness of SBT, including demonstration of translation to practice within organizations and the overall healthcare system.

This chapter begins with a brief discussion of evaluation and its importance in SBT, both today and in the future. Next, the chapter focuses on evaluation of the individual learner, including the differences between formative and summative evaluation and a discussion of self and peer evaluation, followed by an overview of the evaluation of team members during SBTT. A summary of selected SBT and SBTT evaluation instruments is presented. The chapter concludes with a discussion of methods and current tools available for evaluating the simulation activity itself.

EVALUATION IN SBT

Rosen and colleagues (2008) offer an overview of three key concepts for understanding evaluation in SBT: "issues of purpose (i.e., why evaluate?), content (i.e., what to evaluate?), and method (i.e., how to evaluate?)" (p. 353). There are multiple reasons for evaluating SBT, including providing formative and summative feedback to learners, defining key outcomes, validating the usefulness of the training, and demonstrating translation to practice. What to evaluate is often challenging. High-quality simulation design begins with a clear understanding of the learning objectives. These objectives focus on what is to be evaluated. For example, is the focus on individual performance or overall effectiveness or impact on the organization? Performance refers to the "actual behaviors" demonstrated, whereas effectiveness addresses the results of the performance (Rosen et al., 2008). Actual behaviors within SBT are often divided into knowledge, skills, and attitudes (KSAs). These relate to the recognized learning domains, that is, cognitive (knowledge), affective (attitude), and psychomotor (skills). The "how to evaluate" must be determined by the "why" and the "what." Clearly, the tools used to evaluate straight performance versus effectiveness or translation would be quite different. The instrument chosen for assessment or evaluation should reflect the appropriate domain in which the learning has occurred or an integration of all three if appropriate (Kardong-Edgren, Adamson, & Fitzgerald, 2010).

There has been a great deal of attention given to developing evaluation methods and tools to demonstrate that SBT "translates to practice" (Eppich et al., 2011; Rosen et al., 2008; Schaefer et al., 2011). In other words, if the learner performs in a competent manner in the SBT, will this translate into actual clinical practice? Eppich and colleagues (2011) discuss a need to examine SBT and SBTT as "inter-related conceptual" (p. 14) levels of training the individual, team, organization, and system. Translation to practice occurs at the organizational and system levels. Although the current state of evaluation for SBT and SBTT has not reached the level of demonstrating translation, any discussion of evaluation should include it as an ultimate goal. To date, the majority of work related to SBT evaluation has been at the individual learner and team levels, with some work targeting the evaluation of effective simulation design and implementation. We examine these three areas in more detail in the subsequent sections of this chapter.

INDIVIDUAL LEARNER SBT EVALUATION

SBT learner evaluation focuses primarily on the individual's performance and outcomes. Learner evaluation is recognized within the SBT community as an essential component for effective simulation experiences. The International Nursing Association for Clinical Simulation and Learning (INACSL) requires all simulation-based experiences adhering to their published standards for best practice, *INACSL Standards of Best Practice: Simulation*^{SM}, to include participant evaluation. They cite three elements necessary for conducting an "authentic evaluation" from Huang, Rice, Spain, and Palaganas (2015): "(a) determine the intent of the simulation-based experience; (b) design the simulation-based experience to include timing of the evaluation, the use of a valid and reliable assessment tool, and evaluator training required; and (c) complete the evaluation and interpret the results" (p. xxi). INACSL further cites potential consequences for failure to engage in authentic participant evaluation, including:

- Inaccurate assessment
- Poor participant experiences
- Poor learning outcomes, failure to progress
- Inappropriate selection of tools
- Assessment bias (2016, p. S26)

In evaluating learners, it is important to determine desired specific learning outcomes, maintain consistency, and apply standardization in order to be fair and objective with feedback (Motola, Devine, Chung, Sullivan, & Issenberg, 2013). All evaluations of learners begin with the development of clear, measurable objectives for the SBT. Evaluation should always be tightly aligned with the learning objectives. The appropriate choice of the evaluation tool is specific to the measurement of learning outcomes, whether the activity is an individual or group activity. The outcome of the evaluation may be formative, summative, or high stakes, which will be a large determinant of the tool selected. A few of the more well-known SBT evaluation tools are listed in Table 19.1 with brief descriptions.

> **SIMULATION TEACHING TIP 19.1**
>
> Remember to determine what you are evaluating and make sure it is appropriate for the level of the student. Approaches will depend on formative or summative activities. If summative, then you should not give students unfair advantages by cueing or assisting in any way. Are you *evaluating* clinical judgment, competency, psychomotor skills, or critical thinking or *teaching* them? Scenarios in simulation cannot encompass all aspects of a case study, so it is important to define the desired learning outcomes or assessment measures clearly before you begin.

TABLE 19.1
Characteristics of Simulation-Based Team Training Evaluation Instruments

SELECTED CITATIONS	NAME OF INSTRUMENT	CHARACTERISTICS	REQUIREMENTS	MEASURES	OTHER
AHRQ (2014)	TPOT	Observational measurement for team performance	Each specified team behavior is ranked on a 5-point Likert scale; Very poor: 1, Poor: 2, Acceptable: 3, Good: 4, Excellent: 5; for an averaged Team Performance Rating	Team structure, communication, leadership, situation monitoring, mutual support	
Fletcher et al. (2004)	Anesthetists' nontechnical skills	Observational checklist for team performance	Evaluator rates four categories on a 4-point scale; Good: 4, Acceptable: 3, Marginal: 2, Poor: 1, Not Observed: 0	Task management, team working, situation awareness, decision making	
Thomas, Sexton, & Helmreich (2004)	University of Texas Behavioral Marker Audit Form	One-page behavioral rating scale designed for team performance in neonatal resuscitation	Each behavior is rated on observability and frequency	10 behavior markers: information sharing, inquiry, assertion, intentions shared, teaching, evaluation of plans, workload management, vigilance/environmental awareness, teamwork overall, and leadership	Derived from methodologies used in aviation: Line Operations Safety Audit

SELECTED CITATIONS	NAME OF INSTRUMENT	CHARACTERISTICS	REQUIREMENTS	MEASURES	OTHER
Healey, Undre, & Vincent (2004)	Observational Teamwork Assessment of Surgery	Clinical checklist by surgical expert; teamwork behaviors by expert researcher	Clinical checklist is yes or no; behaviors are rated on 7-point Likert scale	Task work and teamwork in three stages: preoperative, intraoperative, and postoperative; teamwork behaviors include communication, leadership, coordination, monitoring, and cooperation	Developed for use in the operating room, not specifically simulation
Adamson et al. (2012); Kardong-Edgren et al. (2010); Todd, Manz, Hawkins, Parsons, & Hercinger (2008)	Creighton Simulation Evaluation Instrument (2008)	A rating tool designed for evaluation of nursing students using simulation	Evaluator scores either a 0 or 1 for 22 specific criteria; example: "Responds to abnormal findings appropriately"	Assessment, communication, critical thinking, technical skills	Modified for use in the NLN high-stakes assessment and NCSBN Simulation Research Study
Lasater (2007); Tanner (2006)	Lasater Clinical Judgment Rubric (2007)	A rubric based on a clinical judgment model by Tanner (2006)	Evaluator rates participant as exemplary, accomplished, developing, or beginning with detailed rubric criteria	Effective noticing, effective interpreting, effective responding, effective reflecting	Has been modified for numeric grading (Ashcraft, et al., 2013)
Mikasa, Cicero, & Adamson (2012)	Seattle University Evaluation Tool (2008)	A tool based on curricular objectives and the American Association of Colleges of Nursing baccalaureate competencies	Evaluator circles observed behaviors that relate to a score from the range of "Below expectations" to "Exceeds expectations"	Assessment, intervention, evaluation, critical thinking/ clinical decision making, direct patient care/communication/ collaboration, professional behaviors	

AHRQ, Agency for Healthcare Research and Quality; NCSBN, National Council of State Boards of Nursing; NLN, National League for Nursing; TPOT, Team Performance Observation Tool.

FRAMEWORKS FOR EVALUATION STRATEGIES

There are several applicable frameworks that support the evaluative process in SBT. These include Kirkpatrick's levels of evaluation, translational science research (TSR) phases, and Miller's pyramid (Adamson, Kardong-Edgren, & Willhaus, 2012; Downing & Yudkowsky, 2009; McGaghie, Draycott, Dunn, Lopez, & Stefanidis, 2011).

Kirkpatrick's Levels of Evaluation

- Level 1 is **reaction**. How satisfied are the learners with the activity? How did they like it? As the lowest level of evaluation, it is usually reflected by self-reporting on surveys, observations, or verbal feedback: "It was fun" or "I didn't like it."
- Level 2 is **learning**. How much did they learn? This level reflects a change in attitudes, skills, or knowledge.
- Level 3 is **behavior**. How has the learner's behavior changed as a result of this activity? Level III relates to a change in behavior and application of what he or she has learned.
- Level 4 is **results**. This relates to a change in practice based on the learning that benefits clients (patients) and/or contributes to a change in the organization with improved outcomes (Adamson, 2014; Downing & Yudkowsky, 2009; Kirkpatrick, 1998; McGaghie, Issenberg, Petrusa, & Scalese, 2010).

TSR Phases

The evaluation of the transfer of the KSAs learned with simulation to patient care and outcomes is appropriate for translational research (Adamson et al., 2012). TSR provides three levels of evaluation:

1. T-1 is the lowest level in relation to simulation activities. It consists of learning in the simulation lab.
2. T-2 is the carryover to patient care.
3. T-3 is that the results of the simulation activity improve patient outcomes. As the name implies, evidence is required to prove the translation to practice, and this requires measurable outcomes at every level. Research design and data collection for the highest level of TSR continue to be a challenge in simulation education (McGaghie et al., 2011).

Miller's Pyramid

Miller's pyramid provides a visual model with "Knows" as the base of the pyramid, followed by "Knows how" and "Shows how." "Does" is the top level of the pyramid (Figure 19.1). The "Shows how" level relates to a demonstration of learning, for example, in objective simulated clinical examinations (OSCEs) or with simulations. The highest level "Does" again relates to transfer to practice in the workplace (Miller, 1990).

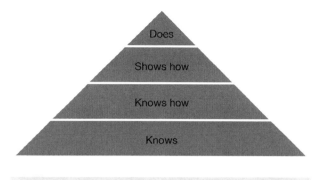

FIGURE 19.1 Miller's pyramid.

Source: Adapted from Miller, G. E. (1990). The assessment of clinical skills competence performance. *Academic Medicine*, 65(9), 63–67. doi:10.1097/00001888-199009000-00045

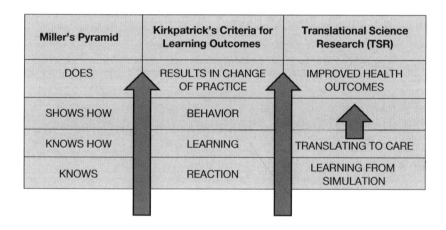

FIGURE 19.2 Selected frameworks for evaluation strategies.

A comparison of the levels, phases, and features of these frameworks confirms that the lowest level of learner evaluation relates to obtaining information and assessing learner reactions. The highest level involves translation to practice and health outcomes. The "in-between" levels, or phases, contain the observation of the learned behavior, that is, performance. Most learner evaluation during SBT, whether formative or summative, is recognized as falling into these "in-between" levels (Figure 19.2).

■ FORMATIVE EVALUATION

Formative evaluation involves the learning process and occurs during or within instruction (Downing & Yudkowsky, 2009). Generally, formative evaluation does not result in a recorded grade or assessment score. Rather, it provides the learners with important feedback to guide them in obtaining appropriate KSAs relative to the study topic. Active learning with simulation promotes an opportunity for formative feedback, particularly regarding the higher level KSAs that encompass critical thinking and competencies (Glynn, 2012; Jeffries, 2012; Tanner, 2006). Formative evaluation of learners "fosters personal and professional development" (INACSL, 2016, p. S26). Tools, such as performance tests, checklists, and pre- and postlearning assessments, are valuable in formative evaluation, enabling deliberate practice toward mastery (Downing & Yudkowsky, 2009; Sando et al., 2013).

SUMMATIVE EVALUATION

Summative evaluation measures the achievement of learning objectives by "summing up" the results of the formative experiences (Downing & Yudkowsky, 2009; Sando et al., 2013). According to INACSL, summative evaluation "focuses on the measurement of outcomes or achievement of objectives at a discreate moment in time" (2016, S26). Summative evaluation generally results in a recorded grade, score, or certification of competence or proficiency. A *"high-stakes" simulation activity* refers to a simulation designed as an assessment tool with an outcome that affects a grade, certification, and has consequences attached to the final rating (Rizzolo, 2014; Sando et al., 2013). There is increasing interest in using simulation not only for training, but also as the basis for learner evaluation. Because a high-stakes evaluation has the potential to lead to significant consequences for the learner (INACSL, 2016) clear objectives and standard, informed measures are critical. In addition, facilitators should never cue the participants or provide information that would affect the evaluation (Wilhaus et al., 2014). According to McGaghie and Issenberg (2009), a major component in developing a simulation-based evaluation is to standardize the "test conditions," that is, the simulation activity, so that the *only* variable in the experience is the learner.

EVIDENCE-BASED SIMULATION PRACTICE 19.1

Brackney, Hayes, Dawson, and Koontz (2017) studied simulation evaluation for senior-level bachelor of science in nursing (BSN) students (*N* = 41) in a Capstone course and National Council Licensure Examination for Registered Nurses (NCLEX-RN™) first-time passing rates. Faculty evaluated students' performance in simulation and the faculty evaluations were strongly correlated with NCLEX-RN success. Specifically, students who were evaluated as "lacking confidence" and who had "flawed skillls" were less likely to pass the NCLEX-RN on the first attempt.

SELF-EVALUATION

Self-evaluation commonly occurs in debriefing after SBT. It can also occur during SBT in which structured feedback is provided. Effective debriefing provides the opportunity to reflect and is a valuable learning experience for the learner. Learning occurs individually during the experience of the simulation and during debriefing (Dreifuerst, 2009). Self-evaluation may be enhanced with recording the simulation activities. Previous self-efficacy studies with nursing students and physicians indicate that abilities may be overrated (Davis et al., 2006; Shinnick & Woo, 2013; Watts, Rush, & Wright, 2009).

PEER EVALUATION

Removing the facilitator from the evaluative process and allowing the participants to evaluate each other has certain benefits. Participants working collaboratively learn from each other and develop the ability to make judgments and give and receive constructive criticism. The success in peer evaluation depends on how the activity is structured to prevent erroneous information, bias, and subjectivity (Rush, Firth, Burke, & Marks-Maran, 2012). Cooperative Learning with Simulation-Based Skills Training (CLSST™) is one method of pairing students with a standardized programmed event menu for peer assessment with scoring. This method alleviates the need for a paper checklist and provides immediate feedback to the participants (Lee, Schaefer, Houck, Walker, & Cason, 2014).

EVALUATION IN SBTT

There are significant challenges in evaluating both the performance and the effectiveness of SBTT. Healthcare teams are complex entities, often comprising ever-changing members in a high-stress environment. The Agency for Healthcare Research and Quality (AHRQ, 2017) defines a *team* as

- Consisting of two or more individuals
- Having specific roles, performing specific tasks, and interacting to achieve a common goal or outcome
- Making decisions
- Possessing specialized knowledge and skill and often functioning under conditions of high workload
- Differing from small groups in that teams embody a collective action arising out of task interdependence

One of the most significant challenges in SBTT evaluation is the need to assess the KSAs of the team members within the context of the team. The team performance and effectiveness must also be considered. If individual team members do not have the KSAs needed to perform the tasks associated with their respective roles, the effectiveness of the team may be impacted. Most of the existing SBTT evaluation tools are observational checklists that focus primarily on the "soft skills" and overall team characteristics rather than outcomes. For example, one of the most used team frameworks is TeamSTEPPS (Team Strategies and Tools to Enhance Performance and Patient Safety), developed by the AHRQ. (Although not an evaluation tool per se, TeamSTEPPS has been used as the foundation for many SBTT evaluation tools.) The four key skills emphasized in TeamSTEPPS are:

1. Leadership
2. Communication
3. Situational monitoring
4. Mutual support

TeamSTEPPS provides a Team Performance Observation Tool (TPOT) that may be used in the evaluation of a team simulation activity. The TPOT uses a 5-point Likert scale to measure team structure, communication, leadership, situation monitoring, and mutual support, and provides a summative team performance rating that is useful in providing feedback (AHRQ, 2014). The TPOT has been modified and used as a specialty instrument for evaluation as the Trauma TPOT (Rice et al., 2016).

A few of the more well-known SBTT tools are listed with brief descriptions in Table 19.1.

CURRENT EVALUATION INSTRUMENTS

Instruments for evaluating individual and team SBT performance continue to be developed and tested. Appropriate feedback and evaluation require valid and reliable tools to avoid subjectivity, bias, and incorrect interpretation of the simulation experience (Motola et al., 2013). Many instruments have been developed without established or reported reliability and validity data (Kardong-Edgren et al., 2010).

- *Validity* relates to the degree that the instrument or tool measures what it is intended to measure, for example, communication skills.

- *Reliability* is the consistency and dependability of the measurement of a particular attribute by the instrument or tool (Polit & Beck, 2012).

More multisite studies are needed to establish validity and reliability of many tools, and choosing a tool that is already developed supports this initiative (Adamson & Kardong-Edgren, 2012). In addition, the importance of facilitator education regarding the appropriate use of an evaluative tool has been established (Parsons et al., 2012; Patton, 2012).

Simulation evaluation instruments vary in design and levels of measurement. As noted in Table 19.1, these may include Likert scales with rankings from 0 to 5, scoring rubrics outlining expected behaviors linked to a score, or dichotomous scales of 0 to 1 (did not meet or met). In deciding the tool most appropriate to use, the most recently reported reliability and validity should be considered in addition to the objective of the evaluation (Adamson & Kardong-Edgren, 2012).

EVALUATING THE SIMULATION ACTIVITY

Another topic within the simulation community involves evaluating the simulation activity itself and the facilitator conducting the SBT. Questions, such as does the activity meet the objectives for which it was designed or is the facilitator effective, are important for improving activities and ensuring quality. There are many ways to evaluate simulation activities, from direct observation by peers or formal to informal surveys and questionnaires. As with other evaluation tools, the surveys and questionnaires used to evaluate the simulation activities should be valid and reliable (Boulet et al., 2011; Jeffries, 2012). It is important to consider instruments or tools with established validity and reliability instead of attempting to develop a new instrument. There are evaluation instruments that exist for each level of evaluation from observation based to haptic sensors that provide objective feedback with touch and pressure sensors (Adamson, 2014).

There are a handful of SBT assessment tools that address facilitator and activity effectiveness. The Simulation Design Scale (SDS) allows the participant not only to self-assess participation, but also to assess the effectiveness of the simulation activity. Another tool, the Educational Practices in Simulation Scale (EPSS), contains elements that assess for best practices in SBT, including active learning, high expectations, diversity in learning, and collaboration (Jeffries, 2012). Debriefing Assessment for Simulation in Healthcare© (DASH©; 2014) is a tool aimed at the evaluation of the debriefing experience following simulation (Center for Medical Simulation, 2014).

SUMMARY

This chapter has explored concepts and tools for evaluating performance and effectiveness of SBT at the individual and team levels, with some discussion related to the need to move to the higher levels of organizational and system impact. Although a variety of SBT, SBTT, and simulation activity evaluation tools exist, there continues to be a need to develop and establish valid and reliable instruments, particularly those that will measure organizational impact and translation to practice (Eppich et al., 2011; Rosen et al., 2008; Schaefer et al., 2011). Outcomes data are needed to determine the overall effectiveness of the SBT, including demonstration of translation to practice within organizations and the overall healthcare system.

CASE STUDY 19.1

An academic medical university is planning an interdisciplinary professional education simulation activity involving medical students, nursing students, physician assistant students, and pharmacology students. The simulation will consist of teams of four, with one from each discipline. The scenarios are designed for specific behaviors, such as effective communication, teamwork and collaboration, procedural skill, and critical thinking. Evaluations consist of facilitator input at debriefing and self-assessment of performance and the activity with an online questionnaire. Results are positive, but the facilitators are determined to improve the evaluative results with peer evaluation and measurement of the achievement of the learning outcomes of effective communication, teamwork and collaboration, procedural skill, and critical thinking.

CASE STUDY DISCUSSION

There are several ways that the facilitators can evaluate the students' performance more effectively. The choice of a rubric could be time intensive and involves an expert from each discipline observing the simulation either in real time, remotely, or by video. Establishing interrater reliability by requiring another faculty member to review the simulation independently is desirable, especially if this type of activity may be used for high-stakes or summative assessments in the future. Programmed menu items allow for assessment while running the simulation and can be assimilated with data retrieval to evaluate the learning for the course overall, to identify knowledge gaps, and to inform curriculum development. Although it is important to evaluate how participants feel about an activity, simulation offers opportunities to evaluate learning in the cognitive, affective, and psychomotor domains.

PRACTICE QUESTIONS

1. Which of the following is the best example of a "high-stakes" simulation activity?

   A. Maintenance of certification requirement for a healthcare profession
   B. Critical care skill development for nurses at the hospital
   C. Medical student physical exam practice
   D. Interprofessional communication assessment for surgical teams

2. A faculty member has asked your advice on how to create an effective learner evaluation for her planned simulation-based training (SBT). Which of the following would you tell her is the **most important** step in this process?

   A. Determine the timing of the evaluation
   B. Identify the learning objectives to be evaluated
   C. Consider the background of the learners
   D. Conduct statistical item analysis to determine reliability

3. Use of a checklist-type evaluation instrument is **most** appropriate for which of the following:

   A. Summative assessment of a student nurse performing the correct steps for inserting a urinary catheter
   B. Summative assessment of a staff nurse's ability to recognize an unstable patient
   C. Formative assessment of a resident's ability to achieve an accurate differential diagnosis
   D. High-stakes evaluation of a medical student's ability to empathically communicate with parents of a critically ill patient

4. The most appropriate type of instrument for measuring the effectiveness of cardiopulmonary resuscitation (CPR) compressions is:

   A. Observation based
   B. Pre- and posttest
   C. Haptic response
   D. Participant feedback

5. Two facilitators are independently rating a summative simulation using an observation instrument. This type of evaluation is known as:

   A. Peer evaluation
   B. Interrater reliability evaluation
   C. Dual evaluation
   D. Rubric evaluation

6. Additional rigorous research and evidence-based practice appraisals are needed to ensure:

   A. Students are satisfied with simulation learning experiences.
   B. Faculty are competent in providing simulation learning experiences.
   C. Simulation is meeting the learners' outcomes.
   D. Simulation is impacting safe patient care.

7. High-quality simulation learning experiences should begin with:
    A. Resource management
    B. Clear learning objectives
    C. Participants in mind
    D. Identification of appropriate technology

8. When choosing an evaluation tool for a simulation learning experience, it should reflect:
    A. The students involved
    B. The technology used
    C. The faculty's expertise
    D. The learning domain

9. Needed simulation research should be focused on which level of evaluation?
    A. Reaction
    B. Leaning
    C. Behavior
    D. Results

10. Which level of translational research is an evaluation of learning "carried over to patient care"?
    A. T-1
    B. T-2
    C. T-3
    D. T-4

REFERENCES

Adamson, K. A. (2014). Evaluation tools and metrics for simulations. In P. R. Jeffries (Ed.), *Clinical simulations in nursing education: Advanced concepts, trends, and opportunities* (pp. 145–163). Philadelphia, PA: Wolters Kluwer, Lippincott Williams & Wilkins.

Adamson, K. A., & Kardong-Edgren, S. (2012). A method and resources for assessing the reliability of simulation evaluation instruments. *Nursing Education Perspectives*, 33, 334–339. doi:10.5480/1536-5026-33.5.334

Adamson, K. A., Kardong-Edgren, S., & Willhaus, J. (2012). An updated review of published simulation evaluation instruments. *Clinical Simulation in Nursing*, 9, e1–e13. doi:10.1016/j.ecns.2012.09.004

Agency for Healthcare Research and Quality. (2014). Team performance observation tool. Retrieved from https://www.ahrq.gov/teamstepps/instructor/reference/tmpot.html

Agency for Healthcare Research and Quality. (2017). Simultion in education: Defining terms. Retrieved from https://www.ahrq.gov/professionals/quality-patient-safety/patient-safety-resources/research/simulation-dictionary/index.html

Ashcraft, A. S., Opton, L., Bridges, R. A., Caballero, S., Veesart, A., & Weaver, C. (2013). Simulation evaluation using a modified Lasater clinical judgment rubric. *Nursing Education Perspectives*, 34(2), 122–26. doi:10.5480/1536-5026-34.2.122

Boulet, J. R., Jeffries, P. R., Hatala, R. A., Korndorffer, J. R., Feinstein, D. M., & Roche, J. P. (2011). Research regarding methods of assessing learning outcomes. *Simulation in Healthcare*, 6, S48–S51. doi:10.1097/SIH.0b013e31822237d0

Brackney, D. E., Hayes, L. S., Dawson, T., & Koontz, A. (2017). Simulation performance and National Council Licensure Examination for Registered Nurses outcomes: Field research perspectives. *Creative Nursing*, 23(4), 255–265. doi:10.1891/1078-4535.23.4.255

Cant, R. P., & Cooper, S. J. (2010). Simulation-based learning in nurse education: Systematic review. *Journal of Advanced Nursing, 66*(1), 3–15. doi:10.1111/j.1365-2648.2009.05240.x

Center for Medical Simulation. (2014). Debriefing Assessment for Simulation in Healthcare (DASH). Retrieved from https://harvardmedsim.org

Chappell, K., & Koithan, M. (2012). Validating clinical competence. *Journal of Continuing Education in Nursing, 43,* 293–294. doi:10.3928/00220124-20120621-02

Davis, D. A., Mazmanian, P. E., Fordis, M., Harrison, R. V., Thorpe, K. E., & Perrier, L. (2006). Accuracy of physician self-assessment compared with observed measures of competence: A systematic review. *Journal of the American Medical Association, 9,* 1094–1102. doi:10.1001/jama.296.9.1094

Downing, S. M., & Yudkowsky, R. (2009). *Assessment in health professions education.* New York, NY: Routledge.

Dreifuerst, K. (2009). The essentials of debriefing in simulation earning: A concept analysis. *Nursing Education Perspectives, 10*(2), 109–114.

Eppich, W., Howard, V., Vozenilek, J., & Curran, I. (2011). Simulation based team training in healthcare. *Simulation in Healthcare, 6*(7), S14–S19. doi:10.1097/SIH.0b013e318229f550

Fletcher, G., Flin, R., McGeorge, P., Glavin, R., Maran, N., & Patey, P. (2004). Rating non-technical skills: Developing a behavioral marking system for use in anesthesia. *Cognition Technology Work, 6,* 165–171. doi:10.1007/s10111-004-0158-y

Glynn, P. (2012). Evaluation of senior nursing students' performances with high fidelity simulation. *Online Journal of Nursing Informatics, 16*(3), 1–12. Retrieved from http://ojni.org/issues

Healey, A., Undre, S., and Vincent, C.A. (2004). Developing observational measures of performance in surgical teams. *BMJ Quality and Safety, 13*(Suppl. 1), i33–i40. doi:10.1136/qshc.2004.009936

Huang, Y., Rice, J., Spain, A., & Palaganas, J. (2015). Terms of reference. In J. Palaganas, J. Maxworthy, C. Epps, & M. Mancini (Eds.), *Defining excellence in simulation programs* (pp. xxi–xxxiii). Philadelphia, PA: Wolters Kluwer.

INACSL Standards Committee. (2016, December). INACSL standards of best practice: Simulation^SM Participant evaluation. *Clinical Simulation in Nursing, 12*(Suppl.), S26–S29. doi:10.1016/j.ecns.2016.09.009

Jeffries, P. R. (2012). *Simulation in nursing education: From conceptualization to evaluation* (2nd ed.). New York, NY: National League for Nursing.

Kardong-Edgren, S., Adamson, K. A., & Fitzgerald, C. (2010). A review of currently published evaluation instruments for human patient simulation. *Clinical Simulation in Nursing, 6,* e25–e35. doi:10.1016/j.ecns.2009.08.004

Kirkpatrick, D. L. (1998). *Evaluating training programs* (2nd ed.). San Francisco, CA: Berrett-Koehler.

Lasater, K. (2007). Clinical judgment development: Using simulation to create an assessment rubric. *Journal of Nursing Education, 46*(11), 496–503.

Lee, F. W., Schaefer, J., Houck, R., Walker, J., & Cason, M. (2014). Cooperative learning in dyads using hybrid task training simulation. Presentation conducted at the International Meeting for Simulation in Healthcare, San Francisco, CA.

McGaghie, W. C., Draycott, T. J., Dunn, F. W., Lopez, C. M., & Stefanidis, D. (2011). Evaluating the impact of simulation on translational patient outcomes. *Simulation in Healthcare, 6,* S42–S47. doi:10.1097/SIH.0b013e318222fde9

McGaghie, W. C., & Issenberg, S. B. (2009). Simulations in assessment. In S. M. Downing & R. Yudkowsky (Eds.), *Assessment in health professions education* (pp. 245–268). New York, NY: Routledge.

McGaghie, W. C., Issenberg, S. B., Petrusa, E. R., & Scalese, R. J. (2010). A critical review of simulation-based medical education research: 2003–2009. *Medical Education, 44,* 50–63. doi:10.1111/j.1365-2923.2009.03547.x

Mikasa, A. W., Cicero, T. F., & Adamson, K. A. (2012). Outcome-based evaluation tool to evaluate student performance in high-fidelity simulation. *Clinical Simulation in Nursing*, e1–e7. doi:10.1016/j.ecns.2012.06.001

Miller, G. E. (1990). The assessment of clinical skills competence performance. *Academic Medicine*, 65(9), 63–67. doi:10.1097/00001888-199009000-00045

Motola, I., Devine, L. A., Chung, H. S., Sullivan, J. E., & Issenberg, S. B. (2013). Simulation in healthcare education: A best evidence practical guide. AMEE Guide no. 82. *Medical Teacher*, 35, e1511–e1530. doi:10.3109/0142159x.2013.818632

Parsons, M. E., Hawkins, K. S., Hercinger, M., Todd, M., Manz, J. A., & Fang, X. (2012). Improvement in scoring consistency for the Creighton Simulation Evaluation Instrument. *Clinical Simulation in Nursing*, 8, e233–e238. doi:10.1016/j.ecns.2012.02.008

Patton, S. K. (2012). A pilot study to evaluate consistency among raters of a clinical simulation. *Nursing Education Perspectives*, 34(3), 194–195. doi:10.1097/00024776-201305000-00013

Polit, D., & Beck, C. (2012). *Nursing research: Generating and assessing evidence for nursing practice* (9th ed., pp. 3–24). Philadelphia, PA: Lippincott Williams & Wilkins.

Rice, Y., DeLetter, M., Fryman, L., Parrish, E., Velotta, C., & Talley, C. (2016). Implementation and evaluation of a team simulation program. *Society of Trauma Nurses*, 23(5), 298–303. doi:10.1097/JTN.0000000000000236

Rizzolo, M. A. (2014). Developing and using simulation for high-stakes assessment. In P. R. Jeffries (Ed.), *Clinical simulations in nursing education: Advanced concepts, trends, and opportunities* (pp. 113–134). Philadelphia, PA: Wolters Kluwer, Lippincott Williams & Wilkins.

Rosen, M. A., Salas, E., Silvestri, S., Wu, T. S., & Lazzara, E. H. (2008). A measurement tool for simulation-based training in emergency medicine: The simulation module for assessment of resident targeted event responses (SMARTER) approach. *Simulation in Healthcare*, 3, 170–179. doi:10.1097/sih.0b013e318173038d

Rush, S., Firth, T., Burke, L., & Marks-Maran, D. (2012). Implementation and evaluation of peer assessment of clinical skills for first year student nurses. *Nurse Education in Practice*, 12, 219–226. doi:10.1016/j.nepr.2012.01.014

Sando, C. R., Coggins, R. M., Meakim, C., Franklin, A. E., Gloe, D., Boese, T., … Borum, J. C. (2013). Standards of best practice: Simulation standard VII: Participant assessment and evaluation. *Clinical Simulation in Nursing*, 9(6Suppl.), S30–S32. doi:10.1016/j.ecns.2013.04.007

Schaefer, J. J., Vanderbilt, A. A., Cason, C. L., Bauman, E. B., Glavin, R. J., Lee, F. W., & Navedo, D. D. (2011). Literature Review: Instructional design and pedagogy science in healthcare simulation. *Simulation in Healthcare*, 6, S30–S41. doi:10.1097/SIH.0b013e31822237b4

Shinnick, M. A., & Woo, M. A. (2013). Does nursing student self-efficacy correlate with knowledge when using patient simulation? *Clinical Simulation in Nursing*, 10(2), e71–e79. doi:10.1016/j.ecns.2013.07.006

Society for Simulation in Healthcare. (2018). *Certified Healthcare Simulation Educator Examination Blueprint, 2018 Version*. Retrieved from http://www.ssih.org/Portals/48/Certification/CHSE_Docs/CHSE_Examination_Blueprint.pdf

Tanner, C. A. (2006). Thinking like a nurse: A research-based model of clinical judgment in nursing. *Journal of Nursing Education*, 45(6), 204–211.

Thomas, E. J., Sexton, J. B., & Helmreich, R. L. (2004). Translating teamwork behaviors from aviation to healthcare: Development of behavioral markers for neonatal resuscitation. *Quality Safety Health Care*, 13, 157–164. doi:10.1136/qhc.13.suppl_1.i57

Todd, M., Manz, J. A., Hawkins, K. S., Parsons, M. E., & Hercinger, M. (2008). The development of a quantitative evaluation tool for simulations in nursing education. *International Journal of Nursing Education Scholarship*, 5, 1–17. doi:10.2202/1548-923X.1705

Watts, W. E., Rush, K., & Wright, M. (2009). Evaluating first year nursing students' ability to self-assess psychomotor skills using videotape. *Nursing Education Perspectives*, *30*, 214–219.

Wilhaus, J., Burleson, G., Palaganas, J., & Jeffries, P. (2014). Authoring simulations for high stakes evaluation. *Clinical Simulation in Nursing*, *10*(4), e177–e182. doi:10.1016/j.ecns.2013.11.006

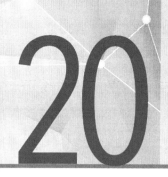

Fostering Professional Development in Healthcare Simulation

MARK C. CRIDER AND MARY ELLEN SMITH GLASGOW

> *Work to become, not to acquire.*
> —Elbert Hubbar

This chapter addresses Domain III: Educational Principles Applied to Simulation (Society for Simulation in Healthcare, 2018).

[LEARNING OUTCOMES]

- Discuss the necessity of professional development in simulation education.
- Describe the role and responsibilities of a simulation leader in an organization.
- Identify methods to disseminate simulation evidence for a wider audience.
- Review the role of simulation educator mentor for novice educators.

■ THE CONTEXT OF PROFESSIONAL DEVELOPMENT

Considering that members of any given profession maintain their professional status at the will of the society they serve, continuous professional expertise development is essential. To maintain professional status, Certified Healthcare Simulation Educators™ (CHSE)™ need to understand their service in the broader context of society.

Sullivan (2005) differentiates professionals from other workers because of their responsibility in providing public goods such as healthcare. Called *civic professionals* (Sullivan), these individuals' work provides added value to the public and are concerned with public values and identity. This then creates the social contract between the profession and the public where the public grants status and authority to the profession for the service it provides within the society. A profession holds the trust of society by maintaining civic contributions to society that remain current and beneficial through the profession's efficient and legitimate self-regulation (Sullivan, 2005). Opportunities for dialogue and scrutiny of the profession by society are expected, and thus the profession is compelled to continue to develop and grow in its civic contributions to society. This is accomplished through professional development activities by members of the profession.

As professionals, faculty and clinicians in a simulation environment develop and maintain specified standards of practice in the provision of simulation healthcare education to healthcare providers through their professional organizations and societies. These standards are developed through ongoing critical analysis of best practices in the field of healthcare simulation and are continuously updated through rigorous scrutiny of the discipline. Such updates are then communicated to members of the profession through professional development activities that allow the CHSE to maintain current in the discipline and meet his or her obligation to society as civic professionals.

STAYING CURRENT AND USING EVIDENCE IN HEALTHCARE SIMULATION

With an understanding of the importance of engagement in professional development by CHSEs it is possible to explore how this can be accomplished by members of the profession. Staying current in practice is a matter of desire and curiosity. As professionals, the CHSE maintains a desire to provide the most effective educational experiences to healthcare providers who have a variety of learning styles. This desire is motivated by a curiosity that propels the CHSE to search for the most current evidence in the practice of the specialty. Keep in mind that evidence supporting development of current professional practice takes a variety of forms, including the development of techniques, interpersonal and intrapersonal skills, and leadership and management skills. Most significant to the professional development of CHSEs is the importance of maintaining communication and support among other CHSEs. Independent, isolated professional development strategies must be further discussed among CHSEs well after the development event. With ongoing collegial support, through professional networking, professional development will directly impact the knowledge and practice of CHSEs (Margolis & Parboosingh, 2015).

Evidence of this is noted by Guillemin, McDougall, and Gillam (2009), who recognized the importance of desire and curiosity in stimulating professional development, particularly in health professions due to the ever-changing healthcare environment. They note that continuing professional development (CPD) provides development of other necessary skills for success as a professional in the healthcare environment, such as communication. Also, as health professionals gain expertise within their discipline there is a need for CPD in areas such as leadership and management. These authors focus specifically on the use of CPD in helping health professionals develop ethically (Guillemin et al., 2009).

Yet focusing professional development on the professional may be limited, as discovered by Heller, Daehler, Wong, Mayumi, and Miratrix (2012). These researchers examined the relationships among professional development, teacher knowledge, practice, and learner achievement in a randomized study of 270 elementary school teachers and 7,000 students in six states. What the authors found was that professional development experiences may provide better educational outcomes when there is integration of learning content, student learning, and teaching. With this understanding, CHSEs are likely to benefit best from professional development activities that go beyond focusing solely on developing the professional, but rather include exploration of knowledge acquisition and learner experiences.

An example of the utilization of evidence specific to the practice of the CHSE is provided by Brink, Back-Pettersson, and Sernert (2012). These authors provided an example of a simulated situation and the use of group supervision as a method in learning in the simulation environment. This was a qualitative study that explored participant perceptions of the simulated, group supervision experience.

Brink et al. found that participants had a sense of security in their engagement of the process, a positive response with collegial dialogue, a direct impact on values and attitudes, and a desire to further develop professional skills. Understanding this evidence, the CHSE can utilize the interventions used by Brink et al. to enhance their own practice in development and provision of simulation scenarios.

Providing another example of the use of evidence to support the professional development of CHSEs, Roche, Pidd, and Freeman (2009) explored the need and use of workforce training in developing skills in health professionals. Although their work focused on drug and alcohol care, the concepts they presented are transferable to the professional development needs of the CHSE, specifically, the need for development to include acquisition of knowledge, attitudes, and skills. As CHSEs it is important to utilize educational skills that are flexible enough to assess, develop, and adjust to any number of individual factors that influence a learner's ability to grow from a simulation experience.

Ricketts and Fraher (2013) recognize the need for the training of healthcare professionals to be in line with reforms in healthcare delivery systems and need for an interprofessional workforce. Thus it is important for CHSEs to develop understanding of organizational structures, systems, and culture, as well as the influence of policies, and strategies that influence working conditions. This knowledge will enhance the CHSE in identifying within organizations opportunities to enhance her or his success within organizations.

PROMOTING AND LEADING EVIDENCE-BASED HEALTHCARE SIMULATION IN AN ORGANIZATION

As mentioned earlier, professional development includes a variety of topics. Understanding that healthcare simulation practices are most likely to occur within organizational systems it is prudent for the CHSE to take advantage of professional development opportunities that enhances understanding of the context within which they practice. It has been noted that organizations can be considered to be social entities involving the interplay of individuals in reaching specified goals (Scott, 2002). In order for CHSEs to succeed within the structures of organizations it is important for them to develop skills to navigate the elements of healthcare organizations.

Mulvey (2013) provided a perspective on the unique interplay among professional practitioners, their professional entities, and the employer as a triad in CPD. The CHSE needs to understand the tensions of all of these in order to effectively obtain and maintain resources, meet professional and organizational accrediting needs, and recruit and engage health professionals. An example of this is provided by Mulvey; the employer focus is on finance, including the cost of training employees, their time away from work, and the coverage needed when the employee is in simulation training. Their other concern is the financial investment and the risk of training an employee who then leaves the organization (Mulvey, 2013). The CHSE needs to understand this fiscal perspective and be prepared to present a cost–benefit analysis within the organization system, shifting the employer's perspective to "what if they stay and they are not trained?" (Mulvey, 2013).

An example of the importance for professional development of CHSE in organizational leadership is provided by Kubitskey et al. (2012). Their study identified that the attrition among teacher participants fell under three general categories:

1. A teaching assignment change

2. Organizational challenges

3. Personal challenges

Understanding these challenges up front provides the CHSE an opportunity to take a leadership role in addressing these during the development of proposals for organizational implementation. Further, this is an example of the utilization of evidence in the development of the CHSE. This study could be easily replicated to provide evidence of the positive outcomes of simulation education, thus supporting the cost-analysis benefits necessary for program sustainability within an organization.

Simmons et al. (2011) provided an example of the impact of an interprofessional educational program. The authors examined the use of five modules in teaching different topics and utilizing a variety of learning methods and teaching strategies. The authors noted the important role of immersion and experiential learning, interprofessional development in supporting practice, and anticipating change in educational and clinical practices. With an understanding of the evidence provided by Simmons et al. the CHSE can articulate to organizational leaders the significant role he or she can play in providing cost-effective educational programming, making a broader impact on patient care.

CULTIVATING AND COMMUNICATING ONE'S PROFESSIONAL DEVELOPMENT EXPERTISE

Continuous self-improvement and learning are essential to improve national health. In order to acquire the requisite competencies, professional development competencies need to be integrated into all levels of health professions' curricula along with the appropriate experiential experiences and mentoring as professional development is critical to advancing health. Healthcare providers need to learn to advocate for patients and engage in *crucial conversations* on behalf of patients in many instances. Crucial conversations are focused on tough issues, the conversations that people normally shy away from. In the professional realm, these conversations concern such issues as safety, productivity, diversity, and quality (Patterson, Grenny, McMillan, & Switzer, 2002). Healthcare simulation is an ideal forum to practice crucial conversations.

Professional development refers to a "positive change process" that healthcare providers experience in role performance, job roles, and a better relationship with colleagues (Ismail & Arokiasamy, 2007). Safety, quality, and excellence underscore the need for healthcare providers to keep their skills and competencies current through ongoing professional development and career advancement (Adeniran, Smith Glasgow, Bhattacharya, & Xu, 2013). The influence of mentorship and self-efficacy on professional development deserves careful consideration. Mentors provide their protégés access to social networks that include sources of knowledge and professional contacts not available through normal channels. Self-efficacy influences how healthcare providers set career goals, which influences not only the initiation of behavior, but also the persistence of behavior in the presence of adversity. Moreover, self-efficacious individuals accept their roles as protégés with greater receptivity and willingness to engage in professional development activities, enhancing their capabilities and competencies (Adeniran et al., 2013).

Self-efficacy as a concept evolved from Albert Bandura's Social Cognitive Theory (SCT) of behavior (Bandura, 1977). SCT contends that individuals learn from the observation of others in a shared social environment. *Learning occurs if the role model is relevant, credible, and knowledgeable.* In the context of mentoring, protégés benefit from mentors who have the expert knowledge, social reference, credibility, and authority leading to empowerment (Bandura, 1977). Self-efficacy is considered one of the most powerful motivational predictors of success in one's career (Spurk & Abele, 2014).

In the context of healthcare simulation, the organizational leader in simulation needs to utilize best practices and maintain currency in the field, as well as serve as a role model. This can be accomplished in a variety of ways:

1. Conferences
2. Professional organizations
3. Continuing education
4. Literature on eimulation
5. Mentors
6. Portfolio development

A list of resources, although not exhaustive, would include:

- The International Nursing Association for Clinical Simulation and Learning inacsl.org
- Society for Simulation in Healthcare www.ssih.org
- International Meeting on Simulation in Healthcare www.simulationinformation.com/events/international-meeting-simulation-healthcare-imsh-2012
- Simulation in Healthcare www.journals.lww.com/simulationinhealthcare/pages/default.aspx
- *Clinical Simulation in Nursing* www.journals.elsevier.com/clinical-simulation-in-nursing/
- *Journal of Simulation* www.palgrave-journals.com/jos/journal/v3/n3/full/jos200910a.html

In addition, there are simulation conferences associated with academic health centers and universities and experts in simulation who can provide consultation. Specific attention to one's professional development in simulation can lead to increased knowledge, skill, and confidence in leading simulation scenarios in an organization. Once mastery is obtained, the simulation expert has a responsibility to share his or her expertise via conferences, journal articles, and playing a mentoring or consultant role.

THE MENTORING ROLE

Mentors support protégés to gain new competencies in a broad spectrum of skills, providing them challenges and opportunities to grow (Lombardo & Eichinger, 2009). Mentors promote learning and competencies that contribute to healthcare provider's vitality and career success. Koberg, Boss, and Goodman (1998) found that those who received mentoring reported higher levels of self-esteem and confidence than nonmentored healthcare professionals. Further, mentoring facilitates critical thinking, a connection to practice supporting professional development that can influence healthcare. This is especially true in the faculty/student role with respect to simulation. Further, Walton, Chute, and Ball (2011) note that faculty who, in their respective roles, function as role models and mentors, also need to use evidence-based teaching in their simulation activities to effectively convey the art and science of simulation. Walton et al. (2011) argue that faculty do not have adequate evidence-based resources on how students learn through simulation. Walton et al. suggests the use of a midrange conceptual model, Negotiating the Role of the Professional Nurse, as this particular model of the professional socialization assists faculty in facilitating students' development during simulation learning activities addressing such concepts as:

1. Feeling like an imposter
2. Trial and error
3. Taking the role seriously
4. Transference
5. Professionalization

Faculty strategies for each concept phase range from: "Validating students' feelings, debriefing with gentleness, role modeling expectations, asking questions about self-improvement and assisting students with visualizing goals" (Walton, Chute, and Ball, 2011, p. 301).

Benner, Sutphen, Leonard, and Day (2010) support a three-pronged approach needed in the professional role. These three attributes (Figure 20.1) are vital in the development of critical reasoning and professional development.

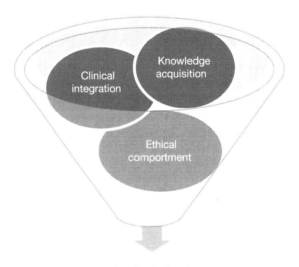

Professional role development

FIGURE 20.1 Benner, Sutphen, Leonard, and Day's three-pronged approach, needed in the professional role.

In addition, fostering the professional development of healthcare providers requires experiential and situated learning, best conducted in a simulated environment, as these individuals must be prepared for the actual clinical situations or crucial conversations marked by uncertainty in the real world (Crider & McNiesh, 2011).

DEVELOPMENT OF THE PORTFOLIO

Packaging one's self to effectively communicate and capture one's work is very important to advancing one's career. The professional portfolio/dossier is one vehicle to display one's work when applying for appointments, certifications, promotions, and tenure. A portfolio or dossier should include sample publications, grant submissions, awards, syllabi, evaluations, simulation scenarios, photos, and recommendation letters. A portfolio or dossier is also a practical way to reflect upon and document one's work with respect to teaching, research, and service. The value of self-reflection of one's work cannot be underscored. The process lends itself to deep self-analysis—it provides a lens for the individual and reviewer to analyze one's accomplishments in the area of simulation (Seldin & Miller, 2009). In recent years, electronic portfolios have come into use in institutions as a means for students to display their work and demonstrate competency related to writing, clinical objectives, and so on. The portfolio should involve the efforts of the individual and the advice of the mentor in order to showcase the candidate's work in the best possible light, in addition to providing the reviewers with insight into the candidate's strengths, accomplishments, and work. Many institutions have requirements for the portfolio in terms of format and content. Typically, a philosophy, one's objectives, examples of work, reflections, and so on are required at some level (Wittmann-Price, 2012).

SUMMARY

The process of professional development is best conducted in the formative years of one's education so healthcare providers can have maximum impact on the profession and health. It is also known that professional development is also largely contextual—different settings will require different expectations and different practices. Therefore, a variety of professional developmental experiences is recommended in the educational journey. Simulation provides a *dress rehearsal* for *real* leadership concerns, crucial conversations, ethical dilemmas, and advocacy issues.

> **SIMULATION TEACHING TIP 20.1**
>
> "Flipping" the classroom may provide time to engage in dialogue with students before/after the simulation experience.
>
> "Ensure that teachers 'think out loud' and make their cognitive 'struggles' with difficult issues visible to students so students can see how one 'thinks like a nurse'" (Valiga, 2012, p. 491). Role model, role model, role model!

CASE STUDY 20.1

Your Role: Colleague Who Takes Advantage of Coworkers

Dr. Sykes is frequently absent due to family obligations and is constantly asking you to cover her simulation healthcare experience, which she is providing to occupational therapy learners. You have worked with her for 3 years but this is getting old. She always has an emergency or excuse. You feel as though she is taking advantage of you.
Note: This case can be adapted for any work setting.
Case Study Objective:
Engage in a crucial conversation with your colleague regarding her behavior.
Checklist
Objectively stated personal experience with concrete examples in a clear, concise manner.
Addressed personal feelings.

- Used "I" statements.
- Remained calm.
- Listened actively.
- Summarized a crucial conversation indicating that he or she would no longer rearrange his or her schedule.

CASE STUDY 20.2

Your Role: Mentor and Faculty Colleague for a Junior CHSE

You are participating in a laboratory session with your colleague, Dr. Pinter, who teaches another section. You note that Dr. Pinter becomes very defensive and sarcastic with learners when they ask what you believe to be appropriate questions. At one point, Dr. Pinter is borderline hostile. You are embarrassed.
Case Study Objective:
Engage in a crucial conversation with your colleague regarding her defensive and sarcastic behavior.
Checklist

- Objectively summarized observations in a private setting
- Explicitly addressed unprofessional behavior
- Used "I" statements
- Remained calm
- Listened actively
- Role modeled appropriate way to respond to questions
- Offered faculty development resources
- Summarized crucial conversation indicating that he or she must maintain a professional demeanor and open/trusting learning environment for students and explained consequences if not maintained.

PRACTICE QUESTIONS

1. The novice healthcare simulation educator needs additional understanding of the governing principle of simulation education when she states:

    A. "Simulation is part of the routine learning for health professionals."
    B. "Simulation assists society."
    C. "Simulation's goal is patient care outcomes."
    D. "Using simulation assists in procedural practice."

2. Developing a social contract includes:

    A. Professionals understanding their roles
    B. Society supporting the profession
    C. Society trusting the works of the profession
    D. Being concerned with public values

3. Simulation standards of practice are developed by:

    A. Experts teaching simulation to novice educators
    B. Critical analysis of best practice
    C. Solidifying practices
    D. Educators maintaining a specific set of skills

4. Continuous professional development (CPD) in simulation assists professionals to increase in:

    A. Career advancement
    B. Debriefing
    C. Communication
    D. Moulage

5. Continuous professional development (CPD) in simulation has been demonstrated to increase:

    A. Learner knowledge
    B. Professional career attainment
    C. Higher fidelity
    D. Critical analysis

6. The graduate students needs a better understanding of continuous professional development (CPD) for healthcare simulation educators when he states that CPD:

    A. "Increases knowledge about systems, structures, and organizational cultures."
    B. "Is not needed to address basic knowledge skills, and attitudes."
    C. "Increases engagement in the learning processes."
    D. "Promotes learning outcomes for teachers and students."

7. Considerations of organizations that healthcare simulation educators should embrace pertain to:

    A. Financial burden
    B. Their career trajectory
    C. Future organizational structure and changes
    D. Personal agendas of management

8. Crucial conversations in professional healthcare situations many times include this subject:

    A. Promotion
    B. Diversity
    C. Compensation
    D. Leadership

9. One of the attributes not included in developing self-efficacy in the simulation learning is:

    A. Relevancy
    B. Credibility
    C. Knowledge
    D. Critical thinking

10. The third step of negotiating a professional role that can be fostered in a simulation scenario is:

    A. Feeling like an imposter
    B. Trial and error
    C. Taking the role seriously
    D. Transference

REFERENCES

Adeniran, R., Smith Glasgow, M. E., Bhattacharya, A., & Xu, Y. (2013). Career advancement and professional development in nursing. *Nursing Outlook*, *61*(6), 437–446. doi:10.1016/j.outlook.2013.05.009

Bandura, A. (1977). Self-efficacy: Toward a unifying theory of behavioral change. *Psychological Review*, *84*, 191–215. doi:10.1037/0033-295x.84.2.191

Benner, P., Sutphen, M., Leonard, V., & Day, L. (2010). *Educating nurses: A call for radical transformation*. San Francisco, CA: Jossey-Bass/Carnegie Foundation for the Advancement of Teaching.

Brink, P., Back-Pettersson, S., & Sernert, N. (2012). Group supervision as a means of developing professional competence within pre-hospital care. *International Emergency Nursing*, *20*(2), 76–82. doi:10.1016/j.ienj.2011.04.001

Crider, M., & McNiesh, S. (2011). Integrating a professional apprenticeship model with psychiatric clinical simulation. *Journal of Psychosocial Nursing & Mental Health Services*, *49*(5), 42–49. doi:10.3928/02793695-20110329-01

Guillemin, M., McDougall, R., & Gillam, L. (2009). Developing "ethical mindfulness" in continuing professional development in healthcare: Use of a personal narrative approach. *Cambridge Quarterly of Healthcare Ethics*, *18*, 197–208. doi:10.1017/S096318010909032X

Heller, J. I., Daehler, K. R., Wong, N., Mayumi, S., & Miratrix, L. W. (2012). Differential effects of three professional development models on teacher knowledge and student achievement in elementary science. *Journal of Research in Science Teaching*, *49*(3), 333–362. doi:10.1002/tea.2100

Ismail, M., & Arokiasamy L. (2007). Exploring mentoring as a tool for career advancement of academics in private higher education institutions in Malaysia. *Journal of International Social Research*, *1*(1), 135–148.

Koberg, C. S., Boss, R. W., & Goodman, E. (1998). Factors and outcomes associated with mentoring among health-care professionals. *Journal of Vocational Behavior*, *53*(1), 58–72. doi:10.1006/jvbe.1997.1607

Kubitskey, B. W., Vath, R. J., Johnson, H. J., Fishman, B. J., Konstantopoulos, S., & Park, G. J. (2012). Examining study attrition: Implications for experimental research on professional development. *Teaching and Teacher Education*, 28(3), 418–427. doi:10.1016/j.tate.2011.11.008

Lombardo, M. M., & Eichinger, R. W. (2009). *FYI for your improvement: A guide for development and coaching* (5th ed.). Minneapolis, MN: Lominger International: A Korn/Ferry.

Margolis, A., & Parboosingh, J. (2015). Networked learning and network science: Potential applications to health professionals' continuing education and development. *Journal of Continuing Education in the Health Professions*, 35(3), 2011–2019. doi:10.1002/chp.21295

Mulvey, R. (2013). How to be a good professional: existentialist continuing professional development (CPD). *British Journal of Guidance & Counseling*, 41(3), 267–276. doi:10.1080/03069885.2013.773961

Patterson, K., Grenny, J., McMillan, R., & Switzer, A. (2011). *Crucial conversations: Tools for talking when the stakes are high* (2nd ed.). New York, NY: McGraw-Hill.

Ricketts, T. C., & Fraher, E. P. (2013). Reconfiguring health workforce policy so that education, training, and actual delivery of care are closely connected. *Health Affairs*, 32(11), 1874–1880.

Roche, A. M., Pidd, K., & Freeman, T. (2009). Achieving professional practice change: From training to workforce development. *Drug and Alcohol Review*, 28(5), 550–557. doi:10.1111/j.1465-3362.2009.00111.x

Scott, W. R. (2002). *Organizations: Rational, natural, and open systems* (5th ed.). Upper Saddle River, NJ: Prentice Hall.

Seldin, P., & Miller, J. E. (2009). *The academic portfolio: A practical guide to teaching, research, and service*. San Francisco, CA: Jossey-Bass.

Simmons, B., Oandasan, I., Soklaradis, S., Esdaile, M., Barker, K., Kwan, D., & Wagner, S. (2011). Evaluating the effectiveness of an interprofessional education faculty development course: The transfer of interprofessional learning to the academic and clinical practice setting. *Journal of Interprofessional Care*, 25(2), 156–157. doi:10.3109/13561820.2010.515044

Society for Simulation in Healthcare. (2018). *Certified Healthcare Simulation Educator Examination Blueprint, 2018 Version*. Retrieved from http://www.ssih.org/Portals/48/Certification/CHSE_Docs/CHSE_Examination_Blueprint.pdf

Spurk, D., & Abele, A. E. (2014). Synchronous and time-lagged effects between occupational self-efficacy and objective and subjective career success: Findings from a four-wave and 9-year longitudinal study. *Journal of Vocational Behavior*, 84(2), 119–132. doi:10.1016/j.jvb.2013.12.002

Sullivan, W. M. (2005). *Work and integrity: The crisis and promise of professionalism in America* (2nd ed.). San Francisco, CA: Jossey-Bass.

Valiga, T. (2012). Nursing education trends: Future implications and predictions. *Nursing Clinics of North America*, 47(4), 423–434. doi:10.1016/j.cnur.2012.07.007

Walton, J., Chute, E., & Ball, L. (2011). Negotiating the role of the professional nurse: The pedagogy of simulation: A grounded theory study. *Journal of Professional Nursing*, 27(5), 299–310. doi:10.1016/j.profnurs.2011.04.005

Wittmann-Price, R. A. (2012). *Fast facts for developing a nursing academic portfolio*. New York, NY: Springer Publishing.

21

The Role of Research in Simulation

JUDY I. MURPHY

If we knew what it was we were doing, it would not be called research, would it?

—Albert Einstein

This chapter addresses Domain III: Educational Principles Applied to Simulation (Society for Simulation in Healthcare [SSH], 2018).

[LEARNING OUTCOMES]

- Discuss the importance of research in simulation for healthcare educators.
- Identify the current state of simulation research.
- Identify gaps in simulation research.
- Discuss research knowledge via case study and practice questions.

Although healthcare simulation has been around for more than 40 years, its movement to the forefront in academe and practice is fairly recent. Simulation literature and research are increasing at an astounding rate. Yet, there are many things that we do not know. This chapter discusses the importance of research in simulation, provides a summary of the current state of the research on simulation, identifies gaps in the literature, and provides teaching tips and application exercises.

One of the hottest topics being debated and studied is "How much clinical time can be substituted with simulation?" Several state boards of nursing have limited the number of hours of simulation that can be substituted for clinical time. In 2010, the National Council of State Boards of Nursing (NCSBN) surveyed 1,729 nursing programs in the United States (Hayden, 2010; Kardong-Edgren, Wilhaus, Bennett, & Hayden, 2012). Sixty-two percent of the programs from all 50 states and the District of Columbia responded. Overall, 87% reported using either high or medium fidelity in their programs. Fifty-five percent used simulation in five or more courses. The response to the question of whether simulation can or should replace clinical time was affirmative by 77% of respondents. Faculty indicated that 25% of clinical time could be replaced with simulation. However, some state boards of nursing require that a specific amount of time be spent in direct care. In Ohio, simulation hours cannot be counted as clinical hours, whereas in Florida, no more than 25% of clinical time can be replaced with clinical simulation. In 2015, a follow-up survey was sent to more than 1,400 prelicensure schools of nursing to identify substitution of simulation for clinical time. A standard substitution ratio for simulation time replacing clinical time does not exist. Thirty-two percent of the schools responded with representation from all states. Reasons for substituting simulation for clinical supervision include value simulation as a teaching methodology (90%) and lack of clinical placements (40%). Seventy-one percent of the schools did not have any Certified Healthcare Simulation Educators™. Simulation training was done by the vendor, continuing education, or a workshop. This survey indicates there is a gap between faculty with expertise with simulation and the need for more faculty development.

Using Weinger's conceptual framework (2010), the pharmacology of simulation to inform simulation research, we still do not know the best dose of simulation needed to get the best response from the learners. The need to answer these questions will be a driving force in simulation research as research findings support the use of simulation, its effectiveness, and its relationship to patient safety. For this review, the current state of the research on simulation is divided into the three components of simulation: prebriefing/orientation, simulation, and debriefing.

PREBRIEFING

According to Standards of Best Practice: Simulation Glossary (International Nursing Association for Clinical Simulation and Learning [INACSL], 2016), *prebriefing* is an information or orientation session immediately prior to the start of simulation-based education (SBE) in which instructions or preparatory information is given to the participants. The purpose of prebriefing is to establish a psychologically safe environment for participants. Suggested activities include reviewing objectives; creating a "fiction contract"; and orienting participants to the equipment, environment, mannequin, roles, time allotment, and scenario (INACSL, 2016). The fiction contract includes confidentiality and believing that the simulation is real.

A concept analysis by Page-Cutrara (2015) "indicates the need for research on the concept of prebriefing to maximize teaching and learning" (p. 335). There is not any consistency in prebriefing and the outcomes of prebriefing have not been well studied.

Prebriefing is important to set the tone and to focus learners on the main objective, which is learning. Healthcare professionals tend to focus on performance outcomes rather than learning. Learners are disappointed if they do not meet their performance expectations. Professional Integrity of Participants Standard (INACSL, 2016) Outlines guidelines and criteria are essential to support mutual respect, professional integrity, and confidentiality. What happens in simulation and debriefing stays in simulation and debriefing. If learners fear that their performance will be discussed outside of simulation, they will be more anxious and will focus on the outcome of simulation rather than learning (Dieckmann, Molin Friis, Lippert, & Ostergaard, 2009).

Anxiety is a common emotion expressed by learners participating in simulation. Cato (2013) found that high learner anxiety related to simulation was associated with fear of making a mistake, being filmed, being observed by faculty and peers, and discriminating between what is real and what is simulation. Preparation was identified as being critically important to build confidence in simulation. Learners in this study requested that they be alerted as to what skills will be used in a simulation in advance so they can practice if needed.

Facilitators to learning from simulation identified by learners include:

> **SIMULATION TEACHING TIP 21.1**
>
> Healthcare simulation educators are usually not aware of recent or past life experiences of learners that may influence how they respond in simulation. Has a loved one been in the intensive care unit (ICU) recently, or has there been a death in the family? Learners need to be briefed early on that simulation may trigger some strong emotions for them. Because research shows that observers learn as much as participants (Jeffries, 2012), learners should be given the option to observe rather than participate in a simulation that may be an emotional trigger.

- Orientation
- Preparation
- Safe environment
- Feedback during debriefing

There is very little research on the effect of prebriefing/orientation on student learning. Cato's recent unpublished doctoral research provides initial evidence as to the importance of adequate preparation prior to a simulation.

SIMULATION

An educational strategy in which a particular set of conditions is created or replicated to resemble authentic situations that are possible in real life. Simulation can incorporate one or more modalities to promote, improve, or validate a participant's performance (INACSL, 2016).

According to the National League for Nursing (NLN) and Jeffries's theoretical framework (updated 2014), simulation has five components:

1. Teacher
2. Participant (changed from student)
3. Educational practices
4. Design characteristics
5. Simulation interventions and outcomes (Ravert & McAfooes, 2013)

The change from *learner* to *participant* was based on the evidence and a review of the literature. *Participant* is more inclusive as it includes demographics, role and responsibilities, attributes, and values. For the purpose of this review, this section focuses on outcomes of simulation. A systematic review of simulation research conducted by Cant and Cooper (2010) provides an extensive evaluation of the evidence behind simulation as an educational tool in nursing. The review includes

12 quantitative studies that compared the effectiveness of medium- to high-fidelity simulations compared to other methods of education, such as lecture, group interaction, case studies, debriefings, or tests. In the medical education literature, Okuda et al. (2009) reported that simulation is an effective means to identify communication errors and poor teamwork. Only one study was a randomized controlled trial; most were pre- and posttest experiments with a comparison group. Seven studies included a validated assessment measure. The authors found that "all 12 studies reported statistical improvements in knowledge, skill, critical thinking ability, and/or confidence after simulation education" (Cant & Cooper, 2010, p. 6). Kirkpatrick's evaluation model (Kirkpatrick & Kirkpatrick, 2006) is used to present examples of research on evaluation. In Kirkpatrick's model, the four levels of evaluation consist of:

1. Reaction
2. Learning
3. Behavior
4. Results

Learner satisfaction and self-confidence (Level 1), both reactions to simulation, are the measures that have been the most heavily researched. Learners' reaction to simulation has been overwhelmingly positive (Jeffries, 2012). According to Chickering and Gamson (1987), learner performance is higher when learners are satisfied with learning experiences. In simulation, students learn to think critically and solve problems in a safe environment. They can make mistakes, from which they will learn without putting patients at risk. The opportunity to be "the nurse" instead of the learner helps to promote self-confidence. In a comparative study, Alfes (2011) found that learners who participated in a simulation were more self-confident than the control group.

Kunst, Mitchell, and Johnston (2016) did an integrative review of mannequin simulation in mental health nursing. Of the 2,034 articles reviewed between 2000 and 2016, only nine met the inclusion criteria for their review. From this research, an increase in learner confidence, self-efficacy in knowledge, and communication was found after the simulations.

Kirkpatrick's learning (Level 2) has been measured in cognitive (Lasater, 2007; Radhakrishnan, Roche, & Cunningham, 2007), affective (Bambini, Washburn, & Perkins, 2009; Schoening, Sittner, & Todd, 2006), and psychomotor domains (Murray et al., 2007; Rosen, Salas, Silvestri, Wu, & Lazzara, 2008). In these simulation studies, significant learning occurred when best practices of simulation were used. Lasater (2007) developed a rubric to measure clinical judgment by scoring learners on a scale that rated

- Noticing
- Interpreting
- Responding
- Reflecting

Learners were rated as beginning, developing, accomplished, or exemplary on this tool.

Radhakrishnan et al. (2007) developed the Clinical Simulation Evaluation Tool (CSET), a clinical performance tool, to measure

- Basic and problem-based assessment
- Prioritization
- Delegation
- Communication
- Interventions and safety

When measuring learning in the cognitive domain, it is important to design the simulation so that learners will be able to demonstrate learning by applying knowledge to make decisions in the scenario.

Evaluation in the affective domain is more subjective. Affective learning and Kirkpatrick's reaction (Level 1) overlap. Many authors have developed both quantitative and qualitative instruments to measure learners' perceptions of simulation. Bambini et al. (2009) measured confidence before and after a simulation. Likewise, Schoening et al. (2006) also measured learners' perceptions of a maternal–child simulation. Although the literature shows (Bandura, 2000; Zimmerman, 2000) that self-efficacy has been a predictor of learners' motivation and learning, simulation research is lacking in making the connection.

Studies in the psychomotor domain measure a range of skills from basic to complex. There is an overlap between the cognitive and psychomotor domain because one must have the knowledge to complete the skill (Adamson, Jeffries, & Rogers, 2012). Instruments to measure performance of medical learners and medical residents were developed by Rosen et al. (2008) and Murray et al. (2007). Both instruments were specifically designed for performance measurement in simulation. Although these psychomotor tools are specific to medical skills, the American Heart Association Basic Life Support (BLS) and Advanced Cardiac Life Support (ACLS) performance tools may be used for research across professions. In a meta-analytic comparative review McGaghie, Issenberg, Cohen, Barsuk, and Wayne (2011) found that simulation-based medical education when combined with deliberate practice was superior to traditional clinical medical education.

Kirkpatrick's last two levels, behavior (3) and results (4), have not been studied as extensively as satisfaction and learning. Behavior measures change in job performance resulting from the learning process, whereas results measure the tangible outcome of the learning process in relation to cost, quality, and efficiency. Collectively, this work is considered translational science (McGaghie, Issenberg, Petrusa, & Scalese, 2010). In the critical review of simulation-based medical education research of McGaghie et al., the researchers found that studies that show transfer to practice outcomes are difficult to design and execute. Some promising work in this regard has been found with medical residents who trained to mastery with central-line insertions in a simulation lab. These residents had significantly less procedural complications in an ICU than those who did not train to mastery in simulation (Barsuk, McGaghie, Cohen, O'Leary, & Wayne, 2009).

Examining the design and pedagogy of simulation as an educational intervention, Schaefer et al. (2011) reviewed the literature from 1990 to 2010. Their review included publications from nursing education, hospital and prehospital domain, virtual reality, task training, and hybrid use of standardized (simulated) patients. They examined the validity and reliability of the simulator and of the performance evaluation tool, the study design, and the translational impact. From their review, they concluded that there is a lack of sufficient well-designed studies to draw consensus. However, they identified well-designed studies that translated to clinical practice and improved patient safety. In a systematic review and meta-analysis done by Cook et al. (2011) they concluded that "technology-enhanced simulation training in health education is consistently associated with large effects for outcomes of knowledge, skills, and behaviours and moderate effects for patient-related outcomes" (p. 978).

In a systematic review of hospital-based simulation in nursing education, Rutherford-Hemming and Alfes (2017) reviewed 224 manuscripts narrowed down to only 65, which met their inclusion criteria from January 2012 to October 2015. They concluded that more randomized control trials with power analysis and validated measurement instruments are needed to improve rigor of findings. Kirkpatrick's Level 4 Outcome results are the gold star of simulation research. However, due to the multiple variables that affect patient outcomes it is difficult to prove that simulation was the primary cause of improvement. Deliberate practice using task trainers with randomized groups is a little easier to correlate to training with Level 4 Outcome (Barsuk et al., 2009).

A valid reliable tool for assessing communication skills is called the Health Assessment Communication Assessment Tool (HCAT; Pagano et al., 2015). This tool was validated by 218 international and interprofessional educators. The average intraclass correlation coefficient was 0.99, simulation is not just about tasks and procedures and teamwork. Simulation can be used for professional development and improved communication skills. This valid reliable measure may spur more research in this area.

In summary, the gaps in simulation research on learning outcomes include the need to explore and quantify sources of measurement error, develop defensible scoring rubrics and methodologies, establish and quantify the relationship between performance in simulation scenarios and in patient care situations, and investigate the impact of implementing high-stakes testing using simulation (Boulet et al., 2011).

DEBRIEFING

According to the INACSL terminology (2016), *debriefing* is a reflective process immediately following the SBE that is led by a trained facilitator using an evidence-based debriefing model. Participants' reflective thinking is encouraged, and feedback is provided regarding the participants' performance while various aspects of the completed simulation are discussed. Participants are encouraged to explore emotions and question, reflect, and provide feedback to one another. The purpose of debriefing is to move toward assimilation and accommodation to transfer learning to future situations (INACSL, 2016).

Participants' reflective thinking is encouraged, and feedback is provided regarding the participants' performance while various aspects of the simulation are discussed. Simulation is the vehicle that takes participants to learning, which is what occurs in debriefing. There are a variety of methods of debriefing, such as

- Plus-delta debriefing
- Advocacy inquiry also known as *Debriefing with Good Judgment*
- Debriefing for Meaningful Learning (DM)

For more detail on these debriefing methods see Chapter 18. Some programs videotape the scenarios and use the videos in debriefing. In a study done by Rossignol (2017), no difference in stress or performance was seen between video-assisted debriefing and oral debriefing. If used properly, showing some critical points in the video can be beneficial but showing the entire video is not helpful (Rossignol, 2017). Stress levels decreased with repeated simulations. According to INACSL Standards of Best Practice: Simulation facilitation, "The facilitator is a trained individual who provides guidance, support, and structure at some or all stages of simulation-based learning including prebriefing, simulation, and/or debriefing" (Decker et al., 2013, pp. S27–S29).

"A facilitator assumes responsibility and oversight for managing the entire simulation-based experience" (INACSL Standards Committee, 2016, p. S16). Although debriefing is a critical component of simulation, the literature indicates there is a need for studies focused on debriefing principles (Neill & Wotton, 2011; Raemer et al., 2011). In a systematic review of the literature in nursing on debriefing, Neill and Wotton found that the format of debriefing varied across institutions; there was no agreement on one developmental framework or on the recommended amount of time spent in debriefing in relation to time spent in simulation. In a review of the medical literature, McGaghie et al. (2010) found that instructor training is an important component of effective simulation debriefing (see Chapter 18). In their review, they found that the instructor and learner did not need to be from the same profession. Gaps in understanding include whether simulation instructors should be certified for various devices, and what the appropriate learning models are for simulation instructors.

Salas, Cooke, and Rosen (2008) found evidence to support that debriefings must be diagnostic and provide a supportive learning environment. The facilitator should

- Be educated on the art and science of leading debriefings
- Focus on just a few critical performance measures during debriefing
- Provide process feedback early and outcome feedback later
- Shorten the delay between task performance and feedback

From the extensive simulation literature in both nursing and medicine, several gaps in our knowledge on debriefing exist. What is the best dose and model of debriefing? Do some methods provide more efficient learning, thus requiring fewer resources and yielding longer lasting results?

RESEARCH

Two research paradigms are described in Table 21.1. These paradigms assume different philosophies in relation to our understanding of reality. Although this chapter is not meant to provide comprehensive information on research frameworks, a review of the basics will help readers see the benefit in both paradigms and how a synthesis of research involving both paradigms enhances our understanding.

> **EVIDENCE-BASED SIMULATION PRACTICE 21.1**
>
> Lasater (2007) investigated nursing students using simulation in a qualitative research study. First-term nursing students using high-fidelity simulation as part of the regular curriculum perceived that it assisted them in the development of clinical judgment.

TABLE 21.1
Research Frameworks

RESEARCH PARADIGM	OVERVIEW	BENEFITS	CHALLENGES
Quantitative	Assumes that reality is objective, measurable, value-free, and unbiased using deductive reasoning.	Uses reliable and valid instruments and clearly describes the population to make results generalizable.	Requires valid and reliable measuring tools. The environment and learner differences may not allow for experimental design.
Qualitative	Assumes that reality is subjective, varying as seen by study participants, value-laden, and biased, using inductive reasoning.	Emerging design provides flexibility to study according to themes identified in the process. A good design used for a pilot study to identify key concepts and variables that may influence outcomes.	Data analysis is labor intensive. Findings may not be generalizable or reproducible in a different environment with a different population.

> **EVIDENCE-BASED SIMULATION PRACTICE 21.2**
>
> Sullivan-Mann, Perron, and Fellner (2009) studied associate degree nursing students' ($N = 53$) critical thinking scores before and after simulation experiences. The tool used was the Health Sciences Reasoning Test (Facione & Facione, 2006). Learners exposed to simulation experienced an increase in critical thinking scores compared to a control group.

> **EVIDENCE-BASED SIMULATION PRACTICE 21.3**
>
> Shapiro et al. (2004) used a mixed-method approach to study simulation with interprofessional students who would respond in an emergency. One group was exposed to simulation education and another was not. The simulation-trained group scored slightly higher in observed behavior and rated the simulation learning experiences as valuable.
>
> Simulation research can be looked at from the overall design perspective or from the type of methods used. So although the reasoning may be inductive or deductive, a mixed-method design in which both qualitative and quantitative methods are used adds to the richness of the data. Until we have valid, reliable tools that can be used across professions, using a mixed-method approach will enhance our understanding of the effect of simulation on learning.

> **EVIDENCE-BASED SIMULATION PRACTICE 21.4**
>
> In a critical review of simulation-enhanced interprofessional education, Palaganas, Brunette, and Winslow (2016) noted that out of 7,062 articles only 54 met the criteria for the review. Ultimately they concluded that the quality of the existing literature is inadequate to identify factors that affect learning using simulation enhanced interprofessional education (IPE).

■ SIMULATION RESEARCH RESOURCES

Keeping Current

One of the most important ways to keep up to date on the research in simulation is by joining one or more of the simulation societies. The two organizations that are most active in simulation research, accreditation, and developing standards of best practice are the INACSL and the Society for Simulation in Healthcare (SSH). Both organizations publish a monthly journal devoted to simulation. The journal articles are peer reviewed and indexed in medical and nursing databases. Other associations that may be helpful include the Association of Standardized Patient Educators (ASPEs) and Simulation Learning, Education and Research Network (SimLEARN). The organizational mission or goals are listed in Table 21.2. All four organizations provide a community of practice in which a group of individuals share a common interest, craft, or profession (Lave & Wenger, 1991).

In 2004, the SSH was established to represent the rapidly growing group of educators and researchers who use a variety of simulation techniques for education, testing, and research in healthcare. The SSH is the organization that provides the certification examination and accredits simulation programs. Programs that comply with core standards and fulfilment of standards applied to one or more of the areas of assessment, research, teaching/education, and/or systems integration are eligible for application. The SSH goal is to lead in facilitating excellence in (multispecialty) healthcare education, practice, and research through simulation modalities.

On July 17, 2009, the acting undersecretary for health authorized the establishment of a national simulation training and education program for the Veterans Health Administration (VHA). Dubbed the "Simulation Learning, Education and Research Network" or SimLEARN, the program is improving the quality of healthcare services for America's veterans through the application of simulation-based learning strategies in clinical workforce development. The program operations and management are aligned with the VHA Employee Education System (EES) in close collaboration with VHA's Office of Patient

> **SIMULATION TEACHING TIP 21.2**
>
> Although I have been using simulation as a teaching/learning pedagogy for more than a decade, I find that I learn something new each time I engage with INACSL, SimLEARN, or SSH. Thus, even for the expert in simulation, these resources provide a place to learn and cocreate simulation knowledge, skills, and best practices (www.inacsl.org/learn/journal).

TABLE 21.2
Simulation Organizations for Healthcare Educators

ORGANIZATION	MISSION/GOALS	PUBLICATION
INACSL	INACSL promotes research and disseminates evidence-based practice standards for clinical simulation methodologies and learning environments. The organization is a community of practice, a place where novice and expert practitioners can network, share ideas, and learn from and with each other about the knowledge, skills, and attitudes necessary for best practices in the use of simulation.	*Clinical Simulations in Nursing*
SSH	The SSH's mission is to improve performance and reduce errors in patient care using all types of simulation, including task trainers, human patient simulators, virtual reality, and SPs. The SSH is a multidisciplinary, multispecialty, international society with ties to many medical specialties, nursing, allied health paramedical personnel, and industry (ssih.org/about-ssh).	*Simulation in Healthcare*
ASPE	ASPE is the international organization of simulation educators dedicated to • Promoting best practices in the application of SP methodology for education, assessment, and research • Fostering the dissemination of research and scholarship in the field of SP methodology • Advancing the professional knowledge and skills of its members • Transforming professional performance through the power of human interaction (www.aspeeducators.org/node/117)	Many web resources; ASPE recently announced its collaboration with MedEdPORTAL to house SP cases. MedEdPORTAL is "A peer-reviewed, open-access journal that promotes educational scholarship and dissemination of teaching and assessment resources in the health professions" (Association of American Medical Colleges, 2018, p.1)
SimLEARN	The SimLEARN is the VHA's program for simulation in healthcare training. Serving the largest integrated healthcare system in the world, VHA's SimLEARN provides an ever-growing body of curricula and best practices that improve healthcare for our nation's Veterans (www.ssih.org/about-ssh)	SimLEARN newsletter

ASPE, Association of Standardized Patient Educators; INACSL, International Nursing Association for Clinical Simulation and Learning; SPs, standardized (simulated) patients; SimLEARN, Simulation Learning, Education and Research Network; VHA, Veterans Health Administration.

Care Services (PCSs) and Office of Nursing Services (ONSs). Although the use of simulation for healthcare training and education is not new to VHA, it has become critical for VHA to develop an integrated approach to better realize the maximum benefits of simulation for VHA staff and the veterans it serves.

These simulation practice communities decrease the learning curve for those new to simulation and help to avoid reinventing the wheel. INACSL, SSH, SimLEARN, and ASPE use the collective expertise of their leaders and membership to advance the science of simulation.

In summary, although simulation is increasingly being used in education and practice, the strength of the evidence is not yet strong. Gaps in the research exist in the orientation, simulation, and debriefing areas. Evidence as to learner satisfaction, self-confidence, and perception of simulation is fairly strong.

Questions that still need to be answered include:

- How much simulation can replace clinical time?
- How much time should be spent in simulation?
- How much time spent in debriefing?
- How do we measure learning from simulation?
- How do we know whether what students learn in simulation is transferred to actual practice?

In order to be up to date on the research, simulation educators and simulation personnel need to stay connected with simulation societies, attend simulation conferences, and read the simulation literature. As this pedagogy continues to diffuse through practice and academia, continued research and lifelong learning will be essential to ensure excellence in simulation.

CASE STUDY 21.1

Mary is an experienced nurse educator, but is new to simulation. One of her students confides that recently she lost a child and is concerned that she might not be able to effectively provide emergency care. Mary tells the learner that the simulation is essential to the course and that she must participate. Does this format follow recommendations of simulation research? How would you counsel Mary to improve her simulation educator skills?

CASE STUDY DISCUSSION

Mary's response does not follow recommendations. As observers who are actively engaged get just as much out of simulation as participants, Mary should give the learner a choice to observe rather than participate in this emotionally charged simulation. Mary should address the possibility of emotional triggers in the orientation/prebrief. Learners should be given the choice to observe rather than participate in the simulation if they think that participation may be too painful.

PRACTICE QUESTIONS

1. Which of Kirkpatrick's levels of evaluation has been *least* heavily researched in simulation?

    A. Level 1, Reaction
    B. Level 2, Learning
    C. Level 3, Behavior
    D. Level 4, Results

2. Which is the best method to utilize to video record a team simulation?

    A. Show the entire video with no comments.
    B. Bookmark while videotaping and show critical points both positive and negative.
    C. Bookmark while videotaping and just show negative points.
    D. Send the video to students to watch on their own.

3. What are the gaps in research? Select all that apply:

    A. Satisfaction
    B. Patient outcomes
    C. Confidence
    D. Valid measuring instruments

4. How does one determine the validity of an instrument?

    A. Content experts review with high correlation of agreement
    B. Piloted on 10 learners prior to use
    C. Colleague review
    D. The instrument measures the correct concepts.

5. A skilled simulation educator plans time in the simulation to include which of the following?

    A. A 10-minute debriefing
    B. Time to watch the entire video
    C. A comprehensive orientation and prebriefing
    D. Ten minutes for students to write a reflection paper

6. What is the gap in faculty simulation expertise identified in the national study of simulation programs? Check all that apply.

    A. Faculty development
    B. Vendor education
    C. Formal education
    D. Lack of Certified Healthcare Simulation Educators

7. Which component of Jeffries theoretical framework was changed?

    A. Facilitator
    B. Student
    C. Design characteristics
    D. Outcomes

8. Which organization offers certification in healthcare simulation education?

    A. International Nursing Association for Clinical Simulation and Learning (INACSL)
    B. Society for Simulation in Healthcare (SSH)
    C. Association of Standardized Patient Educator (ASPE)
    D. American Nurses Credentialing Center (ANCC)

9. From the national survey, what is the amount of simulation that can replace clinical experience?

    A. 20%
    B. 25%
    C. 50%
    D. No evidence supports a particular percentage

10. Which of the following simulation modalities would best fit for a mental health simulation?

    A. A virtual game
    B. A mannequin
    C. A standardized patient\actor
    D. A video

■ REFERENCES

Adamson, K. A., Jeffries, P. R., & Rogers, K. J. (2012). Evaluation: A critical step in simulation practice and research. In P. Jeffries (Ed.), *Simulation in nursing education: From conceptualization to evaluation* (2nd ed.). New York, NY: National League for Nursing Press.

Alfes, C. M. (2011). Evaluating the use of simulation with beginning nursing students. *Journal of Nursing Education*, 50(2), 89. doi:10.3928/01484834-20101230-03

Association of American Medical Colleges. (2018). Explore MedEdPORTAL. Retrieved from https://www.mededportal.org/

Bambini, D., Washburn, J., & Perkins, R. (2009). Outcomes of clinical simulation for novice nursing students: Communication, confidence, clinical judgment. *Nursing Education Perspectives*, 30(2), 79–82.

Bandura, A. (2000). Exercise of human agency through collective efficacy. *Current Directions in Psychological Science*, 9(3), 75–78. doi:10.1111/1467-8721.00064

Barsuk, J. H., McGaghie, W. C., Cohen, E. R., O'Leary, K. J., & Wayne, D. B. (2009). Simulation-based mastery learning reduces complications during central venous catheter insertion in a medical intensive care unit. *Critical Care Medicine*, 37(10), 2697–2701. doi:10.1097/00003246-200910000-00003

Boulet, J. R., Jeffries, P. R., Hatala, R. A., Korndorffer, J. R., Jr., Feinstein, D. M., & Roche, J. P. (2011). Research regarding methods of assessing learning outcomes. *Simulation in Healthcare*, 6(7), S48–S51. doi:10.1097/sih.0b013e31822237d0

Cant, R., & Cooper, S. (2010). Simulation-based learning in nursing education: Systematic review. *Journal of Advanced Nursing*, 66(1), 3–15. doi:10.1111/j.1365-2648.2009.05240.x

Cato, M. (2013, September). *Nursing student anxiety in simulation and its effect on learning*. Paper presented at the National League for Nursing Education Summit, Washington, DC.

Chickering, A. W., & Gamson, Z. F. (1987). Seven principles of good practice in undergraduate education. *AAHE Bulletin*, 39(7), 5–10.

Cook, D. A., Hatala, R., Brydges, R., Zendejas, B., Szostek, J. H., Wang, A. T., ... Hamstra, S. J. (2011). Technology-enhanced simulation for health professions education: A systematic review and meta-analysis. *Journal of the American Medical Association*, 306(9), 978–988. doi:10.1001/jama.2011.1234

Decker, S., Fey, M., Sideras, S., Caballero, S., Rockstraw, L. R., Boese, T., ... Borum, J. C. (2013). Standards of best practice: Simulation standard VI: The debriefing process. *Clinical Simulation in Nursing*, 9(6), S26–S29. doi:10.1016/j.ecns.2013.04.008

Decker, S. I., Anderson, M., Boese, T., Epps, C., McCarthy, J., Motola, I., ... & Lioce, L. (2015). Standards of best practice. *Clinical Simulation in Nursing*, 11(6), 293–297. doi:10.1016/j.ecns.2015.03.010

Dieckmann, P., Molin Friis, S., Lippert, A., & Ostergaard, D. (2009). The art and science of debriefing in simulation: Ideal and practice. *Medical Teacher*, 31(7), e287–e294. doi:10.1080/01421590902866218

Facione, N. C., & Facione P. A. (2006). *Health Sciences Reasoning Test (HSRT): A test for critical thinking skills for health care professionals. Test manual*. Millbrae, CA: California Academic Press.

Hayden, J. (2010). Use of simulation in nursing education: National survey results. *Journal of Nursing Regulation*, 1(3), 52–57. doi:10.1016/s2155-8256(15)30335-5

INACSL Standards Committee. (2016a) INACSL standards of best practice: Simulation^{SM} Simulation glossary. *Clinical Simulation in Nursing*, 12(S), S39–S47. doi:10.1016/j.ecns.2016.09.012

INACSL Standards Committee. (2016b). INACSL standards of best practice: Simulation^{SM} Professional integrity. *Clinical Simulation in Nursing*, 12(S), S30–S33. doi:10.1016/j.ecns.2016.09.010

INACSL Standards Committee. (2016c). INACSL standards of best practice: Simulation^{SM} Facilitation. *Clinical Simulation in Nursing*, 12(S), S16–S20. doi:10.1016/j.ecns.

Jeffries, P. R. (2012). *Simulation in nursing education from conceptualization to evaluation* (2nd ed.). New York, NY: NLN Press.

Kardong-Edgren, S. Willhaus, J., Bennett, J., & Hayden, J. (2012). Results of the National Council of State Boards of Nursing national simulation survey: Part II. *Clinical Simulation in Nursing*, 8, e117-e123. doi: 10.1016/j.ecns.2012.01.003

Kirkpatrick, D. L., & Kirkpatrick, J. D. (2006). *Evaluating training programs* (3rd ed.). San Francisco, CA: Berrett-Koehler.

Kunst, E. L., Mitchell, M., & Johnston, A. N. (2016). Manikin simulation in mental health nursing education: An integrative review. *Clinical Simulation in Nursing*, 12(11), 484–495. doi:10.1016/j.ecns.2016.07.010

Lasater, K. (2007). High-fidelity simulation and the development of clinical judgment: Students' experiences. *Journal of Nursing Education*, 46(6), 269–276.

Lave, J., & Wenger, E. (1991). *Situated learning: Legitimate peripheral participation*. Cambridge, UK: Cambridge University Press.

McGaghie, W. C., Issenberg, S. B., Cohen, E. R., Barsuk, J. H., & Wayne, D. B. (2011) Does simulation-based medical education with deliberate practice yield better results than traditional clinical education? A meta-analytic comparative review of the evidence. *Academic Medicine*, 86(6), 706–711. doi:10.1097/ACM.0b013e318217e119

McGaghie, W. C., Issenberg, S. B., Petrusa, E. R., & Scalese, R. J. (2010). A critical review of simulation-based medical education research: 2003–2009. *Medical Education*, 44(1), 50–63. doi:10.1111/j.1365-2923.2009.03547.x

Murray, D. J., Boulet, J. R., Avidan M., Kras J. F., Heinrich B., & Woodhouse J., (2007). Performance of residents and anesthesiologists in simulation-based skill assessment. *Anesthesiology*, 107(5), 705–713. doi:10.1097/01.anes.0000286926.01083.9d

Neill, M. A., & Wotton, K. (2011). High-fidelity simulation debriefing in nursing education: A literature review. *Clinical Simulation in Nursing*, 7(5), e161–e168. doi:10.1016/j.ecns.2011.02.001

Okuda, Y., Bryson, E. O., DeMaria, S., Jacobson, L., Quinones, J., Shen, B., & Levine, A. I. (2009). The utility of simulation in medical education: What is the evidence? *Mount Sinai Journal of Medicine*, 76(4), 330–343. doi:10.1002/msj.20127

Pagano, M. P., O'Shea, E. R., Campbell, S. H., Currie, L. M., Chamberlin, E., & Pates, C. A. (2015). Validating the Health Communication Assessment Tool© (HCAT). *Clinical Simulation in Nursing*, *11*(9), 402–410. doi:10.1016/j.ecns.2015.06.001

Page-Cutrara, K. (2015). Prebriefing in nursing simulation: A concept analysis. *Clinical Simulation in Nursing*, *11*(7), 335–340. doi:10.1016/j.ecns.2015.05.001

Palaganas, J. C., Brunette, V., & Winslow, B. (2016). Prelicensure simulation-enhanced interprofessional education: A critical review of the research literature. *Simulation in Healthcare*, *11*(6), 404–418. doi:10.1097/sih.0000000000000175

Radhakrishnan, K., Roche, J. P., & Cunningham, H. (2007). Measuring clinical practice parameters with human patient simulation: A pilot study. *International Journal of Nursing Education Scholarship*, *4*, Article 8. doi:10.2202/1548-923x.1307

Raemer, D., Anderson, M., Cheng, A., Fanning, R., Nadkarni, V., & Salvadelli, G. (2011). Research regarding debriefing as part of the learning process. *Simulation in Healthcare*, *6*(Suppl.), S52–57. doi:10.1097/SIH.0b013e31822724d0

Ravert, P., & McAfooes, J. (2013). NLN/Jeffries simulation framework: State of the science summary. *Clinical Simulation in Nursing*, *10*(7), 335–336. doi:10.1016/j.ecns.2013.06.002

Rosen, M. A., Salas, E., Silvestri, S., Wu, T. S., & Lazarra, E. H. (2008). A measurement tool for simulation-based training in emergency medicine: The simulation module for assessment of resident targeted event responses (SMARTER) approach. *Simulation in Healthcare*, *3*(3), 170–179. doi:10.1097/sih.0b013e318173038d

Rossignol, M. (2017). Effects of video-assisted debriefing compared with standard oral debriefing. *Clinical Simulation in Nursing*, *13*(4), 145–153. doi:10.1016/j.ecns.2016.12.001

Rutherford-Hemming, T., & Alfes, C. M. (2017). The use of hospital-based simulation in nursing education—A systematic review. *Clinical Simulation in Nursing*, *13*(2), 78–89. doi:10.1016/j.ecns.2016.12.007

Salas, E., Cooke, N. J., & Rosen, M. A. (2008). On teams, teamwork, and team performance: Discoveries and developments. *Human Factors*, *50*(3), 540–547. doi:10.1518/001872008x288457

Schaefer, J. J., III, Vanderbilt, A. A., Cason, C. L., Bauman, E. B., Glavin, R. J., Lee, F. W., & Navedo, D. D. (2011). Literature review: Instructional design and pedagogy science in healthcare simulation. *Simulation in Healthcare*, *6*(7), s30–s41. doi:10.1097/sih.0b013e31822237b4

Schoening, A. M., Sittner, B. J., & Todd, M. J. (2006). Simulated clinical experience: Nursing students' perceptions and the educators' role. *Nurse Educator*, *31*(6), 253–258. doi:10.1097/00006223-200611000-00008

Shapiro, M. J., Morey, J. C., Small, S. D., Langford, V., Kaylor, C. J., Jagminas, L., … Jay, G. D. (2004). Simulation based teamwork training for emergency department staff: Does it improve clinical team performance when added to an existing didactic teamwork curriculum? *Quality and Safety in Health Care*, *13*(6), 417–421. doi:10.1136/qhc.13.6.417

Society for Simulation in Healthcare. (2018). *Certified Healthcare Simulation Educator Examination Blueprint, 2018 Version*. Retrieved from http://www.ssih.org/Portals/48/Certification/CHSE_Docs/CHSE_Examination_Blueprint.pdf

Sullivan-Mann, J., Perron, C. A., & Fellner, A. N. (2009). The effects of simulation on nursing students' critical thinking scores: A quantitative study. *Newborn and Infant Nursing Reviews*, *9*(2), 111–116. doi:10.1053/j.nainr.2009.03.006

Weinger, M. B. (2010). The pharmacology of simulation: A conceptual framework to inform progress in simulation research. *Simulation in Healthcare*, *5*(1), 8–15. doi:10.1097/sih.0b013e3181c91d4a

Zimmerman, B. J. (2000). Self-efficacy: An essential motive to learn. *Contemporary Educational Psychology*, *25*(1), 82–91. doi:10.1006/ceps.1999.1016

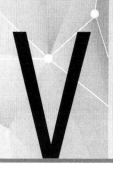

Domain IV: Simulation Resources and Environments

22

Operations and Management of Environment, Personnel, and Nonpersonnel Resources

CAROLYN H. SCHEESE

> *By failing to prepare, you are preparing to fail.*
> —Benjamin Franklin

This chapter addresses Domain IV: Simulation Resources and Environments (Society for Simulation in Healthcare [SSH], 2018a).

[LEARNING OUTCOMES]

- Discuss basic managerial and operational principles associated with delivering simulation activities; management of personnel and nonpersonnel resources.
- Identify ways in which the physical environment can be modified to maximize simulation-based learning, including the use of timelines and checklists.
- Identify common policies, procedures, and practices of an efficient simulation program.
- Discuss effective ways in which one may respond to technical and material issues (e.g., video capture, simulator failures, and material supplies) that may occur in the simulation environment.

This chapter focuses on the management and operations of a simulation center, including the management of personnel and nonpersonnel (space, supplies, equipment, technology, money, etc.) resources. Whether large or small, completely outfitted with the latest high-fidelity technology or an outdated space stocked mainly with task trainers and low- to midfidelity mannequins, there are key operational principles that can apply to almost any setting. This chapter is divided into sections with multiple headings and is intended to serve as a guide and resource, not only to provide sufficient information to aid in passing certification examinations, but also as a resource that you can come back to from time to time so you can improve planning, organizing, managing, and executing simulations in your center.

OPERATIONS MANAGEMENT: WHAT IS OPERATIONS?

Operations management is the process of managing and coordinating all resources—personnel and nonpersonnel—and coordinating and managing them in such a way that they are used efficiently and effectively to meet the goals and mission of the institution. Operations provides the support and infrastructure to get things done; it is considered the business side of simulation. Business operations usually includes four key aspects:

1. The physical space (location)
2. Equipment and supplies (tools)
3. Personnel (people)
4. Policies, procedures, and processes (Peterson, Jaret, & Schenck, 2013)

Operations is the coordination and management of the many support pieces that are required to put a plan into place, and then execute that plan.

SCHEDULING

Scheduling of the space, personnel, and equipment is one of the biggest challenges and headaches of a simulation center because scheduling events involves a complex set of rules and variables. Scheduling involves matching personnel (faculty, students, volunteers, staff, information technology [IT] support, etc.) and nonpersonnel resources (space, technology, mannequins, supplies, etc.) with dates and times. Throughout this section, you will note that scheduled items are referred to as "events." Events can include many things: a simulation scenario, open house, or very important person (VIP) tour; meeting with faculty/instructors; standardized (simulated) patient (SP) training; an objective structured clinical examination (OSCE); skills lab training session; open lab time for students; or center closures to install or maintain equipment. Each of these events is unique, yet all require the coordination of personnel and nonpersonnel resources within a date and time.

Methods to Track Scheduling

Many different methods may be used to schedule and track simulation center activities. Paper-and-pencil office scheduling ledgers are available for a minimal cost and may meet the needs of a small center with just a few activities or events per day. Ideally, keep all various pieces related to an event in one location; having items in multiple locations can be frustrating and lead to lost or missing information critical to the event's success.

Advantages of pen–paper scheduling are that it is inexpensive, portable, and easy to use and update. Limitations to this method include the following:

- Limited access—only one person has access to the ledger at a time
- The ledger may get lost, making it difficult to reconstruct upcoming events
- As a center grows, this system can be time intensive to manage and maintain

- Limited information can be written in the ledger, which may require additional support methods to manage event information, such as the final confirmed date and time, names of students, scenario details, and other resources

Schedules can be maintained through a variety of electronic methods, some of which are free or very low cost, such as Google and Outlook Calendars or homegrown methods, whereas other commercially available event managers and scheduling products may be very costly. The available features vary according to the product. Some advantages of commercial products may include:

- Calendar sharing: Greater access to information related to the simulation center–scheduled events as these products can frequently be shared and may have varying levels of access and privilege for the audience who is viewing the calendar, such as view-only and full-scheduling rights
- The ability to link communication/emails and event information to the scheduled event
- Some systems include the ability to track students, personnel, space, supplies, and equipment to generate detailed invoices reflecting event and center costs
- Some systems house the prework and allow instructor access to student and scenario information remotely
- Some systems allow self-registration and automatic event reminders and allow students and faculty to sign in to the center upon arrival (Scheese, 2013)

Scheduling and maintaining the schedule so that the information is disseminated to the level needed for implementation can take a lot of time. So, although the cost of an electronic event manager may be high, it can potentially generate cost savings by saving time and decreasing frustration as well as increase quality and event consistency (Exhibit 22.1).

EXHIBIT 22.1

Things to Consider When Scheduling

- Mission of the center
- Priorities of the center
- Resource limits (time, personnel, faculty/instructors, space, etc.)
- Personnel (support personnel, faculty, staff, learners/students, volunteers/SPs, etc.)
- Knowledge and skills/skill level
- Availability of personnel and nonpersonnel items
- Nonpersonnel
- Physical space
- Equipment/supplies

SP, standardized patient.

The Scheduler

The individual who is responsible for the scheduling calendar is potentially one of the most powerful individuals in the center. This individual is your public relations officer. He or she is often the first individual with whom your customers interact. He or she is the face of the business, a gatekeeper who can deter or encourage the use of the center by the very manner in which he or she interacts with those who contact the center. How the scheduler's power is used and managed will, to a large extent, determine the accessibility to the center. If someone is unable to schedule an event, or if the hassle factor is too high or negative in nature, customers will go elsewhere. It stands to reason that unless events are scheduled, you would not run events. Understanding your customers and providing good customer service from the very first encounter is essential to sustained success (Scheese, 2013).

> A business absolutely devoted to service will have only one worry about profits. They will be embarrassingly large.
> —Henry Ford

The schedule is a linchpin. The scheduling calendar holds all the information together so that a successful event can occur. A poorly managed schedule creates inefficiencies and frustration for those who use the center as well as those who support the events. An ideal scheduler is detail oriented, good at organizing content and information, proactive, a good communicator, and willingly accepts direction.

Block Scheduling

Block scheduling has been used for many years in operating rooms (ORs) and surgical centers to provide predictability for the end user and the facility (Fei, Meskens, & Chu, 2009). Simulation centers have many common elements with these facilities and may benefit from this method of scheduling events. Block scheduling consists of providing/setting aside a block of days or times for an end user. In this situation, an *end user* could refer to a faculty member, course, class, or pass-off/exam where there is predictability in the need for resources. For example, medical students in your center may have OSCEs every 6 weeks. Scheduling these events out even as far as 1 year in advance makes sense, if supporting the education of medical students is consistent with the center's mission. Using block scheduling, SPs, space, staff, and faculty/instructor support may also be scheduled out into the future and made predictable.

The greater the predictability in the schedule, the easier it is to adjust for minor changes and challenges that come along. Block scheduling is based on the principle that if you schedule your highest priority customers first, you can work the lower priority customers into the vacancies that exist.

First, determine what groups have priority and why. This can be determined by an oversight committee and should be consistent with the center's mission, vision, and values. One method is to classify users into three groups, according to definitions of priority: A, B, and C and to schedule A's first and B's second, followed by C's.

> **CASE STUDY 22.1**
>
> An event that uses SPs will run all day long, 8 hours, for a total of 14 cases. What items should be considered when scheduling this event? Breaks, attire, length and complexity of case, and nature of the case—whether it is invasive or not. SPs have the right to be treated with respect and the right to refuse to continue a simulation experience.

Sharing space and other available resources can be challenging. It takes negotiation and open communication. Like filling a jar with various sizes of rocks, pebbles, and sand, if you put the rocks in first, starting with the largest, followed by the pebbles and last of all the sand, then the jar can hold the maximum amount of material. This principle can be applied to scheduling. Fill the schedule with the largest (priority) users first, then fit your other users around them to maximize the capacity of the center.

Disadvantages: This system can be abused and needs a check-and-balance system to be most effective. You may have some users who schedule block time and then do not use it, especially ones who do not cancel with sufficient notice to schedule other users. Users in the C group may feel frustrated at not getting their first choice or prime slots. Again, ensuring that the scheduling process reflects the mission, vision, and values of the center will help in the decision-making process related to this challenge. One way to deal with this is to reassess your users at regular intervals and reprioritize groups as needed. Clearly established policies, including any non-cancelation fees that may be assessed, will help all parties understand expectations.

First Come, First Scheduled

First come, first served is another philosophy that can be used when scheduling events. Simply put, customers and events are prioritized and scheduled in accordance with when the request is received. Using a hybrid or combination of both block scheduling and first come, first served is another way to manage the schedule. Regardless of the method chosen, it should be consistent with the mission, vision, and values of the center, clearly communicated to the "communities of interest" or "stakeholders," and supported by the policies and procedures of the center.

■ PREPARING FOR DELIVERY OF A SIMULATION EVENT

Preparation and organization are essential to the successful outcome of a simulation experience. Templates may be useful in scheduling events and writing scenarios. Timelines and checklists can be helpful in outlining expectations and organizing events from conception to implementation and final evaluation. Tracking and organizing scenarios can be done electronically, with a physical hard copy, or by a combination of both electronic and hard copies.

Clearly establish timelines and expectations with those who schedule events, so that there is sufficient time for all to prepare for the event (Exhibit 22.2).

> **EXHIBIT 22.2**
>
> **Timeline and Checklist for a New Simulation Event**
>
> **3–6 MONTHS PRIOR TO EVENT**
> - Determine goals/learners/instructor support (overarching concept of event determined).
> - Schedule space and use of any major equipment and supplies needed to support event.
> - Schedule learners/instructors and support personnel.
> - Write scenario/OSCEs.
> - Order needed equipment and supplies.
>
> **6–8 WEEKS PRIOR TO EVENT**
> - Finalize number and begin to schedule SPs.
> - Verify request for ordering of any special supplies.
>
> **4 WEEKS PRIOR TO EVENT**
> - Finalize event/scenario.
> - Review plan with those who will be implementing and modify as needed.
>
> **2 WEEKS PRIOR TO EVENT**
> - Do a "walk-through": Facilitators/instructors and support staff meet together in the space where the simulation will occur and review the scenario and identify and resolve areas of question or concern or that need to be clarified or modified.
> - Train SPs 5 to 10 days prior.
>
> **WEEK OF EVENT**
> - Send reminders to participants and instructors.
> - Review need for and last-minute changes by facilitators/instructors.
> - Preevent evaluation/survey and prework sent out and completed by learners.
>
> **DAY PRIOR/DAY OF**
> - Arrive early.
> - Set up room.
> - Team huddle/preprocedure checklist, verify room setup, and modify as needed.
> - Complete learner postsimulation evaluation and other postwork as assigned.
>
> **FOLLOWING THE EVENT**
> - Debrief all team members—meet to discuss what went well and what can be improved.
> - Revise scenario and document changes as needed.

OSCE, objective structured clinical examination; SP, standardized patient.

Events themselves can also have timelines to aid in keeping the event on time and focused on what matters most. Both simple and complex events can benefit from timelines.

Checklists can be used just prior to when the simulation starts to verify that all items are set up and ready to go, much like the OR uses a checklist for a "time-out" prior to surgery, or the airlines use a preflight checklist (Exhibit 22.3). This checklist can be a part of the "huddle" some centers use. The "huddle" is a short meeting that occurs just prior to starting the simulation to ensure that everyone is ready to go, to ensure a common understanding of the sequence of events, and to answer any questions any member of the team may have (Table 22.1).

TABLE 22.1 Simulation Event Timeline		
TIMELINE	SEQUENCE OF EVENTS	RESOURCES: FACILITATOR AND ROLES
20 min	Orientation to environment Overview and expectations Prework Division of roles	Orient students to simulation room Collect consent from students Review prework, discussion, articles Use PowerPoints with prescenario videos Determine roles Review chart contents/divide into roles
10 min	Scenario 1—Patient needs blood Group B participates in scenario	Group A observational engagement
20 min	Debrief	All facilitators debrief
15 min	Scenario 2—Patient develops acute blood transfusion reaction Group A participates in scenario	Group B observational engagement
20 min	Debrief	All facilitators debrief
5 min	Wrap-up	Closing remarks, handouts, reminder to do postsurvey and confidentiality
Total time = 1.5 hours		

TRACKING CENTER ACTIVITIES

Simulation is expensive. Those who support simulation financially or by other means will want to know how their contributions made a difference. In business, this is referred to as *ROI (return on investment)*. In other words, what was the benefit of the time, energy, and resources put into this event or center as a whole? In order to provide this information to those who invest in the center, it is important to track the usage, productivity, and costs associated with the center. The following are just a few items that can be tracked for each event: number of learners, number of instructors, length of simulation (time/hours), supply costs, equipment and space usage, time required for event setup and breakdown, administrative and support time, and so on. This information can be tracked by individual events and then compiled at the end of the year as a portion of the annual report. Data are invaluable when it comes to asking for continued or additional financial support. It is also important in tracking expenses and depreciating equipment.

EXHIBIT 22.3

Prescenario Checklist

SIMULATION EVENT
- Scenario duration and number
- Sequence of events
- Anticipated end time
- Anticipated breaks/setup changes
- Simulation room number
- Debriefing room number

TECHNICAL ISSUES
- Video/camera setup
- Video debriefing needs
- Electronic files, location
- Smart board needs

MANNEQUIN
- Type
- Preprogrammed/on-the-fly programming
- Position/location
- Moulage
- Fluids
- Name and allergy band

STANDARDIZED PATIENT
- Training/instructions
- Moulage/clothing/attire
- Waiting/staging area
- Props/name and allergy band
- Two-way radio/walkie-talkie
- Time cards/parking validations/meals

(continued)

> **EXHIBIT 22.3 (continued)**
>
> **ROOM SETUP**
> - Equipment
> - Supplies
> - Electronic health record/bedside computer needs
> - Props
> - Bed type/gurney/crib
> - Special needs?
>
> **MEDICATIONS**
> - Label
> - Name
> - Dose
> - Planned med error?
> - Location: Medication refrigerator
> - Medication dispenser programming
>
> **ROLES AND RESPONSIBILITIES**
> - Technical roles/responsibilities
> - Faculty roles/responsibilities
> - Confederate role needed?
> - Adequate resources?
>
> **OTHER?**

Source: Reprinted with permission from Lassche, M., & Scheese, C. (2013). *Effective team work—More than a game of chance*. Poster presentation at the 12th Annual International Nursing Simulation/Learning (INACSL) Resource Centers Conference: Hit the Jackpot with Evidence Based Simulation, Las Vegas, NV.

Annual Report

Preparing and publishing an annual report is a way to report on and evaluate accomplishments, ROI of the center, to relay information to the many communities of interest and stakeholders, and to measure and track progress on goals. Items that may be listed in an annual report include changes in leadership, instructors, or personnel; income and expense reports; purchases of new equipment; grants received and processed; scholarship activities such as manuscripts submitted and published; type and number of presentations; center event utilization rates; and student/learner contact hours.

> **SIMULATION TEACHING TIP 22.1**
>
> The number of students times the number of hours present for a learning activity equals learner contact hours.

Mission, Vision, Values

Businesses (yes, education and simulation can be considered businesses) often create a mission statement to define their purpose and priorities. Many times, but not always, a vision statement and values are also defined. A mission statement is a statement of purpose; it defines the institution's purpose for existence and its focus (Peterson et al., 2013). Vision is the overarching view of purpose—where the company is headed. Key values may also be selected and defined. Examples of values include integrity, quality, collaboration, and so on. Mission, vision, and values help determine what projects to undertake and which ones to decline. Consider defining *why* your simulation center exists. Most likely, it is relatively easy to define *what* your center does and probably not too challenging to explain *how* your center functions and does what it does. However, businesses and individuals that start with *why* tend to be more innovative and flexible and attract a loyal customer base who support them in the long term (Sinek, 2009).

Business Plan

The business plan is like a road map or navigational chart that provides a plan and summaries of information related to that business. This information may include the purpose and organizational structure of the business, company strategy, the existing market place, a marketing plan, a review of finances, and action plans with a timetable. A business plan can be used not only to help establish a business, but it can also be used to help improve operations, efficiencies, or provide a new direction (Fiore, 2005). It takes time and effort to develop a business plan, and it can be challenging because there are many difficult questions that have to be addressed when putting this plan together. However, it is worth the effort and is one of the most important steps you can take for success. A written business plan can help a company stay focused on its purpose (Peterson et al., 2013). Be realistic in establishing a timetable when establishing a new center. Recognize that it takes about 18 months to get a simulation center fully operational (SSH, 2018b). Even once a center has been established, the business plan should be revisited regularly and modified to meet changing needs. The U.S. Small Business Administration (www.sba.gov) has many resources for starting and managing small businesses.

Strategic Plan

A strategic plan is a plan for the future that links present and future operations to the organization's mission, vision, and values. Strategic plans are commonly generated for 3 to 5 years into the future, but can be changed more frequently if the business climate is dynamic or in a rapidly changing environment. Annual and semiannual goals are generated to support and achieve the strategic plan. Strategic plans should be reviewed at least annually. Alterations in the marketplace and other factors, such as changes in an administration with a new direction or goals, may necessitate a change in the strategic plan.

Budget

A budget is a fiscal plan that includes estimated expenses and income for a predetermined amount of time, generally 1 year. Costs must be planned and tracked. However, it is important to realize that a budget is a forecast or plan for the future, and will likely need some flexibility, reassessment, and revisions to account for unforeseen happenings (Marquis & Huston, 2017). Depending on the size of your center, you may have a budget of a few thousand dollars, or in a larger center, your budget may be several million dollars or more. However, the principles of a budget remain the same. Revenue, or money coming in, must not exceed expenses, or money going out. All money coming in and going out must be tracked and accounted for. Costs are usually broken down into personnel and nonpersonnel cost or salary and nonsalary items. A budget should take into account the depreciation of equipment and plan for the replacement of durable equipment. Other considerations include software licensing and upgrades, equipment repair and maintenance, office supplies, and so on. Computers and technology have a very short life span, about 3 to 6 years. A state-of-the-art center, without a plan and budget to consistently and thoughtfully upgrade, repair, and replace old equipment, will quickly become outdated and enter a state of disrepair.

When creating a budget, plan for both current and future costs and needs. Consider the items that you need to request to keep your center going, not just now, but in the future. Work with your finance administrator or chief financial officer (CFO) to see how your institution can set aside money each year for anticipated purchases and to plan for the replacement of simulators, computers, and other technological devices and equipment. Consider the infrastructure; anticipate needs for growth and updates.

Determine the life span of the equipment in your center; then plan for its replacement. Staggering the replacement of some of these items over a few years can help to level out the cost of this in the overall budget. For example, if you have 21 computers that are aging and need to be replaced within the next 3 years, you can budget for seven computers per year for 3 years. This can help to even out the overall budget. Likewise, cameras, mannequins/human patient simulators (HPSs), task trainers, and so on, and their life expectancy need to be considered and put into the budget accordingly.

Capital equipment is generally considered as durable equipment that has a life expectancy of greater than 1 year and exceeds a certain purchase amount. The amount is usually determined by the institution. For example, it might be defined by an institution as $5,000. So anything that costs more than $5,000 would be considered capital equipment and usually has to go through different channels and processes in order to make that purchase. Some institutions require that all capital purchases go out for bid or may require at least three quotes from competing vendors. In simulation, most HPSs fall into the capital equipment request category of the budget. Do not be shy about asking for what you need to run a good program. Recognize that it may take a few budget cycles to get the things you need. Do not give up. Prepare yourself to speak knowledgeably about the proposed purchase and do your research so that you know what features you need and the expected ROI for learners.

> Asking is the beginning of receiving. Make sure you don't go to the ocean with a teaspoon. At least take a bucket so the kids won't laugh at you.
> —Jim Rohn

One thing to keep in mind when considering approving expenses is learning the restrictions on various funds/revenue accounts. For example, money donated to the center may be restricted to a specific purchase, such as a crib, task trainer, or mannequin. Money from grants may also have strict limitations on how it can be spent. In academic institutions, there are many restrictions on what student fees, state funds, or tuition money can purchase. Tracking and accounting for each type of incoming revenue and the requisite expenses are very important. Misuse of funds may result in embarrassment, loss of trust, and even loss of employment.

Equipment and supplies can also be obtained by networking with those in your community who have access to outdated supplies and equipment. This can save a tremendous amount of money for programs that do not have a budget for these items (Lazzara, Benishek, Dietz, Salas, & Adriansen, 2014). Some equipment can be rented; refurbished rather than new items can be purchased at a fraction of the cost.

Simulation centers can obtain their revenue in a variety of ways such as student fees, tuition, grants, donors, usage fees, and so on. Some are for profit, whereas others are nonprofit. A cost recovery center or recharge center is a center that is able to recoup costs by charging fees to users such that it is able to compensate the cost of doing business. Other approaches are called *pay to play*. In order to use the center, you must first agree to pay. Often the payment is received upfront. No matter the source of the revenue stream, in order for a center to be viable, it must be sustainable. Expenses cannot exceed revenue.

PHYSICAL SPACE

As much as possible, organize the physical space of the center so that items are grouped according to similar supplies and convenient to the site or point of use. For example, locate all moulage supplies in the same area, and group all wound dressings or intravenous (IV) supplies together. Organizing the physical space increases efficiency, reduces frustration in not being able to find needed supplies and equipment, and facilitates the ease of tracking the inventory of supplies and equipment. Label everything (Figure 22.1). Supplies for specific scenarios or skills can be organized and placed in containers with their specific inventory sheets/required supply lists and instructions.

Keep reference materials, such as user manuals, policies and procedure manuals, simulation scenarios, skill equipment checklists, and so on, in a common area that can be accessed by all who may need these reference materials. Create logbooks to track capital equipment inventory, periodic maintenance, and repair histories that can be traced to a particular device/piece of equipment such as a specific HPS. This history and tracking information is necessary if a piece of equipment ever malfunctions or needs repairs covered by warranty.

Quick setup guides can be created (or may be available from the manufacturer) and filed in a common area or attached to a device as appropriate. A short-list "quick setup"/"troubleshooting guide" can be written up in bullet points and attached to the equipment/device with clear waterproof tape or laminated and attached as appropriate for the end user. Be sure to include the sales representative's name, phone number, and manufacturer contact information.

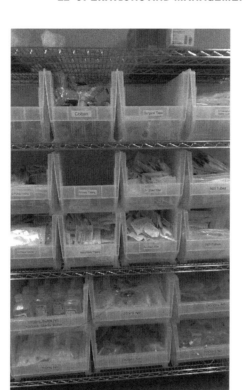

FIGURE 22.1 Shelves of labeled supplies.

Modifying the Environment

Assessing and modifying the physical environment is an important part of setting up a simulation. The physical space of a simulated environment can be modified to create realism. Our senses help us form memory. Sight, smell, sound, and temperature can all be a part of an engaging physical setup for simulation. Moulage can be used to create a more realistic experience for the learner. It can be a wig, a fake scar, vomit, urine, or blood, and so on. Moulage is an art that increases realism. Odors can enhance realism, too. For example, combining lemon juice and finely grated parmesan cheese with food coloring can create not only the appearance of vomit; it also has the odor associated with vomit. Sprays can be purchased that simulate feces, iron tablets can be added to fake blood to create odor, and a small amount of ammonia can be added to fake urine to create a realistic odor (Langford, n.d.). The presence of odors can enhance realism and emotionally engage the learner.

A simulation room at the Winter Institute for Simulation and Research (WISER), the Peter Winter Institute for Simulation in Pittsburgh, Pennsylvania, has several sets of ceiling-to-floor curtains with various images from the environment they want to portray, such as a scene of a big city for a group of emergency medical technicians (EMTs) or a scene of an OR, to help immerse their learners in the physical environment.

The Center for Advanced Medical Learning and Simulation (CAMLS; 2014) in Tampa, Florida, has a trauma OR that projects images on the walls, using sights, sounds, and temperature changes in the environment they wish to recreate to increase realism.

HPSs can be dressed in expected attire, and a few pieces of furniture or relevant objects may be brought into the scenario room. For example, the realism of a disaster scenario may be improved with the use of strobe lights and a fog machine.

A balance between learner goals and costs should be considered. Reviewing the goals and learning outcomes of the simulated event can provide clear guidance as to what is required and what is an unnecessary expense. For example, if there is a scenario that includes a patient-controlled anesthesia (PCA) pump and the center does not own a pump (but could rent one with tubing for a month for $350), reviewing the scenario objectives may help to determine whether it is worth the extra cost of renting the pump. If a key component of the scenario objectives includes the setup and use of the PCA pump, it may be worth the additional cost. If the pump plays a very minor role and the setup and use of the PCA pump are minor, then it may not be worth the extra costs. In its place, a mocked-up pump may work to achieve the learning objectives.

The greater the realism in sights, sounds, smells, and temperature, the easier it is for a learner to engage in the realism of the scenario. The use of prescenario video clips or briefs can be effective engagement tools. Of utmost importance is the willingness of the learner to engage and suspend disbelief no amount of realism can overcome an unwilling participate. However, a highly realistic environment that takes into account all the senses makes it easier to suspend disbelief than it would be otherwise.

POLICIES, PROCEDURE, AND PRACTICES

A policy is a brief description of a plan or standard that is used in decision making. A procedure is the step-by-step process or set of instructions outlining how to implement the policy. Procedures are usually used for complex procedures or for procedures that require detail and quality control. Processes are the manner in which things actually occur. Quality improvement assumes that there is a connection between processes and efficiency or quality care. Process audits can be done to evaluate current inefficiencies and to identify efficiencies (Marquis & Huston, 2017).

Every center should have formally written documents, including organizational structure and policies and procedures to help establish an understanding of expectations for facility users, employees, and the communities of interest/stakeholders. Policies can be either formal (written and sanctioned by a formal authoritative body [governing board or perhaps a guidance or steering committee]) or informal, based on historical actions. Written policy is best, as it allows for transparency and consistency. Writing policies can be very time-consuming and often requires many drafts before a final policy gains approval, is agreed on, and implemented (Exhibit 22.4).

Basic organizational documents include the following:

- Mission, vision, and values
- Organizational chart
- Job descriptions with roles and responsibilities

> **EXHIBIT 22.4**
>
> **Define and Clarify Processes**
>
> - What needs to be done?
> - Who will do it?
> - How will it be done?
> - Are there any costs? How will these be covered?

> **EXHIBIT 22.5**
>
> **Required Documentation for Accreditation**
>
> - Mission and governance
> - Organization and management
> - Facilities, technology, simulation modalities, and human resources
> - Evaluation and improvement
> - Integrity
> - Security
> - Expanding the field
> - Learning activities
> - Qualified educators
> - Curriculum design
> - Learning environment
> - Ongoing curriculum feedback and improvement
> - Educational credit

Source: Adapted from the Society for Simulation in Healthcare. (2014b). Council for accreditation of healthcare simulation programs accreditation standards self-study review. Retrieved from http://www.ssih.org/Accreditation/Full-Accreditation

Core polices should be consistent and support the mission of the facility whether it be research, education/teaching, assessment, or an integration of several of these (Marquis & Huston, 2017; SSH, 2018b).

Basic policies, procedures, and processes include scheduling an event, managing tours, retention and access to video (how long video is retained/archived), resolving customer/communities of interest/stakeholder complaints, hours of operation, access to center and admittance criteria, loaning of equipment and supplies, costs/charges, and many others. Human resource policies and procedures may include dress code, payroll and attendance issues (clocking in, scheduling vacation, calling in sick, etc.), role and expectations, and so on (Marquis & Huston, 2017; SSH, 2018b). Consider developing policies and procedures related to the accreditation requirements. It will provide a good foundation for your center, even if you choose not to go through the accreditation process (Exhibit 22.5).

Physical Security—Locked Up

Simulation centers often contain hundreds of thousands of dollars' worth of equipment and supplies. In order to protect this investment, security systems with alarms should be put into place and policies adopted that can achieve a balance between protecting the valuable assets and allowing entry into the facility in a manner that is consistent with the mission of the center. Some centers allow access to specific users 24/7, whereas other centers greatly restrict access to standard operating hours. For example, medical residents, desiring to improve their skills with laparoscopic surgery, are among those who may want 24/7 access to the equipment and supplies. Their hours are unpredictable and ready access to the center may be required to meet the needs of the user/learner. Clearly established policies and procedures for access and expectations of cleanup, along with proper training on the care and use of the equipment, are essential to preserving the investment and preventing costly repairs or replacements.

Separation of Simulated and Actual Patient Medications, Supplies, and Equipment

Simulation in situ is a simulation done in the actual clinical setting, for example, within an actual OR, emergency room, or critical care unit at a functioning hospital or clinic. This allows for maximum realism as related to the environment. Simulation in situ is particularly valuable in examining processes.

> **CASE STUDY 22.2**
>
> One center used in situ simulation to identify potential problems with a new policy related to responding to a critical patient incident. Through this simulation, they were able to identify equipment and badge-access issues. Another facility used simulation in situ to keep its staff current in responding to codes and other critical patient events. What other applications can simulation in situ have?

When using in situ simulation, there must be a clear separation among actual patient information, equipment, and supplies, and those items used for simulation. Patient safety is of upmost concern. Fake medications and expired or unsterile supplies may be used in simulation, and must be clearly identified "Not for patient use—for simulation use." All simulated medications, supplies, and equipment should be clearly labeled to prevent inadvertent use on an actual patient (Figure 22.2).

Personnel

Personnel or *human capital* are terms that may be used to identify anyone who is employed or volunteers for the simulation center. Personnel is a business's greatest resource because although equipment, supplies, and space (nonpersonnel resources) may depreciate and decline in value over time, personnel can

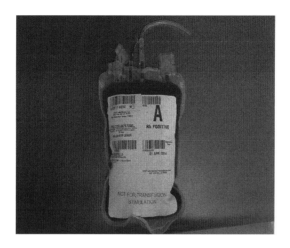

FIGURE 22.2 Labeling props for simulation.

continually improve and increase in value. It is the individual and collective personnel's talents, skills, knowledge, attitudes, and abilities that create the unique nature of each center. Not only are personnel the most valuable asset, they are the most expensive (Lazzara et al., 2014).

Titles, roles, and responsibilities differ from center to center, but support of essential functions remain: managing, planning and preparing, implementing, cleaning up, and evaluating are all required support activities of a simulation event. Each center determines how best to meet the various needs of its unique center accordingly. Some common titles and roles of simulation center personnel may include simulation technology specialists (STSs)/simulation technologists, information technologists, computer support, faculty/instructors, student workers/teaching assistants, administrative support/secretary, simulation coordinators, managers, program directors, operations directors, administration, SPs/patient actors, and so on.

Stakeholders and Communities of Interest

Every simulation center has an impact on individuals and groups in their community. These individuals and groups are called *stakeholders*. Stakeholders can be internal or external. Internal stakeholders include people with a direct vested interest in the success of the center, whereas external stakeholders have an indirect interest in the success of the center due to the actual or potential impact of the center (Exhibit 22.6). Stakeholders can have a variety of goals and vested interests in the center (Marquis & Huston, 2017).

Together (the combination of external and internal stakeholders) these groups are sometimes referred to as *communities of interest*. This term, *communities of interest*, is frequently used in accreditation criteria and by accrediting bodies. These groups are important because they can provide valuable information on how well the center is doing at meeting the expectations of the communities of interest and center goals.

> **EXHIBIT 22.6**
>
> **Examples of Stakeholders in an Academic Healthcare Simulation Center**
>
> | INTERNAL STAKEHOLDERS | EXTERNAL STAKEHOLDERS |
> |---|---|
> | Employees/staff | Local businesses/hiring hospitals |
> | Administration | Accrediting bodies |
> | Financial donors/grantors | Certification agencies |
> | Learners/students | Community leaders |
> | Instructors/faculty | Professional organizations |
> | Board of directors/governing board | Alumni boards |
> | | Malpractice insurance companies |

VARIOUS USERS OF A SIMULATION CENTER

Depending on the physical structure, equipment, and personnel, simulation centers have many opportunities to serve various groups and users. A center can specialize, or expand to fit, several audiences depending on its resources. In healthcare simulation, a center may develop a plan to focus on a wide variety of customer groups or users, including interprofessional education (IPE), continuing education, nurse residency programs, certification pass-offs, research, and medical student and resident training and subspecialty training fellowships.

IPE involves a simulated experience with one or more professions. SPs are individuals who are hired to portray a specific disease or condition with consistency, enabling learners to demonstrate their skills and knowledge of these conditions and diseases. Training, high-stakes testing, or a certification required to obtain or maintain employment are all activities that occur in a simulation center that are events that occur in addition to simulation.

> **SIMULATION TEACHING TIP 22.2**
>
> Evolving to meet the needs of your community can include purchasing equipment and supplies that are representative of those in the clinical settings in which your learners practice. It will decrease reality shock and the amount of time required to transition to the work setting.

Centers may also be used to conduct research, not just research on simulations, but research on equipment and how it interfaces with humans, that is, device testing or as a bench-to-bedside innovation center. Consider ways you can market your center to encourage users, especially those who would benefit from using it off hours.

> A good hockey player plays where the puck is. A great hockey player plays where the puck is going to be.

Managers and Administrators

Managers and administrators have many responsibilities that can keep them on the job and at the office for long hours, especially those who are involved in expansion projects, renovations, mergers, or if they are in the process of bringing an entire new center online. It is not easy to work long hours for extended amounts of time. This can result in fatigue and burnout. Recognize your limitations and ask for the help and support you need. Document your hours and activities, and then review your accomplishments so that you can focus your time and strength on items that have the greatest ROI of time and energy.

Eliminate those items that are not valued and focus on what matters most. Align your goals and efforts with those of administration or the board of directors to avoid a mismatch of expectations and resultant conflict. As new projects are added, assess what can be handed off, simplified, eliminated, or negotiated so that workload and life can be brought back into balance. Learn to say "no." It is far better to focus time and energy in a few essential things than to divide your focus, time, and efforts into many things. Less can be more. Determine your priorities and what is truly essential. Letting go of the nonessential can help to bring energy and balance back into your work and life. Take time to meditate, think, reflect, or read something uplifting each day. Put time and energy into your personal wellness. Invest in yourself, your mind, body, and spirit (McKeown, 2014). Then, support your employees in doing the same.

Be like Switzerland; do not make enemies with anyone. It is a small world, and you never know when a critical and sensitive negotiation or partnership will depend on the relationships you have established and maintained. Do not view others as competitors. Figure out how you can help support the mission of your center. Look at "value added" by using the simulation center and consider it from the customers' or stakeholders' viewpoint: WIFM—What is in it for me? In other words, how it will benefit you (Center for Medical Simulation, 2011).

PERSONNEL AND NONPERSONNEL ISSUES

Personnel issues are any dealings that have to do with human beings. Nonpersonnel issues are concerned with anything that is not human. For example, equipment, supplies, hardware- or software-related items, and so on. Both personnel and nonpersonnel issues have their unique challenges.

Personnel issues may include the following:

- Hiring
- Orienting
- Training
- Coaching
- Counseling
- Termination

Most centers can tap into human resources to assist them in many of these aspects. It is especially important to involve human resources in the hiring, counseling, and termination of employees so as to ensure that the laws and rights of individuals are not violated anywhere in the process. Each region, state, and country can have varying laws and employee rights. Those in human resources generally have the expertise in this area to ensure compliance with local requirements.

The first 90 days of employment are the most important time in helping the new employee understand job expectations and receive orientation and training for his or her position, knowledge, attitudes, and skills. Opportunities for continuing education and personal development support will help to keep the support staff energized about the role they play in supporting the facilitators and improving operations. Institutional review board (IRB) training for support staff involved in research may be necessary.

Leadership Styles and Retention

If you have a high turnover rate (you are not retaining your employees for at least 1–2 years), you are spending a lot of time, money, and energy on recruiting, hiring, orienting, and training employees. It has been estimated in some studies that it costs from several thousand dollars to approximately double the individual's base wage to replace a position (Association of periOperative Registered Nurses [AORN], 2017; Garman, Corbett, Grady, & Benesh, 2008; Tracey & Hinkin, 2008). There are many hidden costs in turnover, including a loss of knowledge and institutional memory. High turnover can result in poor quality and low morale and burnout in existing employees (Porter-O'Grady & Mallock, 2018; Tracey & Hinkin, 2008).

While paying an appropriate wage is important in retaining workers, it is not necessarily the thing that will motivate and engage workers. Hertzberg's motivation-hygiene theory identifies minimum features that must be present in an environment—known as maintenance factors to retain employees, including salary, supervisor, status, personal life, positive working conditions, and job security. These hygiene factors are satisfiers and are necessary to recruit and retain employees. Motivation factors are important in long-term motivation of employees and include opportunities to be involved in meaningful work, to achieve, be recognized, and take on challenges and opportunity for growth (Marquis & Huston, 2015).

The frontline manager is in the best position to affect and implement motivational factors and is really key to retention and employee satisfaction. Transformational leaders have a tremendous impact on an employee's decision to stay in a position (Waldman, Carter, & Hom, 2015), whereas ask-oriented, transactional, laissez-faire, and management by exception leadership styles are used by those who focus primarily on tasks and goal attainment and typically experience higher turnover rates (Cummings et al., 2010).

The attitude leaders have regarding errors can set the tone for the team. Humans make errors. No one is perfect; we all may make mistakes. Some errors are the result of systems and outdated or poor processes. It is important that leaders take the time to review failures and errors with individuals and their team to determine the root cause of problems. Consider, is this a onetime event, caused by human error? Or is there more? Support the well-intended worker with remediation. If the mistake is the result of deliberate carelessness, other steps, such as discipline, should be taken. Recognize that any time something new is tried, there is the potential for error. Error is essential to success. Embracing and recognizing the need to allow for responsible errors and failures as an opportunity to learn and grow is necessary for workers to have confidence that they can be innovative and creative without punishment (Porter-O'Grady & Mallock, 2018).

Counseling and Termination

When counseling an employee or a learner, some common elements should be present. Meet when you are both calm and have sufficient time for the meeting with the employee/learner, clarify and establish expectations, document these expectations, and monitor and revisit as needed. If expectations continue to be met, no further action is required. If expectations are not met, set a meeting during which expectations are again clarified, with documentation of missed expectations/misbehaviors and possible consequences of continued noncompliance, including probable termination/failure. Take time to gain valuable communication skills and tools in difficult conversations by attending relevant workshops and reading books such as *Crucial Conversations: Tools for Talking When Stakes Are High* and *Critical Confrontations* by Patterson, Greeny, McMillian, and Switzler (2011). Talk with a trusted mentor. Be sure to include administration and human resources personnel in these crucial meetings. Do not meet alone with the individual who is hostile or angry. Halt and reschedule. Meetings that turn hostile rarely have a good outcome. Carefully document meeting events, otherwise it can turn into a "he said, she said" scenario that is difficult to prove. Involving another individual can help ensure the message is consistent. He or she can also be there as a neutral party, as protection, or as a witness (Exhibit 22.7).

When Things Do Not Go As Planned: Understanding and Responding to Technical and Material Issues

There is little as unnerving as when you have spent hours preparing the "perfect" simulation, only to have technical difficulties occur and completely throw you off the scenario. Blood pressure cuffs break, HPSs turn off automatically or lose connection, IV pumps go on the blink, and computers or cameras need to be reset. In addition to technology, learners can respond in unexpected ways (Exhibit 22.8).

> It's not the people you fire who make your life miserable. It's the people you don't.
>
> —Dick Grote

EXHIBIT 22.7

Process of Progressive Discipline for Rule Breakers

1. Informal reprimand or verbal admonishment
2. Formal reprimand or written admonishment
3. Suspension from work
4. Involuntary dismissal or termination

Source: Adapted from Marquis, B. L., & Huston, C. J. (2017). *Leadership roles and management function in nursing: Theory and application* (9th ed.). Philadelphia, PA: Lippincott Williams & Wilkins.

> **EXHIBIT 22.8**
>
> **Unexpected Events**
>
> - Technology does not function correctly.
> - The learners misunderstand the objectives of the scenario.
> - The learners have difficulty suspending reality.
> - The scenario is too easy or complex for the learners' stage of education.
> - A learner does something that is not in the scenario and changes the progress or the outcome of the scenario.
> - Debriefing is altered because an unexpected event happened during the scenario.

Source: Adapted from Dieckmann, P., Lippert, A., Glavin, R., & Rall, M. (2010). When things do not go as expected: Scenario life savers. *Simulation in Healthcare, 5*(4), 219–225.

How one chooses to frame or view these situations that can occur from time to time and how one responds to them will have a tremendous impact on the learner and the learning that can take place.

So what is the best way to respond to these unexpected events? It is important to consider this in two phases, immediate and long term. What is the best immediate response during the event and when the learners are present? First, consider the core learning objectives you have for the scenario, and, as much as possible, use the unexpected event to meet the goals.

Scenario lifesavers can be delivered from inside or outside the scenario. Inside-scenario lifesavers use things from within the scenario to influence the learners and the direction the scenario is headed so that they can return to the key learning objectives (Dieckmann et al., 2010).

Dieckmann et al. (2010) suggest that if the unexpected turn of events is a safety issue for the learners or the equipment—such as the possibility of someone being injured with the incorrect use of the defibrillator—you can intervene by making an overhead announcement. This is called a *lifesaver from outside the scenario*. Another approach is to come up with a plausible background story as to why something may have occurred. This is an example of an inside lifesaver, because it is based on something that occurred inside of the scenario.

If the scenario has gone way off course, or there are critical technology failures, consider stopping the scenario and then restarting it so that the core learner objectives can be met. Lifesavers are also discussed in Chapter 5 of this text.

As a debriefer or simulation instructor, take a deep breath and collect your thoughts before you return to debrief the learners. The learners will often mirror the response of the debriefer. If the debriefer is flustered and complains, the learners will quickly pick up on this and join in, and a teaching moment is lost. On the other hand, if the debriefer is composed and positive, the learners can still walk away with a positive learning experience.

> How we choose to see things and respond to others makes all the difference.
>
> —*Thomas S. Monson*

Normalize the feelings of the group—share what it is that groups frequently feel or how they respond in this given situation. Normalizing helps to decrease the feelings of guilt and resistance.

During the debriefing session, as individuals point out the problems that occurred, agree with them quickly. Yes, there was a problem with item A; then quickly bring it back to real life and ask, could that ever happen in the actual clinical setting? Could item A stop working? What actions would be appropriate? What can be learned? Then redirect the group back to the learning objectives. Agreeing with the learners quickly can diffuse the emotion surrounding the situation. Once the emotion is defused, learning can take place (Center for Medical Simulation, 2011).

What is the best long-term response to technical issues? Troubleshoot the item that caused the problem. Determine the cause, and get the item repaired or find a substitute or work around as quickly as possible so that this does not become a common occurrence. Reschedule other events if an acceptable solution is not possible. Include money for technology repairs in the budget. If the unexpected response comes from the learner, edit the scenario to prevent a recurrence.

> **CASE STUDY 22.3**
>
> The HPS suddenly turns off; the monitor has flat lines. The learner notices this, interprets this as a cardiac arrest, and calls a code. What possible responses can you have? What responses can keep you consistent with the key learning objectives?

Troubleshooting Equipment: General Information

When dealing with technology, troubleshooting has some standard steps:

1. Ensure all cable connections are secure.
2. Ensure the device is plugged in/charged.
3. Shut down the device and start it back up again.
4. Refer to the owner's manual for troubleshooting.
5. Call the sales representative/manufacturer.
6. Repair or replace the defective item.

Create a notebook to log all major pieces of equipment: their purchase, service and repairs, and problems. Document everything: date of occurrence, details of event, actions taken, name(s) of individual contacted with number, expected resolution with date, any follow-up, and so on. This record will become particularly useful if you have to make claims on the warranty of an item. Ensuring that all individuals who use the equipment are adequately trained will decrease the problems and breakage of equipment. Again, be sure to budget sufficient funds to repair and replace the equipment.

V DOMAIN IV: SIMULATION RESOURCES AND ENVIRONMENTS

SUMMARY

Effective operation of a simulation center is based on principles of leadership, management of personnel and other resources, policies, procedures, and processes. Additional skills include effective troubleshooting when unexpected events occur and using good judgment in influencing the scenario from inside or outside sources.

PRACTICE QUESTIONS

1. Which of the following leadership styles will most likely result in employee satisfaction?

   A. Transformational
   B. Management by exception
   C. Laissez-faire
   D. Transactional

2. Which words most accurately describe retention? Retention_____.

   A. Is overrated; it is good for business to have a constant turnover of new enthusiastic personnel
   B. Is not something a manager needs focus on
   C. Is an important part of the mission and strategic plan
   D. Is critical in maintaining quality and reducing expenses

3. Which of the following is most important to increase realism and learner engagement in simulation?

   A. Inclusion of actor (standardized [simulated] patient [SP]) and confederates in the scenario
   B. Willingness of the learner to engage in the learning process
   C. Realistic smells, sounds, and images
   D. High-fidelity human patient simulators with voice modulators

4. Which statement most closely reflects the underlying attitude of a transformative leader?

   A. Failure is a way to grow.
   B. Perfection is demanded.
   C. Errors are largely caused by carelessness.
   D. System policies and process rarely need updates.

5. The individual who schedules events (the scheduler) in your simulation center cancels a high-priority user and, in his place, schedules a friend's group (a mid-priority user) in the center. You are the director of the center, and you just received an email complaint from your high-priority user. What initial action is the most appropriate in addressing this situation with the scheduler?

   A. Dismiss the scheduler.
   B. Meet with the scheduler and clarify policy and expectations. Support the scheduler in rectifying the situation.
   C. Immediately place the scheduler on unpaid leave. Meet in a few days after you have straightened everything out.
   D. Stop by the scheduler's office and express your disappointment and frustration.

6. Which method is most likely to be successful for all users in keeping supplies organized in a larger center?

   A. Designate a place for each item and label everything.
   B. Keep secret stashes of hard-to-find items.
   C. Lock supplies in cupboards.
   D. Delegate one contact person as a gatekeeper for all supplies and equipment.

7. When managing supplies and equipment, it is important to _____.

   A. Track equipment repairs and warranty and service agreement information
   B. Track nondurable supplies and equipment for inventory and costs
   C. Determine what supplies and equipment and their costs are used in each scenario
   D. All of the above

8. Which of the following need to be considered in scheduling an event?

   A. Personnel
   B. Mission, vision, and values
   C. Equipment and supplies
   D. All of the above

9. Which one of the following can best help bring balance and effectiveness?

   A. Diligently learn and apply time-management skills.
   B. Consider what is essential and eliminate the nonessential.
   C. Apply the Six Sigma principles in your life.
   D. Never open email first thing in the morning.

10. You are setting up the room for a scenario and notice a piece of equipment is not working correctly. Select the item with the best sequence for troubleshooting and correcting this problem.

    A. Call the sales rep/manufacturer, ensure the device is plugged in/charged, refer to the owner's manual for troubleshooting, shut down the device, and start it back up again.
    B. Ensure all cable connections are secure, repair or replace item, check to see whether the device is plugged in/charged, shut down the device, and start it back up again.
    C. Ensure all connections are secure, shut down the device and start it back up again, refer to owner's manual for troubleshooting, and call rep/manufacturer.
    D. Shut down the device and start it back up again, ensure the device is plugged in/charged, ensure all cable connections are secure, and call the sales rep/manufacturer.

REFERENCES

Association of periOperative Registered Nurses. (2017). How to recruit and retain perioperative nurses amid the nursing shortage: A guide for hospital leaders. Retrieved from https://www.aorn.org/education/facility-solutions/periop-101

Center for Advanced Medical Learning and Simulation. (2014). Surgical and interventional training center. Retrieved from http://www.camls-us.org/

Center for Medical Simulation. (2011, November). *Comprehensive simulation instructor workshop*. Workshop held in Boston, MA.

Cummings, G. G., MacGregor, T., Davey, M., Lee, H., Wong, C. A., Lo, E., ... Stafford, E. (2010). Leadership styles and outcome patterns for the nursing workforce and work environment: A systematic review. *International Journal of Nursing Studies, 47*, 363–385. doi:10.1016/j.ijnurstu.2009.08.006

Dieckmann, P., Lippert, A., Glavin, R., & Rall, M. (2010). When things do not go as expected: Scenario life savers. *Simulation in Healthcare, 5*(4), 219–225. doi:10.1097/SIH.0b013e3181e77f74

Fei, H., Meskens, N., & Chu, C. (2009). A planning and scheduling problem for an operating theatre using an open scheduling strategy. *Computers & Industrial Engineering, 58*(2010), 221–230. doi:10.1016/j.cie.2009.02.012

Fiore, F. F. (2005). *Write a business plan in no time*. Indianapolis, IN: Que.

Garman, A. N., Corbett, J., Grady, J., & Benesh, J. (2005). The hidden costs of employee turnover: Ready-to-use-simulation. *Simulation & Gaming, 36*(2), 274–281. doi:10.1177/1046878104273254

Langford, J. (n.d.). Moulage recipes. Retrieved from http://www.okhealthcareworkforce.com/Conferences/documents/JackieLangford_ArtofMoulage_Recipes.pdf

Lassche, M., & Scheese, C. (2013, June). *Effective team work—More than a game of chance*. Poster presentation at the 12th Annual International Nursing Simulation/Learning (INACSL) Resource Centers Conference: Hit the Jackpot with Evidence Based Simulation, Las Vegas, NV.

Lazzara, E. H., Benishek, L. E., Dietz, A. S., Salas, E., & Adriansen, D. J. (2014). Eight critical factors in creating and implementing a successful simulation program. *Joint Commission Journal on Quality and Patient Safety, 40*(1), 21–29. doi:10.1016/s1553-7250(14)40003-5

Marquis, B. L., & Huston, C. J. (2017). *Leadership roles and management function in nursing: Theory and application* (9th ed.). Philadelphia, PA: Lippincott Williams & Wilkins.

McKeown, G. (2014). *Essentialism: The disciplined pursuit of less*. New York, NY: Currency.

Patterson, K., Greeny, J., McMillian, R., & Switzler. A. (2011). *Crucial conversations: tools for talking when stakes are high and critical confrontations*. New York, NY: McGraw-Hill.

Peterson, S. D., Jaret, P. E., & Schenck, B. F. (2013). How to define operations in your business plan. In Business plan kits for dummies. New York, NY: John Wiley. Retrieved from http://www.dummies.com/how-to/content/how-to-define-operations-in-your-business-plan.html

Porter-O'Grady, T., & Malloch, K. (2018). *Quantum leadership: Sustainable value in health care*. Burlington, MA: Jones & Bartlett Learning.

Scheese, C. (2013, June). *Strategies for a winning hand in scheduling*. Podium presentation at the 12th Annual International Nursing (INACSL), Las Vegas, NV.

Sinek, S., (2009). *Start with why: How great leaders inspire everyone to take action*. New York, NY: Penguin Books.

Society for Simulation in Healthcare. (2014). Council for Accreditation of Healthcare Simulation Programs: Accreditation standards self-study review. Washington, DC: Author. Retrieved from http://www.ssih.org/Accreditation/Full-Accreditation

Society for Simulation in Healthcare. (2018a). *Certified Healthcare Simulation Educator Examination Blueprint, 2018 Version*. Retrieved from http://www.ssih.org/Portals/48/Certification/CHSE_Docs/CHSE_Examination_Blueprint.pdf

Society for Simulation in Healthcare. (2018b). *SSH certified healthcare simulation educator handbook*. Washington, DC: Author. Retrieved from http://www.ssih.org/Portals/48/Certification/CHSE_Docs/CHSE%20Handbook.pdf

Tracey, B., & Hinkin, T. R. (2008). Contextual factors and cost profiles associated with employee turnover. *Cornell Hospital Quarterly, 49*(1), 12–27. doi:10.1177/0010880407310191

Waldman, D.A., Carter, M. Z., & Hom, P. W. (2015). A multilevel investigation of leadership and turnover behavior. *Journal of Management, 41*(6), 1724–1744. doi:10.1177/0149206312460679

23 Accreditation of Simulation Laboratories and Simulation Standards

ANTHONY BATTAGLIA, FABIEN PAMPALONI, AND BETH A. TELESZ

Learning by doing, peer-to-peer teaching, and computer simulation are all part of the same equation.

—Nicholas Negroponte

This chapter addresses Domain IV: Simulation Resources and Environments (Society for Simulation in Healthcare [SSH], 2018).

[LEARNING OUTCOMES]

- Discuss the importance of simulation laboratory accreditation.
- Describe the accreditation standards of the SSH.
- List the nine standards of best practices in simulation of the International Nursing Association for Clinical Simulation and Learning (INACSL, 2014).

As simulation knowledge and theory have evolved, so, too, has the need to provide standards for simulation education. Today, a popular discussion throughout the simulation community is the pursuit of center accreditation to ensure that standards are met. This chapter provides information on the SSH accreditation process and the standards developed by the INACSL and recently revised in 2016. Both organizations are committed to excellence in simulation education. Both organizations are international and sponsor journals that contain up-to-date simulation teaching, research, and practice. SSH supports interprofessional membership and INACSL is a nursing-based organization.

■ ACCREDITATION

The U.S. Department of Education defines *accreditation* as "the status of public recognition that an accrediting agency grants to an educational institution or program that meets the agency's standards and requirements" ([R] 602.3, 1999, p. 1).

In the eyes of the public, accreditation is the promise to consumers that the simulation center in the hospital or educational organization has met the highest quality of standards in order for healthcare students to learn. These standards will ultimately be reflected in the care provided to patients in associated hospitals.

Accreditation promises to put your simulation center in the spotlight, allowing it to be showcased as a premier center of excellence, which will resonate when opening the door for students, family, and public touring events. As a result, learning continuity, best practices, and standardized processes can be anticipated by Certified Healthcare Simulation Educators™ (CHSE™), staff, and learners who use the center. In addition, accreditation will lead to

- Improved learning processes for the student
- Probable ease with budgetary preparedness
- Forecasting benefits
- Anticipated fixed assets
- Improvements in business operations

An understanding of the many benefits of simulation center accreditation can serve as a strong motivator to initiate the process. Improved patient safety is the ultimate outcome of center accreditation, and more studies are needed to support this outcome. One of the major benefits of accreditation is to create stronger opportunities for patient safety efforts that are sustainable through the support of standardized simulation modalities.

Developing a simulation laboratory into one that meets the standards of accreditation places the simulation educators in a mentor capacity. Expect to be the new target for other centers that wish to learn from and with you. This exchange of best practices and effective educational strategies fosters networking and mutual growth. Your center will be considered "a center of excellence" for national and international collaborations that may have never existed.

Once accredited, an observable transformation in CHSEs, learners, and community levels of confidence and belief in the quality of services and educational opportunities will be noted. In a society that has reservations about the care provided in today's hospitals, your center will be considered a highly valid and reliable place where learners want to learn, CHSEs want to advance, and one that the community is proud of. From CHSEs to participants, a growing sense of ownership and enthusiasm will become contagious, and quality-improvement efforts will follow. CHSEs will strive to find ways to continuously make improvements that will contribute to best practices and improved patient safety efforts that serve the center's mission, vision, and values.

> **SIMULATION TEACHING TIP 23.1**
>
> "Accreditation, of course, does not come without determination, dedication and a true investment of time. It is a team effort and involves true commitment," says John O'Donnell, CRNA, MSN, DrPH, professor and director, University of Pittsburgh School of Nursing Nurse Anesthesia Program, associate director and codirector of Research, Winter Institute for Simulation and Research (personal communication, 2014).

To ensure success, Dr. O'Donnell (2014, personal communication) also advises the following:

- Designate a project manager who is highly efficient and organized.
- Determine the area(s) in which your institution best qualifies for accreditation.
- Prepare the appropriate documents to validate the category of accreditation you wish to pursue.
- Understand the accreditation standards in each category in order to select the domain for which your center is best suited for accreditation.
- Practice strong record keeping and progress mapping to prepare for application submission and onsite visits.

Keeping these key principles in mind while reviewing the following standards will open up your pathway to successful accreditation.

THE SOCIETY FOR SIMULATION IN HEALTHCARE

The SSH was established in January 2004 to represent the rapidly growing group of educators, research scientists, and advocates who use a variety of simulation methodologies for education, testing, and research in healthcare. *SSH accredits simulation programs*. As standards and criteria are very specific, most of the following information was directly taken from the SSH guidelines describing the development of a self-study report that must be submitted for the consideration of accreditation.

The self-study report must address the core standards as listed in Exhibit 22.5. In addition, one of the following areas must be addressed: assessment, research, or teaching/education. A fourth area may also be addressed, which is "system integration and patient safety" (SSH, 2014, p. 5). Complete criteria for each area that must be addressed in the self-study can be easily located on the SSH home page (www.ssih.org) using the "Accreditation" tab on the top toolbar of the site and using the "Full accreditation" option to locate the materials needed, which include the following:

- An information guide
- A self-study guide
- Application instructions
- Application form

STANDARDS

Standards are established to promote best practice. Simulation programs that meet established standards provide the public with quality programs that are continuously critiqued and evaluated for best practice. INACSL is an organization devoted to simulation education excellence and has developed best practice standards, which are published and provide an excellent guide for simulation educators.

> **EVIDENCE-BASED SIMULATION PRACTICE 23.1**
>
> "Simulation represents a paradigm shift in health care education. I am pleased that we are able to provide our students with unique learning opportunities in our labs through improved simulation technology, educational methods, practitioner assessment, and patient safety," said Amy Daniels, MS, BSN, RN, CHSE, clinical instructor and interim director of University of Maryland School of Nursing's clinical simulation laboratories.

THE INTERNATIONAL NURSING ACCREDITATION FOR CLINICAL SIMULATION AND LEARNING

In 2011, the Board of Directors at the INACSL presented their first standards for best practices. The mission of INACSL is "to promote research and disseminate evidence-based practice standards for clinical simulation methodologies and learning environments" (INACSL, 2014, p. 1).

The standards of INACSL accreditation were created based on a detailed survey geared toward the needs and importance of maintaining an educational homogeneity among clinical practices. The initial standards were published in August of 2011 and recently revised in December of 2016 as published in an issue of *Clinical Simulation in Nursing* (Volume 12, Issue 12, Supplement, S1–S50). The remainder of this chapter summarizes the most current standards. For a detailed description of each standard, please refer to this reference.

The newly revised standards are as follows (INACSL, 2016):

Simulation^{SM} Simulation Design (INACSL, 2016a)

Simulation^{SM} Outcomes and Objectives (INACSL, 2016b)

Simulation^{SM} Facilitation (INACSL, 2016c)

Simulation^{SM} Debriefing (INACSL, 2016d)

Simulation^{SM} Participant Evaluation (INACSL, 2016e)

Simulation^{SM} Professional Integrity (INACSL, 2016f)

Simulation^{SM} Simulation-Enhanced (INACSL, 2016g)

Interprofessional Education (Sim-IPE) (INACSL, 2016h)

Simulation^{SM} Simulation Glossary

Operations (INACSL, 2017)

STANDARDS OVERVIEW

Simulation^{SM} Simulation Design

This standard outlines the framework for developing effective simulation-based experiences. Its design reflects best practices from adult learning, education, instructional design, clinical standards of care, evaluation, and simulation pedagogy (Lioce, Meakim, Fey, Chmil, Mariani, & Alinier, 2015). This standard focuses on creating simulation-based experiences that are purposefully designed to meet objectives and optimizes achievement of expected outcomes. This standard includes a list of 11 criteria that need to be met in order to exercise best nursing simulation practice. Also, design templates are available to educators who want to apply standardized education (INACLS, 2016a).

Simulation^{SM} Outcomes and Objectives

This standard highlights the importance of creating achievable outcomes that are clearly defined by measurable objectives. Assessment and evaluation of the learning experience in relation to the set learning objectives are necessary to promote best practice. Simulation activities should be used to lead the learner toward the proposed outcomes in a safe and predictable environment. Specific criteria needs to be met in both outcome and objective design (INACSL, 2016b).

Simulation^{SM} Facilitation

This standard describes facilitation methods and presents the key qualities of an effective facilitator. Facilitation methods vary and are dependent on the learning needs of participants and the expected outcomes. A facilitator assumes responsibility and oversight for managing the entire simulation-based experience. Facilitators must be qualified, educated, skilled, and possess the ability to guide, support, and seek out ways to assist learners in successful completion of desired outcomes. "Through the use of facilitation methods, the facilitator's role is to help participants in their skill development and explore their thought processes in critical thinking, problem solving, clinical reasoning, clinical judgment, and apply their theoretical knowledge to patient care in a range of health care settings." For these reasons, facilitator continuing education is essential to maintain skill and for the individual to remain current and effective. This standard consists of five necessary criteria that contain required elements to assist the facilitator in ensuring successful simulation-based experiences. Poor educational consequences may result when this standard is not followed (INACSL, 2016c, p. s16).

Simulation^{SM} Debriefing

The literature supports that essential learning occurs in the debriefing phase of the simulation-based experience. Moreover, the skills of the debriefer are critical to ensure the best possible learning outcomes. This standard describes the significance and background of the debriefing process in simulation-based experiences and supporting criteria with required elements for successful debriefing. It advises that all simulation-based experiences include a planned debriefing session aimed at promoting reflective learning for improvement in future participant performance. There are five necessary criteria to meet this standard. Failure to follow this standard may lead to poor educational consequences to including unsuccessful debriefing sessions and potential uncomfortable experiences for participants (INACSL, 2016d).

Simulation^{SM} Participant Evaluation

This standard advises that all simulation-based experiences require participant evaluation. Formative, summative, high-stakes, and authentic evaluation are assessment types used to determine skill level, competency, and overall performance of the participant. There are four necessary criteria with supporting required elements to meet this standard. If this standard is not followed, poor educational consequences may result to include inaccurate assessment, poor

Simulation^SM Professional Integrity

This standard emphasizes the importance of ethical behavior for all individuals involved in simulation-based experiences. Regardless of one's role or responsibilities, it is important to encourage communication among team members in order to strengthen professional integrity during the somewhat unpredictable simulation-based experiences. The inability to maintain a professional and ethical balance during experiences may cause participants to present altered and biased performance as well as developing a sense of distrust in professional relationships. In order to ensure a proper learning environment, four criteria are necessary to meet this standard (INACSL, 2016f).

Simulation^SM Sim-IPE

This standard's sole purpose is to obtain ultimate learning outcomes while performing interprofessional simulation experiences. Nowadays, healthcare providers from all specialties often collaborate in order to reach a mutual outcome. It is of critical importance that communication, cooperation, and skill sharing are mastered during such collaborations. The Sim-IPE effectively creates learning objectives giving individual the ability to "learn about, from, and with each other to enable effective collaboration and improve health outcome" (INACSL, 2016, p. 31). A list of four criteria is necessary to meet this standard (INACSL, 2016g).

Simulation^SM Simulation Glossary

This standard encourages the use of a consistent terminology throughout simulation experiences, publications, and research. Standardized terminology is used to reduce negative consequences like confusion, misunderstanding, and poor learning outcomes triggered by nonconsistent terminology. A list of more than 60 terms is included in this standard allowing the user to apply proper terminology to future simulation-based experiences (INACSL, 2016h).

Simulation^SM Simulation Operations

This new standard encompasses all components necessary to efficiently and effectively implement simulation-based education (SBE). These components include infrastructure, people, and processes. To successfully fulfill this standard, a skilled professional or qualified team must be appointed to meet six specific criteria. Criteria include, but are not limited to implementing a strategic plan, providing appropriate expertise, maintaining and managing financial resources, and creating policies and procedures. The effective application of this standard will guarantee cohesive simulation operations and improve interprofessional collaboration (INACSL, 2017).

23 ACCREDITATION OF SIMULATION LABORATORIES AND SIMULATION STANDARDS

SUMMARY

The prestigious recognition of accreditation or meeting standards brings a sense of accomplishment to the staff and simulation educators as participants reap the benefits of learning in a simulation center that has gone the distance and has reached either of these remarkable benchmarks. It is time to take your center to the next level and observe the leadership, learners, competitors, and the public marveling at your accomplishment. It is also time to embrace the new and exciting opportunities that will be presented following your certification. Your center will not only gain respect and admiration from the community, but will also enjoy the recruitment, retention, grant funding, and publication opportunities that will follow. This is an exciting time to be a member of the simulation community and to contribute to its success, development, and advancement.

> **CASE STUDY 23.1**
>
> A newly certified healthcare simulation educator is developing a strategic plan for his interdisciplinary laboratory. The laboratory is a converted skills laboratory in a school of physical therapy. The laboratory has been functioning for a year and has one laboratory technician. How would you advise the simulation educator to go about starting the process for SSH accreditation or meeting INACSL standards? What resources would you recommend to him? How long do you think either process should take?

PRACTICE QUESTIONS

1. A simulation educator is developing a self-study report for an accreditation process and is describing a simulation about the goals and responsibilities of a rapid-response team. This should be integrated in standard:
    A. Simulation^{SM} Participant Evaluation
    B. Simulation^{SM} Outcomes and Objectives
    C. Simulation^{SM} Facilitation
    D. Simulation^{SM} Debriefing

2. A simulation educator is developing a self-study report for accreditation and includes a section on personnel qualification; this information should be included in:
    A. Simulation^{SM} Debriefing
    B. Simulation^{SM} Simulation Design
    C. Simulation^{SM} Professional Integrity
    D. Simulation^{SM} Facilitation

3. The U.S. Department of Education (USDE) defines *accreditation* as:
    A. The act or instance of choosing a candidate or organization for election or appointment or honor
    B. An activity that supports or provides active encouragement for the furtherance of cause, venture, or aim

C. The action or process of providing someone or something with an official document attesting to a status or level of achievement

D. The status of public recognition that an accrediting agency grants to an educational institution or program that meets the agency's standards and requirements

4. Accreditation of your Simulation Center is a prestigious recognition that may lead to all of the following EXCEPT:

   A. Decreased student enrollment of the Simulation Lab's educational affiliates
   B. Improved educational experience for students
   C. Forecasting benefits
   D. Improvements in business operations

5. End-of-unit or chapter tests, end-of-term (midterm) exams, and end-of-semester (final) exams are all examples of _____ assessments.

   A. High-stakes
   B. Summative
   C. Self
   D. Authentic

6. When developing an accreditation self-study report, the simulation educator describes a student grievance incident and the due process that led to a resolution. This should be explained in which standard?

   A. Simulation^{SM} Simulation Design
   B. Simulation^{SM} Outcomes and Objectives
   C. Simulation^{SM} Professional Integrity
   D. Simulation^{SM} Security

7. A key ingredient for a successful accreditation process is to have a:

   A. Consultant
   B. Simulation educator
   C. Project manager
   D. Accreditations liaison

8. Simulation programs are accredited by:

   A. International Nursing Association for Clinical Simulation and Learning (INACSL)
   B. International Meeting on Simulation in Healthcare (IMSH)
   C. Certified Healthcare Simulation Educator™ (CHSE™) Independent Accreditors
   D. Society for Simulation in Healthcare (SSH)

9. Best practice is a method that has been generally accepted as superior to any alternatives because it produces results that are supported by research. Which standard incorporates best practice from adult learning?

   A. Simulation^{SM} Simulation Design
   B. Simulation^{SM} Outcomes and Objectives
   C. Simulation^{SM} Facilitation
   D. Simulation^{SM} Debriefing

10. The use of standardized terminology has the goal of reducing negative consequences like confusion, misunderstanding, and poor learning outcomes. What are the accepted sources for terminology in in situ simulation?

   A. Simulation^{SM} Simulation Protocols
   B. Simulation^{SM} Participant Evaluation
   C. Simulation^{SM} Professional Integrity
   D. Society for Simulation in Healthcare's *Healthcare Simulation Dictionary*

■ REFERENCES

International Nursing Association for Clinical Simulation & Learning. (2014). Mission statement. Retrieved from http://www.inacsl.org/i4a/pages/index.cfm?pageid=3278

INACSL Standards Committee. (2016a). INACSL standards of best practice: Simulation^{SM} Simulation design. *Clinical Simulation in Nursing*, 12(S), S5–S12. doi:10.1016/j.ecns.2016.09.005

INACSL Standards Committee. (2016b). INACSL Standards of Best Practice: Simulation^{SM} Outcomes and objectives. *Clinical Simulation in Nursing*, 12(S), S13–S15. doi:10.1016/j.ecns.2016.09.006

INACSL Standards Committee. (2016c). INACSL standards of best practice: Simulation^{SM} Facilitation. *Clinical Simulation in Nursing*, 12(S), S16–S20. doi:10.1016/j.ecns.2016.09.007

INACSL Standards Committee. (2016d). INACSL standards of best practice: Simulation^{SM} Debriefing. *Clinical Simulation in Nursing*, 12(S), S21–S25. doi:10.1016/j.ecns.2016.09.008

INACSL Standards Committee. (2016e). INACSL standards of best practice: Simulation^{SM} Participant evaluation. *Clinical Simulation in Nursing*, 12(S), S26–S29. doi:10.1016/j.ecns.2016.09.009

INACSL Standards Committee. (2016f). INACSL standards of best practice: Simulation^{SM} Professional integrity. *Clinical Simulation in Nursing*, 12(S), S30–S33. doi:10.1016/j.ecns.2016.09.010

INACSL Standards Committee. (2016g). INACSL Standards of Best Practice: Simulation^{SM} Simulation-enhanced interprofessional education (sim-IPE). *Clinical Simulation in Nursing*, 12(S), S34–S38. doi:10.1016/j.ecns.2016.09.011

INACSL Standards Committee. (2016h). INACSL standards of best practice: Simulation^{SM} Simulation glossary. *Clinical Simulation in Nursing*, 12(S), S39–S47. doi:10.1016/j.ecns.2016.09.012

INACSL Standards Committee. (2017). INACSL Standards of Best Practice: Simulation^{SM}: Operations. *Clinical Simulation in Nursing*, 13(12), 681–687. doi:10.1016/j.ecns.2017.10.005

Lioce, L., Meakim, C. H., Fey, M. K., Chmil, J. V., Mariani, B., & Alinier, G. (2015). Standards of Best Practice: Simulation Standard IX: Simulation Design. Clinical Simulation in Nursing, 11(6), 309–315.

Society for Simulation in Healthcare. (2014). *Council for accreditation of healthcare simulation programs accreditation standards self-study review*. Washington, DC: Author. http://www.ssih.org/Accreditation/Mid-Cycle-Accreditation

Society for Simulation in Healthcare. (2016). *Healthcare simulation dictionary*. Washington, DC: Author. Retrieved from http://www.ssih.org/dictionary

Society for Simulation in Healthcare. (2018). *Certified Healthcare Simulation Educator Examination Blueprint, 2018 Version*. Retrieved from http://www.ssih.org/Portals/48/Certification/CHSE_Docs/CHSE_Examination_Blueprint.pdf

U.S. Department of Education. (1999). *Federal aid. Citations: (R)602.3*. Retrieved from http://ifap.ed.gov/regcomps/doc3983_bodyoftext.htm

24

Practice Test

RUTH A. WITTMANN-PRICE, LINDA WILSON, AND SAMUEL W. PRICE

1. Learners in a simulation laboratory who have a cognitive or physical disability receive:

    A. Special equipment
    B. More time
    C. Reasonable accommodations
    D. An individual educator

2. The key concept of debriefing is to:

    A. Critique the event
    B. Identify peer interaction
    C. Build consensus
    D. Develop improvement strategies

3. The simulation educator understands that the best way to present a situation to a cohort of healthcare learners is to:

    A. Schedule specific time during each semester.
    B. Have students sign up on their own.
    C. Use simulation as a remediation tool.
    D. Integrate simulation throughout the curriculum.

4. For which of the following is videotaping most appropriate?

    A. Interviewing a patient (standardized/simulated patients) for professional development
    B. Megacode in Advanced Cardiac Life Support (ACLS)
    C. Medication administration
    D. Intraosseous vascular insertion

5. According to Kern et al. (2009), the initial step in curriculum development to include in simulation is (Chapter 15):

    A. Needs assessment
    B. Learner assessment
    C. Choosing the appropriate environment
    D. Establishing learning objectives

6. The novice simulation educator needs additional understanding when she states the following is a protection of students' ethical, legal, and regulatory rights in a simulation laboratory:

    A. Having codes of conduct
    B. Maintaining fair evaluation processes
    C. Having consent to record
    D. Implied consent for picture taking

7. Which research method should be used to measure mastery learning?

   A. Validated checklists
   B. Multiple choice test
   C. Peer critique
   D. Focus group

8. The novice simulation educator needs further understanding when she states a mode of simulation includes:

   A. Live scenarios
   B. Virtual learning
   C. Constructive theory
   D. Task trainers

9. What was Rossignol's (2017) conclusion when she compared oral debriefing to video-assisted debriefing (Chapter 21)?

   A. Video-assisted debriefing is better.
   B. Oral debriefing is better.
   C. There is no significant difference between oral and video-assisted debriefing.
   D. Repeated simulations increase psychological stress.

10. In the medical education literature, simulation is a reliable tool for assessing which of these?

    A. Clinical outcomes
    B. Teamwork and communication
    C. Patient outcomes
    D. Knowledge

11. Interprofessional education (IPE) is a form of:

    A. Experiential learning
    B. Behavioralism
    C. Deliberate practice
    D. Self-directed learning

12. When combined with simulation-based medical education, which teaching method improves skills acquisition?

    A. Deliberate practice
    B. Didactic content
    C. Case studies
    D. Mock codes

13. Simulation educators understand that the purpose of formative evaluation is to provide:

    A. A grade for the activity
    B. Information for prebriefing
    C. Constructive feedback
    D. A pass/fail for the clinical skill

14. The Certified Healthcare Simulation Educator™ observes the students missing an important assessment during a scenario and has the mannequin cough so the students listen to lung sounds. According to Meller (1997), this element of activity is a(n) (Chapter 14):

    A. Passive element
    B. Active element
    C. Interactive element
    D. Transference

15. Feedback is a process used in debriefing to:

    A. Provide a grade for the student.
    B. Identify remediation needs.
    C. Consider the student successful or unsuccessful.
    D. Promote desirable student development.

16. Professional conduct expected from a hired standardized patient (SP) includes:

    A. Articulation skills
    B. Knowledge of evaluation processes
    C. Emotional intelligence
    D. Honesty

17. A new educator has developed a simulation scenario for his critical care course and after the scenario the educator should undertake the following activity first:

    A. Write another simulation scenario on a topic of interest.
    B. Evaluate the students' feedback about the scenario.
    C. Determine the methods of evaluation to be used.
    D. Develop a schedule for the simulation activities.

18. An asset to using part-task trainers is:

    A. They are lightweight.
    B. They are disposable.
    C. They are small and store easily.
    D. They are cost-effective.

19. In planning the simulation event, the exper4inced simulation educator understands that:

    A. Student skills should all be at an acceptable level
    B. Scenarios that are difficult and challenging will produce better discussion in debriefing
    C. Topic areas should include common scenarios
    D. Activities that will help meet student learning outcomes usually work the best

20. A nurse educator is developing goals for the simulation activities to be included in her course. A goal written in the affective domain is:

    A. "Learners will demonstrate the correct technique for inserting an intravenous catheter."
    B. "Learners will demonstrate the correct technique for administering intramuscular medications."

C. "Students will demonstrate empathy for the patient and family members."
D. "Learners will understand the steps of checking tube feeding residuals."

21. The following would be an example of a high-stakes simulation laboratory evaluation:

    A. Performing an end-of-course pass/fail objective structured clinical examination (OSCE)
    B. Completing one of four didactic tests given throughout the semester
    C. Deliberate practice of Foley catheter insertion in open laboratory hours
    D. A simulation scenario about a cardiac infarction that is recorded for review

22. The new simulation educator needs additional understanding of curriculum development when she states:

    A. "I need to identify every place where I can get resources."
    B. "This curriculum needs to be evaluated in an ongoing fashion."
    C. "I am positive that we have political support for this simulation curriculum."
    D. "We can address implementation barriers as they arise."

23. The healthcare simulation educator understands that the four main core competencies for interprofessional collaborative practice include the following:

    A. Leadership
    B. Evidence-based practice
    C. Reflection
    D. Communication

24. In an advocacy-inquiry debriefing session the simulation educator correctly starts a process improvement when he states:

    A. "I am concerned because I noticed the team took four minutes to organize themselves."
    B. "The team took too long to organize themselves."
    C. "Let's list what went well and what needs improvement."
    D. Can you all tell me as a group what took you so long?

25. During a formative evaluation with a student after a simulation scenario about patient safety, the best response from the debriefer would be:

    A. "Not identifying the patient could result in you eventually losing your license."
    B. "Your lack of safety in patient identification fails you."
    C. "Understanding patient safety is my priority."
    D. "Can you think of how to increase patient safety in the next scenario."

26. The most effective simulation method to teach intravenous (IV) insertion would be:

    A. Using a standardized patient
    B. Using a part-task trainer with a standardized patient
    C. Using a high-fidelity mannequin
    D. Using a peer who is role-playing

27. During a simulation scenario a student starts to have an anxiety attach and stands against the wall as if immobile. The best recourse for the simulation educator in this scenario is:

   A. Stop the scenario and ask the student to come out then continue.
   B. Continue the scenario and provide feedback to the student individually immediately after.
   C. Give the other students a "life saver" to focus their attention on the student having the anxiety attach.
   D. Stop the scenario and debrief the group.

28. One of the primary reasons to integrate simulation throughout a curriculum is to identify:

   A. Skill attainment
   B. Missing procedures
   C. Knowledge gaps
   D. At-risk students

29. The Certified Healthcare Simulation Educator™ takes great care to make a patient wound on a part-task trainer look real. This will increase:

   A. Physical fidelity
   B. Psychological fidelity
   C. Environmental fidelity
   D. Equipment fidelity

30. Standardized patients (SPs) should come out of character when:

   A. The student makes an error.
   B. The student requests further information.
   C. The student is finished.
   D. The student asks the SP to come out of character.

31. The Certified Healthcare Simulation Educator™ prebriefs the student by allowing him or her to view and touch the mannequins. This will increase:

   A. Physical fidelity
   B. Psychological fidelity
   C. Environmental fidelity
   D. Equipment fidelity

32. The novice Certified Healthcare Simulation Educator™ needs additional orientation when she states:

   A. "Increased realism will ensure the learning outcomes."
   B. "Realism should be created within a safe environment."
   C. "Realism increases the fidelity of the simulation scenario."
   D. "Realism may assist the students to better understand the situation."

33. The concept of deliberate practice builds on the understanding that:

   A. People will keep trying to get things right.
   B. Deliberate practice will lead to perfection.
   C. Repeated behaviors will become automatic habits.
   D. Every attempt provides new understanding.

34. The Certified Healthcare Simulation Educator™ understands that one of the main core competencies for interprofessional collaborative is:

    A. Leadership
    B. Responsibility
    C. Reflection
    D. Demonstration

35. The novice simulation educator needs a better understanding of the role of standardized/simulated patients when he states:

    A. "They can grade the student."
    B. "They can provide feedback."
    C. "They can be scripted."
    D. "They can display emotions."

36. Microethical situations can be simulated and include all of the following except:

    A. Borderline medication administration practices
    B. Poor infection control practices
    C. Breeches in confidentiality
    D. Sexual misconduct

37. The following is an example of basic a "sandwich" feedback approach:

    A. "You did a good patient assessment and need to improve on both heart sounds and lung sound stethoscope placement."
    B. "The heart sound stethoscope placement was incorrect so let us review, but the lung sound stethoscope placement on the standardized patient was correct."
    C. "You did an overall thorough patient head-to-toe assessment but need practice in lung sound stethoscope placement, but your heart stethoscope placement was fine. "
    D. "Let us consider going over the placement of your stethoscope for the heart sounds one more time."

38. In order to create a simulation scenario that appropriately uses the concept of "as if" it should:

    A. Have increased fidelity.
    B. Contain moulage.
    C. Contain believable information.
    D. Use a complex care case.

39. Simulation scenarios can evaluate students in all learning domains. One student states during a debriefing that he felt as if there was an ethical issue when the feeding tube was inserted in the patient. The domain that is reflected in this student's learning is:

    A. Cognitive
    B. Psychomotor
    C. Internalization
    D. Affective

40. The Certified Healthcare Simulation Educator™ writes a student learning outcome, "At the end of this scenario the students will demonstrate correct sterile technique." This student learning outcome is written in which domain?

    A. Cognitive
    B. Psychomotor
    C. Internalization
    D. Affective

41. Using a TeamSTEPPS approach, the simulation scenario should teach the CUS principles, which are:

    A. Concerned, Uncommunicated, Strategies
    B. Cognitive, Uncomfortable, Safety
    C. Cognitive, Uncommunicated, Scenario
    D. Concerned, Uncomfortable, Safety

42. The Certified Healthcare Simulation Educator™ writes a student learning outcome, "At the end of this scenario the students will describe correct sterile technique." This student learning outcome is written in which domain?

    A. Cognition
    B. Psychomotor
    C. Internalization
    D. Affective

43. One of the most important professional development pieces about simulation for faculty is:

    A. Working the mannequins
    B. Developing scenarios
    C. Understanding debriefing
    D. Learning how to troubleshoot

44. Common team problems identified during simulation include all of the following except:

    A. Lack of role understanding
    B. No plan to correct mistakes
    C. Lack of evaluation for the team effort
    D. Lack of leadership

45. The Certified Healthcare Simulation Educator™ understands that the four main core competencies for interprofessional collaborative practice include:

    A. Leadership
    B. Delegation
    C. Values
    D. Demonstration

46. A student gets upset during a team-based simulation scenario and raises her voice. The Certified Healthcare Simulation Educator™ debriefs her and discusses the behavior with her in order to promote which of Wong and Driscoll's (2008) affective learning domains (Chapter 14)?

    A. Receiving
    B. Valuing
    C. Internalizing
    D. Organizing

47. In planning to use standardized patients for simulation, the experienced nurse educator knows that it is important to:

    A. Provide orientation and training for the people involved.
    B. Recruit only trained actors to serve as standardized patients.
    C. Ensure that the actors are paid prior to the simulation day.
    D. Provide an exact script for the actors to follow.

48. To identify potential issues and problems that may occur with new simulation activities, the nurse educator should:

    A. Seek the input of students who will be participating.
    B. Ask other faculty whether they can foresee any problems.
    C. Conduct a run-through or field test of the new simulation.
    D. Ask for suggestions from practice partners.

49. When prescreening standardized patient actors, the Certified Healthcare Simulation Educator™ should collect:

    A. A reference
    B. A curriculum vitae (CV)
    C. Application
    D. Video of acting skills

50. When observing a debriefing led by a novice educator, the experienced nurse educator would need to intervene when which statement is made?

    A. "Help me to understand why you did this."
    B. "How do you think the group did overall?"
    C. "You know this is the wrong way to do this."
    D. "Can you tell me what you were thinking at this time?"

51. In planning to teach the students intravenous (IV) insertion, the nurse educator elects to use the computer-generated, three-dimensional (3-D) IV program to allow learners to practice the skill. This is an example of what type of simulation modality?

    A. High fidelity
    B. Virtual reality
    C. Task trainer
    D. Standardized patient

52. When discussing advantages of simulation, the nurse educator would not include which statement?

A. "Simulation can substitute for some clinical hours in difficult-to-find specialty areas."
B. "Simulation is useful in helping students to experience uncommon clinical situations."
C. "Simulation can help students to develop confidence before entering the hospital setting."
D. "Simulation is something that can be done at the last minute if needed for makeup days."

53. A simulation educator is developing an interprofessional simulation experience involving physicians, registered nurses, emergency medical technicians (EMTs), and licensed practical nurses. Which standard's guidelines would the educator have to follow in order to reach learning outcomes shared by all specialties?

A. Simulation^{SM} Simulation Design
B. Simulation^{SM} Outcomes and Objectives
C. Simulation^{SM} Professional Integrity
D. Simulation^{SM} Simulation-Enhanced Interprofessional Education (Sim-IPE)

54. The Simulation^{SM} Debriefing standard contains the following learning goals except:

A. Facilitate reflection on individual and team performance to achieve targeted performance improvement.
B. Facilitate appropriate critical thinking, clinical judgment, reasoning, reflection, and reflective thinking.
C. Recognize unprofessional and unethical behavior during simulation and take steps to abate it.
D. Allow facilitation to be modified based on assessed participant needs and the impact of the experience.

55. Components of team training include leadership, and that role specifically includes which key component:

A. A shared understanding
B. Delegation
C. Balance of work
D. Mutual trust

56. The Certified Healthcare Simulation Educator™ understand that the four main core competencies for interprofessional collaborative practice include the following:

A. Teamwork
B. Delegation
C. Prioritization
D. Demonstration

57. Simulation can be a reliable method of evaluation when:

A. There are effective evaluation tools.
B. When simulation educators videotape students.
C. Students understand the purpose of simulation.
D. When students pass an objective test on the content learned in simulation.

58. When using simulation to understand students' perceptions, the experienced nurse educator would choose:

    A. Objective structured clinical exams (OSCEs)
    B. Self-reporting surveys
    C. Skills checklists
    D. Direct questioning

59. What statement by the nurse educator would indicate that she has a poor understanding of designing simulation activities?

    A. "I will have students arrive at 0700 a.m., and we will see how long the simulation takes."
    B. "I will schedule small groups of learners for each simulation activity."
    C. "I will have the course faculty help develop objectives for the day."
    D. "I will bring each group of students in for pre-briefing."

60. When discussing plans for a simulation day with his mentor, the new nurse educator demonstrates lack of knowledge about simulation modalities by stating:

    A. "Intravenous (IV) arms are a great use of low-fidelity simulation."
    B. "High-fidelity mannequins can be used effectively with new nursing students."
    C. "A task trainer can be effective in teaching new skills."
    D. "Debriefing is an effective method for evaluating skill acquisition with task trainers."

61. The simulation educator gets the same results with six different groups of students using a newly made skills checkoff list for skill attainment of second year physical therapy students. The simulation educator understands this supports the interments:

    A. Credibility
    B. Validity
    C. Reliability
    D. Content

62. The best description of a simulation educator who is a transformational leader is:

    A. "She moves people toward the future by providing us with what simulation can do for learners."
    B. "She organizes the simulation laboratory so it is easy for students to learn."
    C. "She supports faculty by developing scenarios that depict hard-to-get student clinical experiences."
    D. "She is excellent at scheduling the simulation experiences needed for learners throughout the semester."

63. A key concept of interprofessionality is:

    A. Constant knowledge sharing
    B. Leadership ability
    C. Delegation of tasks
    D. Prioritization of interventions

64. Debriefing should create a climate of:
    A. Mutual respect
    B. Straightforwardness
    C. Shared perspectives
    D. Psychological safety

65. The best description of a simulation educator who is a transactional leader is:
    A. "She moves people toward the future by providing us with what simulation can do for learners."
    B. "She organizes the simulation laboratory so it is easy for students to learn."
    C. "She provides the resources needed so simulation educators can be creative."
    D. "She keeps the mission of the simulation laboratory learning environment in focus as meetings."

66. What level of proficiency is the Certified Healthcare Simulation Educator™ displaying when he uses a life saver that assists students to stay on track when the students demonstrate the first indication that they will deviate from the student learning outcomes:
    A. Advanced beginner
    B. Competent
    C. Proficient
    D. Expert

67. National studies have demonstrated that student learning outcomes in healthcare programs are:
    A. Negatively impacted by overuse of simulation
    B. Positively impacted by the use of simulation
    C. Not significantly affected by simulation
    D. Obscured by simulation learning experiences

68. The reason that simulation laboratories are an appropriate place for diversity training is:
    A. Standardized patients (SPs) can pretend to be of any ethnicity or race.
    B. Mannequins can be altered with moulage to look like a minority patient.
    C. Learners do not bring their social determinant's into the laboratory space with them.
    D. It is safe space where learning can take place for all under the guidance of experienced simulation educators.

69. When healthcare students negotiate the role of a professional they begin by:
    A. Feeling like an imposter
    B. Using trial-and-error methods to learn
    C. Start understanding the seriousness of the role
    D. Gain confidence and socialize into role

70. When a healthcare learner enters a simulation scenario and stops for a moment to observe the surroundings and the placement of the patient in the room, this student demonstrates socialization in the form of a(n):

    A. Understanding
    B. Expert
    C. Modulation frame
    D. Primary frame

71. When a healthcare learner enters a simulation scenario and reflects on a past simulation experience, the socialization is in the form of a(n):

    A. Understanding
    B. Expert
    C. Modulation frame
    D. Primary frame

72. The novice simulation educator needs additional understanding when he states:

    A. "Minority students will do just as well in simulation because they are apt to join in like everyone on else."
    B. "Minority students can feel marginalized in the learning environment."
    C. "Minority students need to feel as if they belong in the scenario with everyone else."
    D. "Minority students may have more difficulty succeeding due to social determinants."

73. A student receives time and a half during classroom testing. During and evaluative scenario in the simulation laboratory students have to read the patient's case history. The student who is accommodated in the classroom should:

    A. Be referred to the student services Americans With Disabilities Act (ADA) officer
    B. Be provided with time and half to read the case
    C. Be held to the same clinical standards as all students
    D. Be provided a private testing time

74. The goal of interprofessional education (IPE) is to:

    A. Have people understand each other's role.
    B. Make the working environment more congenial.
    C. Provide different perspectives about patient care.
    D. Provide safe patient care.

75. When simulation educators discuss how students learn, store, and recall information, they are referring to:

    A. Worldviews
    B. Philosophies
    C. Teaching theories
    D. Learning theories

76. The simulation educator writes the following objective: "At the end of this simulation experience the learner will correctly demonstrate intravenous insertion." When reading this objective, it is understood that the simulation educator is using:

   A. Constructivism
   B. Behaviorism
   C. Scaffolding
   D. Realism

77. A simulation educator begins the session by asking the students to recall information from the previous session a week ago in order to assist them to gain new related knowledge. The simulation educator is using which educational theory?

   A. Constructivism
   B. Behaviorism
   C. Scaffolding
   D. Realism

78. According to adult learning theory, which of the following learning preferences attributes is not associated with students in the simulation laboratory:

   A. Self-directedness in instruction
   B. Motivation to learn
   C. Independence in decision-making
   D. Seeking out theoretical knowledge

79. The novice simulation educator needs a better understanding when he states:

   A. "Simulation can be used for pharmacology practice."
   B. "Using simulation for basic science is difficult."
   C. "Practicing skills is done well using part-task trainers."
   D. "Crisis management can be taught effectively with simulation."

80. A simulation educator is asking the standardized patients (SPs) for feedback about the learner's performance and skills. The simulation educator is using which educational philosophy?

   A. Constructivism
   B. Behaviorism
   C. Scaffolding
   D. Realism

81. A learner is trying over and over to gain skill placing a nasogastric tube on a part-task trainer. The student is displaying which concept in Kolb's experiential learning theory?

   A. Concrete experience
   B. Abstract conceptualization
   C. Reflective observation
   D. Active experimentation

82. The novice simulation educator needs a better understanding of scenario learning objectives when he states:

    A. "It is basically to get students to make up clinical hours."
    B. "It is to understand taking a health history on a patient."
    C. "It is to understand patient teaching."
    D. "It is to understand the proper physical assessment techniques."

83. A learner is watching the scenario of cardiac arrest on a patient and a resuscitation effort and chooses to be the "recorder" for the event. The student is displaying which concept in Kolb's experiential learning theory?

    A. Concrete experience
    B. Abstract conceptualization
    C. Reflective observation
    D. Active experimentation

84. An example of closed-loop communication is:

    A. "Did you get a regular heart rhythm?"
    B. "Please provide the patient with a shock."
    C. "Please let me know what you heard me say about the treatment plan."
    D. "Are you going to tell me what you would like first?"

85. A learner approaches the simulation educator the day following a scenario that she participated in and tells the educator she has been thinking about her responses and thinks they could have been communicated better. The student is displaying which concept in Kolb's experiential learning theory?

    A. Concrete experience
    B. Abstract conceptualization
    C. Reflective observation
    D. Active experimentation

86. During a simulation scenario, a student performs skills on the mannequin and reacts and changes directions appropriately when the cardiac monitor strip is different. The student is displaying which concept in Kolb's experiential learning theory?

    A. Concrete experience
    B. Abstract conceptualization
    C. Reflective observation
    D. Active experimentation

87. A simulation educator is debriefing learners and provides them with Internet resources and poses questions that stretch their current knowledge base to consider different approaches. The simulation educator is using which learning theory?

    A. Constructivism
    B. Behaviorism
    C. Scaffolding
    D. Realism

88. The novice simulation educator needs a better understanding of Kneebone's essential elements for successful simulation when he states simulation should:

    A. "Allow for deliberate practice."
    B. "Can include experiences as close to real life as possible."
    C. "Be learner-centered."
    D. "Encourage students to learn skills using peer-tutoring."

89. A tool that shows validity between the simulation educator's responses and expectations is said to have:

    A. Content validity
    B. Construct validity
    C. Face validity
    D. Predictive validity

90. Reflective debriefing techniques encourage the standardized patients (SPs) to understand the student's:

    A. Frame of reference
    B. Social determinants
    C. Prior learning
    D. Role and responsibilities

91. The effective application of the Simulation℠ Simulation Operations standard will guarantee the following:

    A. Reduced engagement of the simulation team
    B. Variability in student performance in the simulation lab
    C. Successful advancement of the simulation program director
    D. Improve interprofessional collaboration

92. An effective method of studying for the Certified Nurse Educator (CNE) examination is:

    A. Reviewing the Society for Simulation in Healthcare (SSH) website
    B. Reading the handbook
    C. Establishing a peer study group
    D. Asking others about test specifics

93. During a scenario using a part-task trainer haptic body part and a computer to insert a central line, students ask why they need the leg and torso when they can see them on the computer. The simulation educator's best answer is:

    A. "It is to get you to visualize the anatomy in three dimensions (3-D)."
    B. "So students understand where to place the line."
    C. "To get the real feel of the puncture site."
    D. "To further demonstrate the technique."

94. Standardized patient instructions should include:

    A. Being flexible and telling the student what they feel
    B. Sharing personal experiences
    C. Answers to questions that may be asked
    D. Going off script at will

95. Using moulage is appropriate for:
    A. Promoting simulation as a learning experiences
    B. Meeting objectives
    C. Increasing realism
    D. Decreasing student anxiety

96. Closed-loop communication includes:
    A. Eye contact
    B. Team members of different disciplines
    C. Technology
    D. Repeating what was said

97. The "B" in situation, background, assessment, and recommendation (SBAR) communication reminds one to remember:
    A. The assessment findings
    B. The patient's medications
    C. The blood test results
    D. The patient's healthcare history

98. During standardized patient case development by a novice simulation educator, the mentor realizes more understanding is needed when the educator prioritizes the:
    A. Setting
    B. Standardized patient role
    C. Student role
    D. Timing

99. When simulation evaluation checklists are subjective it is helpful to use:
    A. Two evaluators
    B. Descriptions
    C. The student's input
    D. The standardized patient's input

100. The "S" in situation, background, assessment, and recommendation (SBAR) communication should be succinctly used for:
    A. Introduction
    B. Healthcare history
    C. Prescription recommendation
    D. Symptoms

25 Answers and Rationales to End-of-Chapter Practice Questions

■ CHAPTER 2 PRACTICE QUESTIONS

1. The most important element(s) of the simulation certification test for educators is (are):

    A. Professional values and capabilities—NO, although this is very important, it is not the largest percentage of questions on the certification examination.
    B. Managing simulation resources—NO, although this is very important, it is not the largest percentage of questions on the certification examination.
    C. Engaging in scholarship activity—NO, although this is very important, it is not the largest percentage of questions on the certification examination.
    D. Education and assessment of learners—YES, this is the main reason why simulation learning experiences exist and it is the largest percentage of questions on the certification examination.

2. The healthcare simulation educator understands that acting as a role model at all times in the simulation laboratory is an expectation under the simulation certification examination criteria of:

    A. Professional values and capabilities—YES, these need to be constantly role modeled for student learning.
    B. Managing simulation resources—NO, it is listed under the professional values criteria.
    C. Engaging in scholarship activity—NO, it is listed under the professional values criteria.
    D. Education and assessment of learners—NO, it is listed under the professional values criteria.

3. The simulation educator is facilitating learning in the simulation laboratory for a group of healthcare students. The students are in a complex situation and have adjusted their plan of care according to the physical, psychological, and social needs of the patient. The simulation educator understands that the students are at which novice-to-expert level:

    A. Novice—NO, they would need to follow rules.
    B. Advanced beginner—NO, they would need to recognize patterns.
    C. Competent—NO, they can plan but not with flexibility.
    D. Proficient—YES, can modify as they move along in a situation.

4. The novice simulation educator needs additional understanding about the impact of simulation when he states:
   A. "Simulation should be used for difficult to find clinical learning experiences."—NO, this is true it can be used for hard to acquire experiences.
   B. **"Students who use large percentages of simulation will not be able to perform as well in clinical practice."—YES, this is not true as demonstrated by evidence.**
   C. "Simulation can assist educators to teach professional values and standards."—NO, simulation can assist student to learn affective behavior.
   D. "Simulation should not be limited if it meets the students' learning outcomes."—NO, this is true as long as student learning outcomes are met simulation is a great learning modality.

5. The simulation educator is at a general faculty meeting and describes how simulation can be used as a recruitment tool for the university. The simulation educator is demonstrating which simulation certification examination criteria of professional values and capabilities:
   A. Mentorship—NO, this occurs on usually a one to one basis for personal or professional growth.
   B. Role modeling—NO, this is done so students understand the professional roles in healthcare.
   C. Leadership—NO, this is usually a situation when the person is doing something that assists a group to move to a goal.
   D. **Advocating—YES, the educator is advocating the use of simulation.**

6. One of the affective learning domains that simulation has been effectively used for is:
   A. Risk-management control—NO, this is not a usual behavior addressed in simulation laboratories for students.
   B. **Cultural humility—YES, simulation is a good place to learn about diversity and respect.**
   C. Emotional adjustments—NO, this is not a usual behavior addressed in simulation laboratories for students.
   D. Personality categorizing—NO, this is not a usual behavior addressed in simulation laboratories for students.

7. A simulation educator rearranges the simulation space to depict a plane crash in order to teach triage. The simulation educator is guided by which simulation certification examination criteria:
   A. Professional values and capabilities—NO, this has to do more with affective human attributes.
   B. **Managing simulation resources—YES, environment comes under resources.**
   C. Engaging in scholarship activity—NO, this has to do with professional growth and career advancement.
   D. Education and assessment of learners—NO, this is the actual teaching and learning that takes place in the environment.

8. A simulation education team from an academic setting is presenting at a national conference. The educators are encouraging which simulation certification examination criteria by their work:
   A. Professional values and capabilities—NO, this has to do more with affective human attributes.
   B. Managing simulation resources—NO, this has to do with environment.
   C. Engaging in scholarship activity—YES, this has to do with professional growth and career advancement.
   D. Education and assessment of learners—NO, this is the actual teaching and learning that takes place in the environment.

9. The simulation educator has taught a group of students in the simulation laboratory for the past three semesters and has watched them develop their health assessment skills. The students now complete physical examinations from head to toe and understand that a finding in one patient may translate to the same healthcare issue in other patients they examine. The simulation educator understands that the students are at which novice-to-expert level in preforming physical examinations:
   A. Novice—NO, they would need to follow rules.
   B. Advanced beginner—YES, they recognize patterns.
   C. Competent—NO, can plan but not with flexibility.
   D. Proficient—NO, cannot modify as they move along in a situation.

10. The simulation educator presents a 5-year strategic plan for the simulation laboratory at a general faculty meeting. The simulation educator is demonstrating which simulation certification examination criteria of professional values and capabilities:
    A. Mentorship—NO, this occurs on usually a one to one basis for personal or professional growth.
    B. Role modeling—NO, this is done so students understand the professional roles in healthcare.
    C. Leadership—YES, this is planning for the future.
    D. Advocating—NO, the educator is planning for the future.

CHAPTER 3 PRACTICE QUESTIONS

1. Simulation educators understand that beside skills simulation can enhance the student's:
   A. Intrapersonnel and interpersonnel communication—YES, These can be enhanced with simulation.
   B. Cognitive test answering—NO, this is didactic learning.
   C. Test-taking skills—NO, this is didactic learning.
   D. Concept mapping—NO, this is used in clinical learning.

2. The novice simulation educator needs a better understanding of simulation principles when she states:
   A. "Simulation is safe space for learning."—NO, this is correct.
   B. "Simulation can be less anxiety provoking."—NO, this is correct.
   C. "Simulation is uncontrolled."—YES, this is incorrect, simulation should be a controlled environment.
   D. "Simulation teaches safe patient care."—NO, this is correct.

3. Which of the following is not considered a goal in the use of simulation?
   A. Provide standardization for evaluating a student's strengths and weaknesses—NO, this is a strength.
   B. Having participants reflect on their thoughts and feelings—NO, this is a strength.
   C. Widen the gap between theory and practice—YES, it closes the gap.
   D. Discovery learning—NO, this is a strength.

4. Which of the following reasons to become simulation certified is not correct?
   A. Personal accomplishment and professional competence that can result in tangible and intangible benefits—NO, this is correct.
   B. Ability to develop well-designed interdisciplinary scenarios for the purpose of enhancing collaboration and communication—NO, this is correct.
   C. Publish about effective uses of simulation in nursing education—NO, this is correct.
   D. It is mandated in order to conduct any simulation experience with nursing students—YES, this is not correct.

5. In which stage do the participants get oriented to the environment and obtain information on the scenario?
   A. Designing—NO, this is the first stage done by the simulation educator.
   B. Planning—NO, this is the second stage done by the simulation educator.
   C. Implementation—YES, it is done in this stage.
   D. Postsimulation—NO, this is the last stage done by the simulation educator.

6. The simulation educator is in the process of completing a written scenario for a simulation experience and you have just identified the objectives. The simulation educator now needs to decide on the evaluation tool to be used to evaluate the participants. This describes which simulation stage?
   A. Designing—YES, this is the stage in which it is completed.
   B. Planning—NO, this is the stage of setting up the scenario and is done after selecting a tool.
   C. Implementation—NO, this is when the scenario takes place.
   D. Postsimulation—NO, this is after the scenario is over.

7. The simulation educator is conducting a simulation using both a high-fidelity simulator as the patient and a standardized participant who is acting as a concerned and agitated family member. Which method of simulation is being used?

    A. Task trainer—NO, this is just using a part-task trainer.
    B. Human patient simulators—NO, this is just using a human patient simulator (HPS).
    C. Hybrid simulation—NO, this is using two things for one objective.
    D. Mixed simulation—YES, because not only will the participant learn how to effectively care for the patient but also how to deal with family members appropriately and respectfully.

8. A good test-taking strategy is to:

    A. Skim the references—NO, the references need to be read thoroughly.
    B. Just do a review course—NO, a review courses and studying.
    C. Do as many questions as possible—YES, this will help with the test.
    D. Ask friends what was on the test—NO, this cannot take the place of studying.

9. The simulation educator asks the following question on a test: "Identify the best type of simulation for developing interpersonal skills" and the answer is "standardized patients." This question is at what level of Bloom's taxonomy?

    A. Understanding—NO, this is application of the right simulation equipment.
    B. Applying—YES, this is applying the right simulation equipment.
    C. Comprehending—NO, this is application of the right simulation equipment.
    D. Analyzing—NO, this is application of the right simulation equipment.

10. The simulation educator understands that certification is a process that:

    A. Travels with nurses through their careers—NO, it must be renewed every 3 years.
    B. Can be revoked if wrong-doing is noted in a career—NO, it is earned.
    C. Is good for 3 years—YES, it needs renewal every 3 years.
    D. Tells others that you are proficient—NO, it designates expertise.

CHAPTER 4 PRACTICE QUESTIONS

1. An important quality needed in mentors to engage novice simulation educators is:

    A. Expert knowledge—NO, although this is important it is not the most important attribute.
    B. Enthusiasm—YES, they need to engage the novice.
    C. Delegation skills—NO, although this is important it is not the most important attribute.
    D. Prioritization skills—NO, although this is important it is not the most important attribute.

2. A simulation educator who is requesting assistance of the manufacturer of the high-fidelity mannequin is probably on which level of expertise?

   A. Novice—YES, this usually occurs on the novice level.
   B. Advanced beginner—NO, this level is more advanced and can troubleshoot.
   C. Competent—NO, this level is more advanced and can troubleshoot.
   D. Proficient—NO, this level is more advanced and can troubleshoot.

3. A simulation educator's "comfort zone" includes:

   A. High-fidelity mannequin use—NO, this is not the necessary element.
   B. Low-fidelity mannequin use—NO, this is not the necessary element.
   C. Content that is familiar—YES, this places educators in their comfort zone.
   D. Environments that are familiar—NO, this is not the necessary element.

4. Expert simulation educators understand that sometimes the best learning experiences for students include the following:

   A. Coaching through the scenario—NO, this may not allow students to think on their feet.
   B. Minimal interventions—YES, this allows students to critically think.
   C. Just-in-time instructions—NO, this is saving them form their own mistakes at times.
   D. Clear prebriefing content review—NO, this is helpful but minimal intervention will encourage them to make clinical decisions.

5. A mentor for simulation educators should be in which stage of development?

   A. Advanced beginner—NO, they should be more advanced.
   B. Competent—NO, they should be more advanced.
   C. Proficient—NO, they should be more advanced.
   D. Expert—YES, this stage provides the best mentorship.

6. During a scenario a mannequin unintentionally "dies." The simulation educator can expert which type of student reaction?

   A. Physiological effects—YES, evidence tells us that there are physiological effects.
   B. Emotional effects—NO, this is possible but there is no current evidence.
   C. Cognitive effects—NO, this is possible but there is no current evidence.
   D. Social effects—NO, this is possible but there is no current evidence.

7. A good learning resource for novice simulation educators is:

   A. Observation—NO, although this is good it is not the best way to get a novice up and running in simulation.
   B. Trial and error—NO, although this is good it is not the best way to get a novice up and running in simulation.
   C. Reading how-to books—NO, although this is good it is not the best way to get a novice up and running in simulation.
   D. Training sessions by simulation organizations—YES, there are many good training sessions form reputable organizations.

25 ANSWERS AND RATIONALES TO END-OF-CHAPTER PRACTICE QUESTIONS

8. One of the keys to developing simulation educator leaders is to determine:
   A. Who has seniority?—NO, this not always the best person.
   B. Who is interested?—YES, the person who is interested is more likely to engage.
   C. Who is technically savvy?—NO, this not always the best person.
   D. Who is the best didactic or clinical educator?—NO, this not always the best person.

9. Student engagement in simulation is most influenced by:
   A. Time of day—NO, although this may have something to do with engagement it is not the main element.
   B. Attitudes of instructors—NO, although this may have something to do with engagement it is not the main element.
   C. Frequency of exposure—NO, although this may have something to do with engagement it is not the main element.
   D. Appropriate content—YES, the student must be familiar with the content in order to engage.

10. A simulation educator is collaborating on the development of a scenario. The simulation educator is most likely in which stage of development?
    A. Novice—NO, this level is not to that point yet.
    B. Advanced beginner—NO, this level is not to that point yet.
    C. Competent—YES, it is at this level that simulation educators can start to develop scenarios.
    D. Proficient—NO, the simulation educator is already doing this task.

■ CHAPTER 5 PRACTICE QUESTIONS

1. The simulation educator observes a student crying after the death of a cardiac victim portrayed by a mannequin in the scenario. The simulation educator understands that this can happen because simulation is a:
   A. Social practice—YES, simulation is a social practice and students bring experiences with them.
   B. Learning experience—NO, a learning experience does not have to be upsetting.
   C. Emotionally charged situation—NO, a learning experience does not have to be upsetting.
   D. Unpredictable—NO, simulation can be does not have to be unpredictable.

2. Simulation learning activities lend themselves to a better understanding of human diversity because
   A. There are faculty who can adjust scenarios—NO, this is not a diversity concept.
   B. Many laboratories have diverse mannequins—NO, this is good but not the main necessity.
   C. It is a reflective learning environment—YES, learners reflect on what they learn.
   D. There are standards that should be met—NO, standards do not teach humility.

3. Student learning styles are important to understand so educational methodologies can reflect students' preferences. The simulation educator should be aware that a simulation scenario is most likely best suited for learners preferring which style?

   A. Visual—NO, this appeals to learners who like graphics.
   B. Read/write—NO this appeals to learners who prefer to read.
   C. Aural—NO, these are auditory learners.
   D. Kinesthetic—YES, normally you can demonstrate something in a scenario.

4. A simulation educator is facilitating learning about a procedure and one of the learners has difficulty following the steps. The learners may be displaying characteristics of which learning type?

   A. Tactile—NO, this is a learner who learns by movement and hands-on activity.
   B. Intuitive—NO, this type of learner likes problem solving.
   C. Global—YES, this type of learner is creative and spontaneous.
   D. Reflective—NO, this learning style is open to reviewing and thinking about information learned.

5. Many simulation educators are baby boomers or generation Xers and learners are millennials. One of the learning strategies that millennials respond positively to is:

   A. Modular learning—NO, this is more for baby boomers.
   B. Lecture before the scenario—NO, this is more for baby boomers.
   C. Independent problem solving—NO, this is more for baby boomers.
   D. Group activities—YES, millennials like to work in groups to solve problems.

6. Grasha's teaching styles describe simulation educators who have different approaches. The best approach an educator can have with a group of learners in a simulation scenario is:

   A. Expert—NO, this does not assist in learner reflection.
   B. Formal—NO, this may be viewed as unapproachable.
   C. Demonstrator—NO, this is not needed all the time.
   D. Facilitator—YES, this style helps the students to discover their own learning.

7. A simulation educator provided students with a topic for the simulation for the following day and asks them to research the patient's care. According to Quirk, which teaching style is this?

   A. Assertive—NO, this is someone who gives information.
   B. Suggestive—YES, this style has the students look up information.
   C. Collaborative—NO, this is a coordinated problem solving method.
   D. Facilitator—NO, the is when educators challenge students to reflect and learn.

8. The novice simulation educator is reviewing her teaching effectiveness characteristic outlined by Kelly (2008) and needs further review when she states that _____ is included as a trait of an effective teacher.

   A. Feedback—NO, this is a trait.
   B. Communication—NO, this is a trait.
   C. Knowledge—NO, this is a trait.
   D. Sensitivity—YES, this is not a trait.

25 ANSWERS AND RATIONALES TO END-OF-CHAPTER PRACTICE QUESTIONS

9. Culturally diverse learners have social determinants that place them at risk. Among those determinants is
   A. Lack of friends—NO, this is not one of the prominent risk factors.
   B. Family members who understand education—NO, this is not one of the prominent risk factors.
   C. Lack of diverse faculty—YES, this is a factor or a barrier to success.
   D. Peer support—NO, this is not one of the prominent risk factors.

10. Lifesavers are sometimes needed in a scenario to promote positive learning and to:
    A. Decrease emotions—NO, this is not their main goal.
    B. Understand health and illness concepts—NO, this is not their main goal.
    C. Reach the learning outcomes—YES, they are used to refocus the group.
    D. Developed a care plan for the patient—NO, this is not their main goal.

■ CHAPTER 6 PRACTICE QUESTIONS

1. Which of the following is the overarching domain identified for interprofessional education (IPE)?
   A. Interprofessional collaboration—YES, this is the overarching domain.
   B. Team communication—NO, it is interprofessional collaboration.
   C. Interprofessional teamwork—NO, it is interprofessional collaboration.
   D. Scope of practice—NO, it is interprofessional collaboration.

2. The simulation educator overhears a participant of the interprofessional education (IPE) experience raising her voice loudly and stating an order to someone in a different discipline without addressing this person by name. The simulation educator would best handle this situation initially by:
   A. Exploring the action observed in the debriefing following the case—YES, this should be done through discussion and reflection.
   B. Ignoring the behavior and focusing on the medical management of the case—NO, it should be addressed.
   C. Reporting the participant to her supervisor for remediation—NO, it should be dealt with in debriefing.
   D. Stopping the scenario, removing the participant, and restarting the scenario—NO, in debriefing.

3. The most common cause of error in authentic patient care is which of the following?
   A. Lack of knowledge—NO, this is not the reason.
   B. Inadequate resources—NO, this is not the reason.
   C. Lack of communication—YES, this is what causes most errors.
   D. Lack of leadership—NO, this is not the reason.

4. Experiential learning includes components of:
   A. Laboratory experimentation—NO, this is not usually used in experiential learning.
   B. Surface memory acquisition—NO, this is not used in experiential learning.
   C. Active participation—YES, this is used in experiential learning.
   D. Didactic education—NO, this is not usually used in experiential learning.

5. The goal of all the Institute of Medicine (IOM) reports is:
   A. Better patient care—YES, this is the ultimate goal.
   B. Reduction of healthcare retirements—NO, this is not the goal.
   C. Increasing technology knowledge—NO, this is not the goal.
   D. Decreasing healthcare errors—NO, this is not the goal, but it is what started the IOM's concern.

6. The essence of interprofessional education (IPE) is:
   A. Cooperation—NO, this is part of IPE.
   B. Knowing scopes of practice for each role—NO, this is part of IPE.
   C. Collaboration—YES, this is the essence and what will lead to better patient care.
   D. Meeting accreditation standards—NO, this is not part of IPE.

7. The Interprofessional Education Collaboration (IPC) program places mutual respect in which core competency?
   A. Values and ethics—YES, this is the standard where these are placed.
   B. Roles and responsibilities—NO, it is not contained within this standard.
   C. Communication—NO, it is not contained within this standard.
   D. Teamwork—NO, it is not contained within this standard.

8. The Interprofessional Education Collaboration (IPC) program places relationship building into which core competency?
   A. Values and ethics—NO, it is not contained within this standard.
   B. Roles and responsibilities—YES, these reside within this standard.
   C. Communication—NO, it is not contained within this standard.
   D. Teamwork—NO, it is not contained within this standard.

9. The Interprofessional Education Collaboration (IPC) program places expressing one's knowledge and opinion ino which core competency?
   A. Values and ethics—NO, it is not contained within this standard.
   B. Roles and responsibilities—NO, it is not contained within this standard.
   C. Communication—YES, this is part of effective communication.
   D. Teamwork—NO, it is not contained within this standard.

10. The Interprofessional Education Collaboration (IPC) program places integrating knowledge into which core competency?
    A. Values and ethics—NO, it is not contained within this standard.
    B. Roles and responsibilities—NO, it is not contained within this standard.
    C. Communication—NO, it is not contained within this standard.
    D. Teamwork—YES, this is a component of teamwork.

CHAPTER 7 PRACTICE QUESTIONS

1. Participation in ethical simulation experiences is important for healthcare professionals because they can assist participants to:

    A. **Develop moral reasoning and recognize professional values.—YES, this is the correct answer because the goal of enacting ethical scenarios is to provide opportunities to develop moral reasoning and enhance professional values.**
    B. Learn to work out healthcare problems in a neutral way.—NO, working out problems in a neutral way may not always be possible or necessary.
    C. Focus on the negative aspects of the healthcare professions.—NO, working out ethical situations does not require a focus on negative aspects of other healthcare professions.
    D. Rationalize behavior when making moral decisions.—NO, rationalization may not be a positive behavior, in fact it can be used to convince one's self that a decision is appropriate, when in fact, it may not be.

2. A student is participating in a summative simulation activity and has failed in an area that has been identified as a "critical element." It is clearly stated in the testing guidelines that if a student misses a "critical element," the student must fail the exam. The evaluator is rationalizing that the student's omission is an oversight, and therefore the student should not be failed. What is the best action for the simulation leader/manager?

    A. Leave it alone as the faculty are the experts.—NO, the faculty may be content experts, but the simulation manager has the responsibility to ensure that testing procedures are followed.
    B. Call in an administrator to lead the discussion about the situation.—NO, the simulation leader/manager should be able to lead this discussion.
    C. Inform the evaluator that their behavior will be reported to administration.—NO, this does not help figure out a solution to the current problem and "passes the buck" to someone else.
    D. **Lead a discussion of the situation, identifying the policy and ramifications if the omission is ignored.—YES, the simulation leader/manager is responsible for ensuring that testing procedures are followed.**

3. You are completing a summative testing session with students in an educational program. The testing session is about to start, but one of the faculty evaluators is not present because of traffic issues. She has phoned in and will be at least 60 minutes late. The Simulation Center leader/manager's best decision is to:

    A. Have the students wait until the faculty evaluator can arrive.—NO, although this may have to be an eventual outcome, if at all possible, try to keep the process moving along so students focused and less anxious.
    B. Step in as a substitute evaluator until the faculty member arrives.—NO, this is not appropriate if you do not have the subject matter expertise.
    C. **Call in a substitute faculty evaluator with similar content expertise and testing training.—YES, if there is another person available with the content expertise who is also aware of the testing process and has been trained, this will help prevent undue student stress.**
    D. Inform the students that they will have to return and be tested on a different day.—NO, although this could be an eventual outcome, if at all possible, allowing the students to participate in the testing for which they have prepared is best.

4. A student is participating in a simulation scenario and must give a medication. The correct calculation to give the patient should have been 0.5 mL of the medication and the student drew up and administered 0.6 mL. During debriefing the student's response is that it was not a big deal because it was only 0.1 more milliliters than the desired dose of the medication. The facilitator's best response should be:

    A. Well, it was not a critical medication, but next time please be more cautious.—NO, any medication error is considered serious.

    B. Any medication error is ethically important and should be considered serious.—YES, medication administration is a microethical situation that requires positive ethical behavior.

    C. All medications should be given using the five rights of medication administration.—NO, although this may be accurate, it does not include the ethics associated with medication errors.

    D. If this were real life, this would be considered inappropriate and an event report would need to be completed as soon as possible.—NO, although this may be accurate, it does not include the ethics associated with medication errors.

5. A group of educators is creating an end-of-life scenario. In addition to creating the details about the patient and family, what other considerations related to designing the simulation are critical to make the scenario appropriate for the participants?

    A. Standards of care and culture of the region should be considered.—YES, as the world becomes more global, there is an increased need for cultural and ethical training appropriate to the culture of the region and standards of care for the profession.

    B. Family-centered care is an essential element of the simulation design.—NO, this is not essential to all simulation design.

    C. The scenario must be based on a real-life situation.—NO, although this can be helpful, it is not required.

    D. The scenario must include all healthcare disciplines.—NO, although this can be helpful, it is not required.

6. A student is in the hall discussing the last simulation scenario with her peers. She states that the standardized patient had HIV and was being told for the first time about the disease. The healthcare simulation educator overhears the conversation. The appropriate action by the healthcare simulation educator would be to

    A. Ask the students to take the conversation into a private room—NO, the conversation should be stopped.

    B. Call the student who was discussing the patient later and explain that her conversation breeched confidentiality—NO, stop the conversation right away.

    C. Stop the conversation and explain that it breeches confidentiality—YES, this should be the learning moment.

    D. Explain to the students that if it were a real patient this would be a Health Insurance Portability and Accountability Act (HIPAA) violation—NO, this is a violation because students should treat each scenario as if it were real.

25 ANSWERS AND RATIONALES TO END-OF-CHAPTER PRACTICE QUESTIONS

7. A healthcare student states that he has had a bad day and does not want to participate in the simulation scenario that is scheduled. The healthcare simulation educator should:

   A. Remind him of the code of conduct to act professionally at all times.—YES, healthcare workers need to be ready for work when they arrive.
   B. Excuse him for the day.—NO, this is not teaching professionalism.
   C. Have him observe the scenario.—NO, this is allowing unprofessionalism.
   D. Tell him he can make it up by writing a response to a case study.—NO, this is not equivalent.

8. The healthcare simulation educator wants to determine the intravenous administration competency level of junior healthcare students and then develop a module for remediation for identified weaknesses. This is an example of:

   A. Summative evaluation—NO, it is not the end evaluation.
   B. Ongoing assessment—NO, it does not say it will be repeated.
   C. Competency-based simulation—NO, this is determined at the end (summative).
   D. Formative evaluation—YES, there is a remediation and expectation for improvement.

9. Graduates from a healthcare educational program see an advertisement for the educational organization on a billboard with their pictures in it from a simulation experience. The students did not give consent for the pictures to be used as external advertisements. This is an example of:

   A. Free trade—NO, this is not part of academia.
   B. Extended use of educational material—NO, this has to be stated to the student.
   C. Lack of consent—YES, they should have consented to other possible uses.
   D. Academic freedom—NO, this has to do with teaching subjects to students.

10. An example of a microethical situation embedded in a simulation scenario would be:

    A. Administering the wrong medication to a patient that causes an allergic reaction—NO, this is a major event.
    B. Forgetting to wash hands before touching a patient—YES, this is something that is simple but has great implications.
    C. Forgetting to identify the patient—NO, this is a major event.
    D. Leaving a Foley in all night that was supposed to come out the evening before—NO, this is a major event.

CHAPTER 8 PRACTICE QUESTIONS

1. The healthcare simulation educator identifies which common problem during a team-based scenario in which a student does not adequately check a patient's carotid pulse before beginning cardiopulmonary resuscitation (CPR) and another student begins to assist the first student with CPR?

   A. The group does not understand that each team member has a unique role.—NO, students may be within their scope of practice.
   B. There was a lack of clear role definition resulting in confusion.—NO, students are assuming traditional CPR roles.
   C. There was no plan in place to use when errors occur.—YES, the error was allowed to continue and involve other team members.
   D. There is no method to use to measure individual or team performance.—NO, evaluation is not mentioned.

2. Which student is participating in deliberate practice? The student who is:

   A. Thinking about his mistakes and trying again—YES, this is the critical reflective piece associated with deliberate practice.
   B. Doing a task over and over again without a break in between—NO, this does not permit critical reflection.
   C. Reading up on the task that he is about to perform—NO, this is not practice.
   D. Discussing the task with the healthcare simulation educator—NO, this is also not practice.

3. The student understands the goal of crises resource management when she states:

   A. "I should keep trying to figure out the correct patient intervention."—NO, crises resource management is a state of awareness of what resources can be used in a serious situation.
   B. "The team members need to provide each other with direction and I will do the intervention."—NO, in crises resource management there is no time to wait for direction.
   C. "I should request help as soon as possible when a serious situation occurs."—YES, part of crises resources management is calling for backup.
   D. "I should flex my role during a serious situation and do what is needed."—NO, knowing roles and scope of practice is part of crises resource management.

4. The healthcare simulation educator realizes a student needs additional team training when he states:

   A. "When I become uneasy about an intervention being done, I will say something."—NO, this is something that should be done in team learning.
   B. "My only role is to remain at the bedside and calm the patient and family members."—NO, this is not being flexible within the team.
   C. "Patient safety includes both physical and psychological safety."—YES, the team goal is patient safety.
   D. "Understanding CUS provides me with more autonomy as a practitioner."—NO, this is true it provides each member autonomy.

25 ANSWERS AND RATIONALES TO END-OF-CHAPTER PRACTICE QUESTIONS ■ 363

5. During a simulation scenario, the team leader provides orders to another member who requests clarification of the medication dosage. This is an example of:
   A. Situation, background, assessment, and recommendation (ISBAR) communication—NO, the "R" in ISBAR refers to recommending an intervention.
   B. Reflective practice communication—NO, this is not a communicative style.
   C. TeamSTEPPs communication—NO, this is not a communicative style.
   D. Closed-loop communication—YES, clarifying is part of closed-loop communication.

6. The student demonstrates the proper method of using introduction, situation, background, assessment, and recommendation (ISBAR) communication in a simulation scenario when he states
   A. "I know you can give me an order to help."—NO, this is not a recommendation.
   B. "The current vital signs are 99-92-24-86/40."—YES, this is an assessment piece.
   C. "The past health history of this patient includes all of the following…"—NO, this is not necessary for the situation (usually).
   D. "The referrals made so far for this patient's discharge are…"—NO, this is not necessary for the situation (usually).

7. Having a high-fidelity mannequin that can close its eyes during a simulator simulation is an example of what kind of fidelity?
   A. Physical fidelity—NO, this has to do with the room and space.
   B. Functional fidelity—YES, this has to do with what the equipment can do.
   C. Task fidelity—NO, this has to do with how real the intervention is to reality.
   D. Psychological fidelity—NO, this has to do with the affective situation of the scenario.

8. What type of experiential learner would a student be if, during a simulation scenario, he decides to try a new innovative intervention because the patient's condition is worsening using traditional methods?
   A. Convergent—NO, this is decision making.
   B. Divergent—YES, this is trying something creative.
   C. Assimilator—NO, this is applying inductive reasoning.
   D. Accommodator—NO, this is adapting to a situation.

9. The healthcare simulation educator allows a learner to repeat a procedure as many times as she would like. Studies demonstrate that "perfect practice" assists students to:
   A. Memorize procedures.—NO, this is not recommended for deep learning.
   B. Provide efficient patient care.—NO, efficient care is not as important as safe care.
   C. Increase self-confidence.—YES, it increases satisfaction and confidence.
   D. Decrease healthcare errors.—NO, studies do not demonstrate this to date.

10. During a simulation scenario, a member of the team who has been actively engaged in the care of the patient quickly recognizes a change in the patient's condition, calls for rapid response, delegates tasks to the other team members, and administers prescribed medications before the patient's condition deteriorates. Which of Kolb's learning styles is this learner demonstrating?

   A. Converger—YES, this person is a decision maker.
   B. Diverger—NO, this is not using creativity.
   C. Assimilator—NO, this is not applying inductive reasoning.
   D. Accommodator—NO, this is not adapting to a situation, it is taking the lead.

■ CHAPTER 9 PRACTICE QUESTIONS

1. When considering to use moulage in a simulation scenario, which is the most effective use of time and effort when preparing the moulage for a simulation session.

   A. Concentrate on the wounds or representation of the illness to save time and reduce the cost of the simulation—NO, this is not the most effective focus to increase realism.
   B. Strike the best balance between effort on the principle illness or wounds wardrobe and the scene staging to provide the best authenticity—YES, this is the best method to increase the effectiveness of the scenario.
   C. Concentrate on the patient, clothing and monitor settings as that is all the student will focus on—NO, this is not the most effective focus to increase realism.
   D. Spend most of the time and effort on developing charting materials and wound characteristics that can be documented—NO, this is not the most effective focus to increase realism.

2. The degree to which the moulage in a simulation scenario is important to how the learner performs because authenticity will

   A. Shock or jar the learner into paying attention to the simulation and give cues for use in the simulation—NO, this is not the objective of using moulage.
   B. Resonate with the learner and their sense of fun and playing along with the simulation—NO, this is not the objective of using moulage.
   C. Keep the learner on their toes and thinking ahead to the next realistic surprise—NO, this is not the objective of using moulage.
   D. High level of authenticity has an impact on the learner's emotional arousal and engagement in the learning activity—YES, learning engagement will increase the learner reaching the objectives of the scenario.

3. It is important to teach the standardized patient to protect/preserve the moulage because

   A. It is extremely expensive.—NO, this is not the most important reason.
   B. It has to be perfect.—NO, it does not have to be perfect to meet the learning objectives.
   C. It is very time consuming to apply.—YES, it takes time and effort to redo it if it is not preserved.
   D. It is a work of art.—NO, this is not the most important reason.

25 ANSWERS AND RATIONALES TO END-OF-CHAPTER PRACTICE QUESTIONS ■ 365

4. Two advantages of using moulage on standardized patients (SPs) are
   A. Most standardized patients see moulage as fun and make the day of simulation more enjoyable and they do not mind coming in early to prepare.—NO, SPs should be paid for their professional time.
   B. The SPs can be taught to care for and protect the moulage before and during the session as well as assisting with cleanup after the session.—YES, they should be taught to respect the moulage so it lasts for all learners.
   C. The anatomy of the SPs is very similar to the mannequins so appliances fit well and the adhesives work better on the SPs.—NO, the anatomy of a live actor is not similar.
   D. SPs usually do not move much so the appliances tend not to fall off and the dyes in moulage do not stain the SPs.—NO, SPs many times have to move to produce realism in the scenario.

5. When starting out working with moulage the best type of kit to begin with is one that
   A. Contains one of each of the most commonly used makeups as well as a varied assortment of application tools—NO, this is not the most important criteria.
   B. A professionally designed set with an organized case to carry and separate moulage used for manikins from supplies used on standardized patients (SPs)—NO, this is not the most important criteria.
   C. A kit assembled from the sale items at the makeup shop to keep the cost down in spite of the quality—NO, quality matters for both SPs and mannequins.
   D. Matches the expertise of the user and provides enough variation to meet the objectives of the simulation while growing with the increased experience of the moulage artist—YES, it must meet the objectives of the simulation experience.

6. The most accurate statement regarding odors is
   A. They are always required as they help to involve all the senses in a simulation.—NO, they are not always required.
   B. They are wild and uncontrollable and must be used with caution only as the scenario dictates.—YES, once used they are difficult to reduce so they need to be used with caution and thought.
   C. They are easy to find in the correct quantity and quality so that anyone can apply them during the scenario.—NO, they are not always easy to find and the quality is not easy to control.
   D. Involving multiple senses does not affect learner engagement so odors are not necessary.—NO, they do effect the learner's perception of the scenario.

7. When considering the recipe for vomit the moulage artist should keep in mind
   A. Including some real food products as they can increase the gag factor and do not have any cautions to worry about—NO, this is not the most important element to creating vomit and producing the gag factor is not necessary.
   B. Choosing the visual representation to match the simulation learning points and carefully cleaning up to minimize unwanted growth and contamination in the lab—YES, meeting the objectives is important as well as infection control.

C. Paying attention to the liquid content so that the resulting mixture is soupy and will run easily down the mannequin's face and neck—NO, this is not the most important element.
D. The possible blockage of the airway and choking of the mannequin—NO, this is not the most important element if it is not a scenario objective.

8. Which items and materials that are found in the kitchen are good for use in moulage?
   A. Chocolate syrup—NO, this is not the only material that may be effective.
   B. Cherry pie filling—NO, this is not the only material that may be effective.
   C. Clear gelatin—NO, this is not the only material that may be effective.
   D. All of the above—YES, they all may be used but careful cleanup must also be considered.

9. Which would be the best choice to make a bruise on a mannequin?
   A. Oil based makeup with high concentrations of red dye—NO, oil based and red dye is difficult to remove.
   B. Wax crayons heated to soften them—NO, it looks too artificial and blending is more difficult.
   C. Cream-based theatrical makeup—YES, this will remove without damaging the plastic.
   D. Blue and purple crushed grapes—NO, this may stain permanently.

10. What is the best source to acquire makeup for your kit?
    A. Local drug store—NO, this may not have the correct products needed.
    B. Local grocery store—NO, this may not have the correct products needed.
    C. Local theater supply store—YES, this is most likely to contain products that can be easily removed.
    D. National department store—NO, this may not have the correct products needed.

■ CHAPTER 10 PRACTICE QUESTIONS

1. A simulation educator is planning a simulation to practice therapeutic communication. What type of simulation is most effective for the focus of this scenario?
   A. Human patient simulator (HPS) simulation—NO, this is using mannequins.
   B. Computer-based simulation—NO, this is computer oriented and not person oriented.
   C. Standardized patient (SP) simulation—YES, there will be a real person involved.
   D. Virtual reality—NO, this is computer oriented and not person oriented.

2. A simulation educator has hired a new group of standardized patients (SPs) who have minimal or no previous experience. During the training session the majority of the SPs state they are not comfortable with providing feedback. The simulation educator should

25 ANSWERS AND RATIONALES TO END-OF-CHAPTER PRACTICE QUESTIONS ■ 367

    A. Provide videos for the SPs to review from previous simulations—NO, this may not be the most effective method to teach feedback techniques.
    B. Provide each SP with a book on feedback methods—NO, this may not be the most effective method to teach feedback techniques.
    C. Provide the SPs extra time to practice and role-play—NO, this may not be the most effective method to teach feedback techniques.
    D. Provide an education and training session on feedback methods for the SPs—YES, providing education will be the best method to ensure that the SPs understand appropriate and beneficial feedback.

3. When developing a standardized patient (SP) simulation scenario the SP can portray what types of roles?

    A. Patient—NO, not just patients.
    B. Family member—NO, not just family members.
    C. Health professional—NO, not just health professionals.
    D. All of the above—YES, SPs can portray any role.

4. What is the required length of time for the standardized patient (SP) training session?

    A. 1 hour—NO, there is no set time that works for all scenarios.
    B. 2 hours—NO, there is no set time that works for all scenarios.
    C. 4 hours—NO, there is no set time that works for all scenarios.
    D. The specific training time is based on the complexity of the case—YES, complex scenarios take longer.

5. During a simulation scenario, the learner, completing the assessment, proceeds to gag the patient with a tongue depressor. The patient should

    A. Not do anything—NO, this does not give the immediate feedback necessary.
    B. Run out of the exam room—NO, this is over dramatization.
    C. Scream—NO, this is over dramatization.
    D. State, "I do not want you to do that to me."—YES, this is an appropriate response.

6. During a standardized patient (SP) scenario, the SP notices the learner chewing gum. The SP should

    A. Do nothing—NO, this is an unprofessional behavior.
    B. Make a note on the student checklist—YES, this should be brought to the learner's attention by the SP so they learn from the experience.
    C. Ask the learner why they are chewing gum—NO, confronting the learner may interrupt the scenario.
    D. Notify the simulation educator—NO, this can be dealt with during feedback.

7. An educator is interested in learning how to write a standardized patient (SP) scenario. Which is the best method for the simulation educator to provide this training?
   A. Give the educator a book on SP simulation—NO, this may not answer all their questions.
   B. Give the educator a simulation case they can copy—NO, this may not answer all their questions.
   C. Provide the educator with a book, a sample case and meet with the educator—YES, this will provide the most comprehensive education and provide time for questions.
   D. Provide the educator with some helpful websites on SP simulation—NO, this may not answer all their questions.

8. The standardized patient (SP) is reviewing the list of learners assigned to their room prior to the simulation experience. The SP notices that one of the names on the list is someone they might know personally. The SP should
   A. Do nothing—NO, the scenario may be interrupted if the student knows the SP.
   B. Put a note on the checklist—NO, the scenario may be interrupted if the student knows the SP.
   C. Notify the simulation educator after the simulation—NO, the scenario may be interrupted if the student knows the SP.
   D. Notify the simulation educator immediately—YES, so assignments can be altered.

9. At the completion of an assisted suicide simulation, the simulation educator notices several of the learners crying. The simulation educator should
   A. Gather the learners together for a debriefing session—YES, the emotions need to be debriefed.
   B. Do nothing—NO, the emotions need to be debriefed.
   C. Notify the primary contacts for the learners—NO, this is inappropriate and a violation of the learners right to privacy in education (Family Educational Rights and Privacy Act [FERPA]).
   D. Revise the scenario—NO, it may not be a scenario issue it may be level of student or prebriefing issue.

10. Following a simulation experience a learner comes out of the room and appears very upset. The simulation educator should
    A. Escort the learner out of the simulation lab—YES, first remove the learner from the stimuli.
    B. Notify the primary contact for the learner—NO, this is inappropriate and a violation of the learners right to privacy in education (Family Educational Rights and Privacy Act [FERPA]).
    C. Take the learner aside and speak to them privately—NO, it is better to debrief the learners together and not to single out one student.
    D. Speak to the standardized patient (SP)—NO, the SP may not be the issue.

25 ANSWERS AND RATIONALES TO END-OF-CHAPTER PRACTICE QUESTIONS

■ CHAPTER 11 PRACTICE QUESTIONS

1. One assessment advantage afforded though hybrid simulation is:
   A. It combines interprofessional groups in a single training program.—NO, this is not assessment.
   B. It is primarily used for formative versus summative assessment.—NO, it could be used for both types of assessment.
   C. Assessment can be done by a trained standardized participant.—YES, a standardized participant can assist in the evaluation process.
   D. Debriefing is optional because scores are given by the standardized participant.—NO, debriefing is needed.

2. The simulation venue:
   A. Is the best place to conduct debriefing—NO, this is done after the simulation and in a different location.
   B. Generates different processes and expectations—NO, this should be completed before the simulation.
   C. Dictates the types of scenario used—YES, it must be logical and fit the environment.
   D. Always utilizes standardized participants—NO, it does not have to use standardized participants.

3. Psychological fidelity occurs when:
   A. The risks experienced through the simulation closely approximate what is experienced in real life.—YES, it would produce the same feelings.
   B. Patient safety measures are ensured.—NO, it pertains to the learners.
   C. The learners experience "psychological safety."—NO, it is more about realism.
   D. The simulation educator adheres to the training objectives.—NO, this should be done, but this does not ensure psychological fidelity.

4. A standardized participant:
   A. Can be a faculty member who plays the part of a clinician in a scenario—YES, this may work well for some scenarios.
   B. Is another term for *standardized patient*—NO, this is not the same individual.
   C. Is a simulated patient participating in a standardized examination—NO, this is still acting as a standardized patient not participant.
   D. Cannot reliably assess skills because they are too involved with the scenario to pay attention to the learners—NO, this is not true they can give good feedback to the learners as perceived by a patient.

5. Physical fidelity is compromised when:
   A. The raters are not adequately trained.—NO, this should not effect the environment.
   B. When the simulation is cut short.—NO, this should not effect the environment.
   C. The learners are required to take excessive risks.—NO, this should not effect the environment.
   D. A patient condition cannot be realistically simulated.—YES, there is no way to get around this and it will compromise physical fidelity.

6. To assess skills, it is recommended that the raters:
   A. Develop the clinical skills checklists to be used.—NO, this is evaluative only.
   B. Always participate in the scenarios.—NO, the raters need to observe.
   C. Know how to perform the skill being assessed, and practice assessing it.—YES, practicing assists learning.
   D. Develop quality-assurance practices.—NO, this should be done, but does not actually assess skills.

7. Which one of the following is not a role for standardized participants:
   A. Standardized patient—NO, this is a role if they are trained to assume it.
   B. Standardized family member—NO, this is a role.
   C. Standardized test developer—YES, this is done by faculty.
   D. Simulated clinician—NO, this is a role.

8. Hybrid simulation requires the simulation educator to:
   A. Be proficient in all modes of simulation.—YES, because more than one mode is used and in different combinations.
   B. Understand the principles and practices of test development.—NO, this does not guarantee that the simulation educator understands hybrid simulation.
   C. Debrief the learners after scenarios.—NO, all simulations require debriefing or feedback.
   D. Manage all technical problems that may arise.—NO, this may be the role of the technician.

9. A standardized patient educator:
   A. Manages the simulation scenario—NO, this may be done by a technician.
   B. Services the mannequins—NO, this may be done by a technician.
   C. Creates standardized patient (SP) cases and trains SPs to participate in hybrid simulation—YES, this is part of the role.
   D. Analyzes performance assessment data—NO, this is completed by the simulation educator.

10. One of the best ways to educate faculty about how simulation works is to:
    A. Conduct ongoing faculty development webinars.—NO, this is not active participation.
    B. Show videos of actual simulation sessions.—NO, this is not active participation.
    C. Observe simulations.—NO, this is not active participation.
    D. Participate in simulations.—YES, this demonstrates the importance of learning in a hands-on environment.

CHAPTER 12 PRACTICE QUESTIONS

1. The simulation educator is deciding on the modality of simulation to use to present a set of skills to interprofessional healthcare learners. The first consideration should be:

    A. The cost of the equipment needed—NO, although this is a consideration it is not the first priority.
    B. The learning level of the students—NO, although this is a consideration it is not the first priority.
    C. How the learning outcomes are met—YES, he or she should ask whether the simulation matches the goals or the student objectives or learning outcomes.
    D. How the students responded during a previous simulation—NO, although this is a consideration it is not the first priority.

2. A simulation educator would like to **increase fidelity** related to cardiac arrest response. The best simulation method to accomplish this would be:

    A. Using a part-task trainer (PTT) of a torso—NO, this is still low fidelity.
    B. Using a standardized simulated patient—NO, this does not work for cardiopulmonary resuscitation.
    C. Using a computer program in "real life"—NO, this increases fidelity but not as much as high-fidelity mannequin.
    D. Using a mannequin that is fully equipped—YES, this is high fidelity.

3. The novice simulation educator needs further understanding when he states:

    A. "A part-task trainer (PTT) can only be used for simple procedures."—YES, this is not true it can be used for complex tasks.
    B. "PTT can be used in hybrid form."—NO, this is true.
    C. "PTT are at times more durable."—NO, this is true.
    D. "PTT may jeopardize suspending disbelief."—NO, this is true.

4. A simulation educator is developing a haptic hybrid skill station. In order to do this she will need:

    A. A part-task trainer (PTT) and a mannequin—NO, this does not ensure the correct tactile stimuli.
    B. Two PTTs—NO, this does not ensure the correct tactile stimuli.
    C. A PTT and a computer—NO, this does not ensure the correct tactile stimuli.
    D. A PPT with the feel of real anatomy—YES, this will create haptic simulation.

5. An element to consider when using part-task trainers (PTTs) in the simulation laboratory is:

    A. They are always easy to move.—NO, this makes them easier to use.
    B. They are usually less expensive.—NO, this makes them easier to use.
    C. They may have to be replaced.—YES, when they are worn they will have to be replaced.
    D. They are usually durable.—NO, this makes them easier to use.

6. To increase fidelity using a part-task trainer (PTT) the simulation educator may consider using a PTT with:

   A. **A standardized patient—YES, this is a good way to increase fidelity.**
   B. Another PTT—NO, this is not the best way to increase fidelity.
   C. A high fidelity mannequin—NO, this is not the best way to increase fidelity.
   D. A virtual environment—NO, this is not the best way to increase fidelity.

7. Part-task trainers (PTTs) are considered

   A. High fidelity—NO, they are low fidelity when used alone.
   B. **Low fidelity—YES, they are considered low fidelity.**
   C. Midfidelity—NO, they are low fidelity when used alone.
   D. Are not classified—NO, they are low fidelity when used alone.

8. Simulation educators understand the usefulness of part-task trainer (PTT) mainly because they are:

   A. Easy to obtain and use—NO, they still have to be ordered and paid for.
   B. Anatomically exact—NO, they are not exact.
   C. Travel well—NO, most of them not all do travel well.
   D. **Have been around many years—YES, this gives support to their usefulness.**

9. Using part-task trainers (PTTs) decreases the risk of:

   A. **Replacing expensive equipment—YES, this is a concern.**
   B. Mistakes in procedures—NO, mistakes can still occur.
   C. Simulation burnout—NO, burnout can still occur.
   D. Test anxiety—NO, they will not decrease anxiety.

10. When a part-task trainer (PTT) needs repair the simulation coordinator should:

    A. Use special chemical to clean it well.—NO, this may occur but will not repair the PTT.
    B. Order a new one because they are inexpensive.—NO, this may occur but trying to read the instructions would be a good first step.
    C. Take it apart and check functionality.—NO, this may occur but trying to read the instructions would be a good first step.
    D. **Read the manufacturer's instructions.—YES, always follow manufacturer's instructions.**

■ CHAPTER 13 PRACTICE QUESTIONS

1. The novice simulation educator needs additional understanding when he states virtual reality (VR) platforms:

   A. **"Are designed for distance education learners"—YES, VR platforms can be used by in-class learners also.**
   B. "Can be three-dimension (3-D) to enhance immersion"—NO, this is true.
   C. "Are a mechanism to teach teamwork"—NO, this is true.
   D. "Provide an opportunity for students to manipulate equipment"—NO, this is true.

2. Virtual worlds (VW) provide the learner with all the following elements *except:*

   A. Dynamic feedback—NO, VWs provide feedback.
   B. Increased attentiveness—YES, this is not one of the identified attributes.
   C. Creativity—NO, VWs do enhance the learner's ability to be creative.
   D. Decreased anxiety—NO, this is something that VWs can provide to learners.

3. The main objective of using a virtual patient (VP) in virtual worlds is to:

   A. Entertain while learning—NO, this is not the main objective of this learning platform.
   B. Practice clinical decision making—YES, this is main objective.
   C. Practice skills—NO, this is not the main objective of this learning platform.
   D. Encourage creatively—NO, this is not the main objective of this learning platform.

4. Serious gaming is a method of learning delivery that is associated with which educational theory?

   A. Behaviorism—NO, this theory has to do with observable behavior.
   B. Realism—NO, this theory implies science can explain all components of learning.
   C. Emancipatory—NO, this theory is about social justice.
   D. Constructivism—YES, this theory is learner-centered and encourages students to create knowledge.

5. A novice simulation educator is designing a virtual world, which of the following concepts should not be included:

   A. There should be a sense of immersion for the participant.—NO, this is needed.
   B. Real world scenarios should be replicated.—NO, this can be beneficial.
   C. No opportunities for social networking are provided so as to keep students on track.—YES, there can be networking for collective knowledge.
   D. Learners should be allowed to experiment in the scenario.—NO, experimentation helps build knowledge.

6. The primary purpose of a serious game is to:

   A. Allow entertainment to lower stress.—NO, this is not the purpose.
   B. Design the learning experience so only one response is correct.—NO, this is restricting learning.
   C. Meet educational and professional goals.—YES, this is the overall purpose.
   D. Create the game using a one-dimensional approach.—NO, it is more than one-dimensional.

7. The professor wants to design a scenario on the proper method to use for intubation. Which platform is the best choice for this learning experience?

   A. Second Life—NO, this does not provide hands-on.
   B. Task trainer—YES, this will assist to teach a skill.
   C. Voki—NO, this is not the best method to teach a skill.
   D. SimTab—NO, this is not the best method to teach a skill.

8. The design of a simulation or serious game based on Vygotsky's theory would include:

    A. **An opportunity for social interaction between learners—YES, this is a major part of the theory.**
    B. Recall of previously learned information—NO, experimentation is a part of the theory.
    C. Development of an avatar by the instructor—NO, this should be done by the student.
    D. Application of Maslow's hierarchy of needs—NO, this would cause it to be linear.

9. When developing a serious game, the first action the teacher must perform is which of the following?

    A. Determine the platform to use to design the game.—NO, this is not the first step.
    B. Require students to have taken a computer course on using the technology.—NO, this is not the first step.
    C. Conduct a debriefing about the experience.—NO, this is not the first step.
    D. **Develop objectives for the activity.—YES, this is where learning starts and provides an assessment mechanism.**

10. During the action phase of the multi-user virtual environment (MUVE) the learner does which of the following?

    A. Creates her or his avatar.—NO, this is in the beginning or preparation phase.
    B. Watches videos to familiarize him- or herself with the requirements for the activity.—NO, this is in the beginning or preparation phase.
    C. **Interacts in the environment created in the simulation.—YES, this is implementation.**
    D. Discusses what he or she has learned during the game or simulation.—NO, this is happens after the experience or the debriefing phase.

CHAPTER 14 PRACTICE QUESTIONS

1. A healthcare simulation educator is developing a scenario for a student to learn newborn care and would like to use the constructivist theory as the foundation. The best method would be:

    A. Have the student repeat a newborn assessment several times to get procedures correct.—NO, this reflects behaviorism or procedural knowledge that is demonstrated.
    B. **Use a newborn mannequin that simulates an active newborn and have the student approach the assessment without interfering and discuss later.—YES, this is allowing the student to build knowledge.**
    C. Develop a scenario that changes the newborn's status if an assessment is performed wrong.—NO, this is a stimulus-response method or behavioralism.
    D. Change the newborn's status to mimic a healthy newborn if the assessment is done correctly.—NO, this is a stimulus-response method or behavioralism.

25 ANSWERS AND RATIONALES TO END-OF-CHAPTER PRACTICE QUESTIONS ▪ 375

2. The student needs additional understanding when he states, "A constructivist approach to this scenario includes…" the following:

   A. "Using the material we learned yesterday and applying it today."—NO, this is correct, it is building knowledge on what is known.
   B. "Starting with what we know about this situation and then assessing the patient."—NO, this is correct, it is building knowledge on what is known.
   C. "Approaching the patient as if we have no information."—YES, there is no knowledge to build upon.
   D. "Relating what is similar in this case to other cases we have worked through."—NO, this is correct, it is building knowledge on what is known.

3. During a team-based simulation scenario, one student takes the lead and approaches the patient first and takes a blood pressure when the mannequin talk the group that she feels lightheaded. This student who takes the blood pressure is displaying which of Kolb's learning styles?

   A. Concrete experience (CE)—NO, this is not built from reality.
   B. Abstract conceptualization (AC)—NO, this is not thinking about what to do.
   C. Reflective observation (RO)—NO, this is actively doing something.
   D. Active experimentation (AE)—YES, this is using hands-on practice to learn.

4. The simulation healthcare educator has developed a simulation scenario based on the scaffolding learning theory and presents it to a group of students. The students are provided with an explanation of the case that becomes increasingly difficult. The group was unable to formulate a cohesive plan for the patient. One of the learning elements missing may have been:

   A. Instructor presence—NO, this healthcare simulation educator does not necessarily need to be present.
   B. Realism—NO, realism should not interfere with decision making.
   C. Constructive feedback—YES, this may be a missing element.
   D. Knowledge—NO, they may have the knowledge but not know how to apply it.

5. Guided by social learning theory, the healthcare simulation educator demonstrates to a student who has low self-efficacy how to insert chest tubes correctly. The principle that the healthcare simulation educator is using is:

   A. Mastering experience learning—NO, this student is inactive.
   B. Vicarious experience learning—YES, the healthcare simulation educator is demonstrating so the student is learning vicariously.
   C. Verbal persuasion—NO, the healthcare simulation educator is not verbally encouraging.
   D. Modulating psychological state—NO, the psychological state of the student was not addressed.

6. One of the healthcare students was previously an emergency medical technician (EMT) and during a simulation prebriefing she states that she would like to advance her splinting skills. The student is demonstrating which type of educational concept?

A. Pedagogy—NO, this is the method instructors teach passive, younger students.
B. Realism—NO, this does not apply in this situation, it is a state not a learning process.
C. Behavioralism—NO, this is demonstrating learning through behavior.
D. Andragogy—YES, this is taking charge of one's learning and building on experience.

7. The new healthcare simulation educator needs additional information when she lists Kneebone's (2005) simulation learning principles as (p. 63):

   A. It should occur in a safe environment.—NO, this is true and a needed element.
   B. Tutors should be available to learners.—NO, this is true also.
   C. Principles are teacher centered.—YES, Kneebone's simulation learning is student centered.
   D. They should mimic real life.—NO, this is also one of the recommendations.

8. Kirkpatrick's (1998) simulation learning principles are orderly and once learning is achieved the healthcare simulation educator should expect the students to:

   A. Display a reaction.—NO, this is the first step.
   B. Describe results.—YES, this is the last step—taking the knowledge and applying it to actual patients.
   C. Continue to learn.—NO, this is the second step "learning."
   D. Demonstrate the behavior.—NO, this is the third step.

9. The last step of Doerr and Murray's (2008) simulation teaching–learning process is:

   A. Debriefing—NO, this is the third step.
   B. Transference—YES, this is the last step—taking the knowledge and applying it to actual patients.
   C. Developing learning outcomes—NO, this is the first step.
   D. Creating the situation—NO, this is the second step.

10. A simulation educator is developing student objectives/learning outcomes and would like to assess students at the application level. Which objective/learning outcome would best fit the application level?

    A. Observe the hybrid simulation procedure.—NO, observation is not application.
    B. Discuss the clinical decision for starting cardiopulmonary resuscitation.—NO, verbalization is not application.
    C. Decide on the priority intervention.—YES, this is applying knowledge and making a clinical decision.
    D. Evaluate the intervention's effect.—NO, the application is already complete.

CHAPTER 15 PRACTICE QUESTIONS

1. The expert simulation educator understands that integrating simulation throughout the curriculum involves:

   A. Resources—YES, simulation programs need resources and administrative support.
   B. A new building—NO, this is not necessary.
   C. High-fidelity equipment—NO, this is not necessary.
   D. Staff approval—NO, this is not necessary, faculty and administrative approval is needed.

2. The first step in integrating simulation throughout a curriculum should be to:
   A. Acquire equipment.—NO, this is a later step.
   B. Develop student learning outcomes.—NO, this is a later step.
   C. Discuss the best learning environment.—NO, this is a later step.
   D. Perform a needs assessment.—YES, this is the first step to determine feasibility.

3. The novice simulation educator needs better understanding when she states that learning goals need to be established in the following domain:
   A. Psychomotor—NO, this domain should be addressed.
   B. Cognitive—NO, this domain should be addressed.
   C. Empathetic—YES, this is not a learning domain.
   D. Affective—NO, this domain should be addressed.

4. The final step of developing an integrative simulation curriculum is:
   A. Evaluation—YES, the outcomes of using simulation should be assessed.
   B. Teaching methods—NO, this is in the process of using simulation.
   C. Developing student learning outcomes—NO, this is an initial step.
   D. Discussing the mission—NO, this is the very first step.

5. The novice simulation educator understands deliberate practice when she states:
   A. "It has the goal of developing perfect skills."—NO, the goal is to get better at skills.
   B. "It is a method to evaluate and grade students."—NO, it is to allow students to practice.
   C. "It is a method to ensure appropriate formative evaluation."—NO, it is not an evaluative mechanism, it is just for practice.
   D. "It is a method to use to practice skills to become better at doing them."—YES, this is exactly what it describes.

6. A student who is practicing insertion of central lines on a task-trainer is learning mainly in which domain?
   A. Affective—NO, this is the attitudinal domain.
   B. Psychomotor—YES, this is an example of hands-on training.
   C. Cognitive—NO, this is the thinking domain.
   D. Psychosocial—NO, this is not a learning domain.

7. A scenario in which a student is telling family members "bad news" about a patient is developing skill in which domain?
   A. Affective—YES, this is the attitudinal domain.
   B. Psychomotor—NO, this is hands-on.
   C. Cognitive—NO, this is the thinking domain.
   D. Psychosocial—NO, this is not a learning domain.

8. A student who is calculating the correct morphine dosage in a simulation to complete a patient-controlled analgesic (PCA) pump setup is developing skill in which domain?

    A. Affective—NO, this is the attitudinal domain.
    B. Psychomotor—NO, this is not hands-on practice.
    C. Cognitive—YES, this is the thinking domain.
    D. Psychosocial—NO, this is not a learning domain.

9. A simulation principle that is followed by educators is:

    A. Educational goals should match the simulation type.—YES, there should be congruency.
    B. Always use the lowest simulation type to accomplish a task.—NO, this is not always followed.
    C. The more real the environment, the better the learning outcome will be.—NO, realism doesn't just include the environment it also includes the scenario itself and the roles demonstrated.
    D. All students should be exposed to all simulation types.—NO, this is not necessary to reach learning goals.

10. A summation educator has used an evaluation tool for three different groups and the scores are inconsistent. The simulation educator concludes the tool lacks:

    A. Content validity—NO, this refers to the measurement of the tool's appropriateness and comprehension.
    B. Face value—NO, this refers to the tool measuring what it was made to measure.
    C. Construct validity—NO, this refers to the test measuring what the educator wants to measure.
    D. Relatability—YES, this is a tool that works consistently to evaluate a concept and content.

CHAPTER 16 PRACTICE QUESTIONS

1. A new educator is planning to include simulation in his medical–surgical course. To begin the planning process, the educator should first:

    A. Write a simulation scenario on a topic of interest.—NO, this is more advanced.
    B. Assess the needs of the learners in the course.—YES, this can be done by allowing learners to self-identify their needs or by the educator, who should consider student learning outcomes.
    C. Determine the methods of evaluation to be used.—NO, this is more advanced.
    D. Develop a schedule for the simulation activities.—NO, this is more advanced.

2. In planning the simulation, the educator should give priority to including:

    A. Skills that students have requested—NO, this may not fulfill the objectives.
    B. Scenarios that are difficult and challenging—NO, these may not be at the correct level of learning.

C. Topic areas recommended by clinical faculty—NO, these may not meet the course objectives.
D. **Activities that will help meet student learning outcomes—YES, simulation should be relevant to the course and assist learners in achieving the student learning outcomes.**

3. A simulation educator is developing goals for the simulation activities to be included in her course. The best example of a goal is:
   A. "Learners will demonstrate the correct technique for inserting a nasogastric tube."—NO, this is a skill.
   B. "Learners will demonstrate the correct technique for administering enteral medications."—NO, again this is a skill.
   C. **"Simulation activities will enable learners to demonstrate their knowledge and skills with nasogastric tubes."—YES, this describes the expected outcome at the end of the teaching–learning process.**
   D. "Learners will demonstrate the correct technique for checking tube-feeding residuals."—NO, this is a skill.

4. In developing objectives for a simulation exercise planned for her course, the simulation educator should write objectives that are
   A. **Measurable and relevant—YES, in addition, objectives should be short-term, appropriate for the level of the learner, and measuring a single behavior.**
   B. Broadly written and long-term—NO, they should be measurable.
   C. Complex and difficult to achieve—NO, they should be achievable.
   D. Vague and intangible—NO, they should be specific.

5. A simulation educator elects to use formative evaluation to evaluate student learning following simulation activities. The best example of a method of formative evaluation is to:
   A. Administer a survey at the end of the simulation.—NO, this is summative.
   B. Include questions on the next exam that address the simulation objectives.—NO, this is summative.
   C. **Encourage learners to give return demonstrations following skill demonstrations.—YES, formative evaluation is done during the learning activity; it is used to facilitate learning.**
   D. Include simulation skills as part of the end-of-semester evaluation tool.—NO, this is summative.

6. When planning an evaluation method that will provide the learner with constructive critique for improvement and the opportunity for self-reflection, the simulation educator should select?
   A. Observation—NO, this does not provide feedback.
   B. Surveys—NO, this does not provide feedback.
   C. Skills checklists—NO, this does not provide feedback.
   D. **Debriefing—YES, this is particularly effective following high-fidelity simulations; it provides learners with the opportunity to process what they have learned.**

7. When using simulation to document competencies, the experienced simulation educator would choose an evaluation tool that is valid and reliable such as:
   A. **Objective structured clinical exams (OSCEs)—YES, OSCEs have been used extensively in medical schools and have been shown to be a valid assessment tool.**
   B. Self-reporting surveys—NO, validity has not been ensured.
   C. Skills checklists—NO, validity has not been ensured.
   D. Debriefing—NO, validity has not been ensured.

8. What statement by the simulation educator would indicate that she has a good understanding of designing simulation activities?
   A. "I will have students arrive at 8:30 a.m., and we will see how long the simulation takes."—NO, this is poor planning.
   B. **"I will schedule small groups of learners for each simulation activity."—YES, simulation activities are more effective when learners are placed in smaller groups.**
   C. "I will have the adjunct clinical faculty develop objectives for the day."—NO, this should be done by the simulation educator.
   D. "I will bring a large group of students in to get them all done at one time."—NO, large groups should be broken down into smaller learning groups.

9. When discussing plans for a simulation day with his mentor, the new simulation educator demonstrates evidence of his knowledge of simulation modalities by stating:
   A. "IV arms are a great use of high-fidelity simulation."—NO, they are low fidelity.
   B. "High-fidelity mannequins have limited use with new nursing students."—NO, they can be programmed at the correct learning level.
   C. **"A task trainer can be effective in teaching new skills."—YES, task trainers are often used for procedural training and the practice of skills.**
   D. "Debriefing is an effective method for evaluating skill acquisition with task trainers."—NO, task practice does not call for debriefing.

10. Which statement by the novice simulation educator would need to be corrected by the simulation coordinator?
    A. "A skill station designed for a review can be self-directed."—NO, it needs instruction.
    B. "A basic skill station could be monitored by a senior level or graduate student."—NO, it can be an undergraduate if it is basic.
    C. "An adjunct clinical instructor can teach a skill within their expertise."—NO, they should teach the correct method.
    D. **"The lab technician will serve as content expert for the high-fidelity simulation."—YES, although lab personnel or technicians can run the high-fidelity simulator, a content expert who has advanced knowledge and skill related to the scenario should be monitoring the simulation and leading the debriefing.**

25 ANSWERS AND RATIONALES TO END-OF-CHAPTER PRACTICE QUESTIONS ■ 381

■ CHAPTER 17 PRACTICE QUESTIONS

1. The novice simulation educator who is going to facilitate a debriefing needs further understanding when she:
   A. Observes the entire simulation—NO, it is important that the debriefer observes the entire simulation.
   B. Takes notes on observations during the simulation—NO, it is important for the debriefer to take notes to help facilitate the debriefing.
   C. Has an experienced debriefer with her—NO, to be an effective debriefer the educator should have training and experience in debriefing.
   D. Starts debriefing students one at a time—YES, all students should be debriefed together.

2. A simulation educator is very new to the debriefing process. Which method of debriefing might be easier for the educator to start with?
   A. Debriefing with Good Judgment—NO, this type of debriefing requires specific training to be done effectively.
   B. Case Study Debriefing—YES, all educators are familiar with case study reviews so this is a good type of debriefing for the inexperienced debriefer.
   C. Debriefing for Meaningful Learning—NO, this type of debriefing requires specific training to be done effectively.
   D. Advocacy Inquiry—NO, this is not a method of debriefing but instead a technique used with Debriefing with Good Judgment.

3. Ideally, the length of the debriefing time should be:
   A. 5 minutes—NO, the debriefing is supposed to be longer than the simulation encounter.
   B. Half the time needed to complete the simulation—NO, the debriefing is supposed to be longer than the simulation encounter.
   C. Equal to the time needed to complete the simulation—NO, the debriefing is supposed to be longer than the simulation encounter.
   D. Double the time needed to complete the simulation—YES, this will allow enough time to facilitate reflection in the learners.

4. The debriefing method in which the simulation educator facilitates the identification of what went well compared to what can be changed next time is called:
   A. Debriefing with Good Judgment—NO, this type of debriefing does not facilitate a discussion of what went well and what should be changed next time.
   B. Case Study Debriefing—NO, this type of debriefing does not facilitate a discussion of what went well and what should be changed next time.
   C. Debriefing for Meaningful Learning—NO, this type of debriefing does not facilitate a discussion of what went well and what should be changed next time.
   D. Plus Delta—YES, this type of debriefing facilitates a discussion of what went well and what should be changed next time.

5. The debriefing method in which the simulation educator focuses on defusing, discovering, and deepening is called:
   A. Plus Delta—NO, this type of debriefing facilitates a discussion of what went well and what should be changed next time.
   B. Debriefing with Good Judgment—NO, this debriefing focuses on a non-judgmental approach to debriefing uses the simulation educator as a patient advocate by asking questions using "I" and referring to the patient (advocacy).
   C. 3-D Model of Debriefing—YES, the 3-D Model of Debriefing focuses on defusing, discovering, and deepening.
   D. Debriefing for Meaningful Learning—NO, this method of debriefing focuses on fostering student reflective thinking and learning; socratic questioning; principles of active learning; and E5 Model: Engage, Explore, Explain, Elaborate, Evaluate, Extend.

6. The simulation educator wants to learn how to be an effective debriefer. The best method to learn debriefing is to:
   A. Read a book about debriefing.—NO, this is not effective because the debriefer does not get any experience or feedback.
   B. Practice with an experienced debriefer.—YES, this is the best way to learn debriefing because you will learn and practice debriefing techniques and get feedback from the experienced debriefer.
   C. Watch a video of a debriefing session.—NO, this is not effective because the debriefer does not get any experience or feedback.
   D. Attend a lecture on debriefing.—NO, this is not effective because the debriefer does not get any experience or feedback.

7. How does a simulation educator select the best debriefing method to use?
   A. Review all available methods of debriefing—NO, it is important to review all available methods of debriefing.
   B. Compare each debriefing method with your personal educational philosophy—NO, it is important to compare each debriefing method with your personal educational philosophy.
   C. Test out each type of debriefing method—NO, it is important to test out each type of debriefing method.
   D. All of the above—YES, because you should do all of the above to select the best debriefing style for you.

8. Which debriefing method includes a technique called *Advocacy Inquiry*?
   A. Plus Delta—NO, Plus Delta does not use a technique called *Advocacy Inquiry*.
   B. Debriefing with Good Judgment—YES, Debriefing with Good Judgment uses a technique called *Advocacy Inquiry*.
   C. 3-D Model of Debriefing—NO, the 3-D Model of Debriefing does not use a technique called *Advocacy Inquiry*.
   D. Debriefing for Meaningful Learning—NO, Debriefing for Meaningful Learning does not use a technique called *Advocacy Inquiry*.

9. The debriefing environment should be:
   A. Comfortable with seats for everyone—YES, the debriefing location should be a comfortable environment.
   B. A location away from where the simulation took place—YES, the debriefing location should be away from where the simulation took place.
   C. A safe environment—YES, the debriefing environment should be a safe environment where the learners feel safe to share information.
   D. All of the above—YES, the debriefing environment should be all of the above.

10. The simulation educator's role in the debriefing process is that of:
    A. Educator—NO, the educator's role in the debriefing process is that of facilitator.
    B. Researcher—NO, the educator's role in the debriefing process is that of facilitator.
    C. Evaluator—NO, the educator's role in the debriefing process is that of facilitator.
    D. Facilitator—YES, the educator's role in the debriefing process is that of facilitator.

CHAPTER 18 PRACTICE QUESTIONS

1. Feedback is
   A. Another term for *debriefing*—NO, it is different.
   B. A tool of debriefing—YES, it occurs congruent with debriefing.
   C. Is best delivered when something positive is said first—NO, it can be something positive or negative.
   D. A process of self-reflection—NO, it should spur self-reflection.

2. Preparing the learner for debriefing:
   A. Helps teach the learner how to debrief.—NO, this is not their role.
   B. Is optional.—NO, preparation should be done.
   C. Is required.—NO, it should be done.
   D. Helps the learner to participate more effectively in the process.—YES, it provides orientation to the process.

3. Debriefing is an advanced standardized patient (SP) core competency because:
   A. Not every SP is capable of providing feedback.—NO, many are not trained.
   B. It is more difficult than communication assessment.—NO, it is a communication assessment process.
   C. It is more use than just giving feedback.—NO, feedback is complex also.
   D. Debriefing is arguably the most complex activity for SPs to master.—YES, it needs additional training.

4. The reason standardized patients (SPs) provide feedback on communication is:
   A. **They are arguably in the best position to judge, and therefore debrief, the communication quality of the learners.—YES, they were part of the process and understand the objectives.**
   B. It is easier to evaluate communication than the physical examination.—NO, communication is difficult to evaluate.
   C. They are trained to do it.—NO, not all are trained.
   D. They are trained to assess communication.—NO, not all are trained.

5. One of the best ways to debrief the physical examination is:
   A. Telling the learner directly what he or she did incorrectly—NO, this may shut them down to learning.
   B. Showing leaners how the physical exam should be performed—NO, the learner needs to practice.
   C. **Asking the candidate to retry the exam and correct as necessary—YES, this assists learning.**
   D. The standardized patient (SP) should never debrief the physical examination—NO, this is not true.

6. The advantage of using Pendleton's Rules for debriefing is:
   A. **It helps both the standardized patient (SP) and the learner prepare for debriefing by listing positive performance as well as what could have been done differently.—YES, it shows both the good and what needs improvement and thereby balances the assessment.**
   B. It is an easy technique for SPs to remember.—NO, this is not the reason.
   C. Research shows it is an effective debriefing process.—NO, this is true, but not the only reason.
   D. Learners like to get both positive and negative feedback.—NO, learners usually do not like negative feedback.

7. To ensure standardized patient (SP) debriefing quality:
   A. Give the SP feedback about their debriefing.—NO, there should be a systematic method.
   B. Ask SPs to self-assess their work.—NO, there needs to be oversight to ensure quality improvement.
   C. Question them about their knowledge of debriefing.—NO, this is not the most objective method.
   D. **Use a debriefing quality-assurance checklist to note SP behaviors.—YES, this will assist the evaluation process to be objective.**

8. Empathy is important to the debriefing process because:
   A. **It helps the SP understand the learner's frame of reference.—YES, it assists the standardized patient (SP) to understand the learner's reaction or actions.**
   B. It demonstrates that the SP is a warm and caring person.—NO, this is not necessary in all learning situations.
   C. It creates psychological safety for the learner.—NO, this is not the objective of all simulation scenarios.
   D. It is an important adult learning approach.—NO, it is not part of the Knowles adult learning theory.

9. Reflective debriefing models:
   A. Promote positive learning.—NO, it can be negative.
   B. Are always appropriate.—NO, it may not always be appropriate depending on the debriefer, learner, and situation.
   C. Get the learners to self-assess their work so that in actual practice they can self-correct their performance.—YES, and this is the most important learning consequence.
   D. Get the standardized patients (SPs) to reflect on the quality of the learner's work.—NO, it is to get the learner to reflect.

10. One disadvantage of using the sandwich style of feedback is:
    A. It makes learners passive recipient's of the debriefer's information.—YES, it is passive.
    B. It does not work as well as reflective feedback.—NO, it can work well.
    C. It does not work well with physical examination debriefing.—NO, it can work well.
    D. It puts the debriefer in charge of what to discuss.—NO, the learner can discuss issues also.

CHAPTER 19 PRACTICE QUESTIONS

1. Which of the following is the best example of a "high-stakes" simulation activity?
   A. Maintenance of certification requirement for a healthcare profession—YES, this is evaluative.
   B. Critical care skill development for nurses at the hospital—NO, this is a learning experience.
   C. Medical student physical exam practice—NO, this is a learning experience.
   D. Interprofessional communication assessment for surgical teams—NO, this is a learning experience.

2. A faculty member has asked your advice on how to create an effective learner evaluation for her planned simulation-based training (SBT). Which of the following would you tell her is the **most important** step in this process?
   A. Determine the timing of the evaluation.—NO, although this is important, knowing the objectives of the evaluation is paramount.
   B. Identify the learning objectives to be evaluated.—YES, this is the most important and first step.
   C. Consider the background of the learners.—NO, although this is important, knowing the objectives of the evaluation is paramount.
   D. Conduct statistical item analysis to determine reliability.—NO, although this is important, knowing the objectives of the evaluation is paramount.

3. Use of a checklist-type evaluation instrument is **most** appropriate for which of the following:
   A. **Summative assessment of a student nurse performing the correct steps for inserting a urinary catheter—YES, this is procedural.**
   B. Summative assessment of a staff nurse's ability to recognize an unstable patient—NO, there are too many variables and the variables do not always follow a sequence.
   C. Formative assessment of a resident's ability to achieve an accurate differential diagnosis—NO, there are too many variables and the variables do not always follow a sequence.
   D. High-stakes evaluation of a medical student's ability to empathically communicate with parents of a critically ill patient—NO, there are too many variables and the variables do not always follow a sequence.

4. The most appropriate type of instrument for measuring the effectiveness of cardiopulmonary resuscitation (CPR) compressions is:
   A. Observation based—NO, this may not tell depth.
   B. Pre- and posttest—NO, this is for knowledge not for demonstration.
   C. **Haptic response—YES, this is the best measurement.**
   D. Participant feedback—NO, this cannot be done on a person and the participant doing CPR may not be the best judge.

5. Two facilitators are independently rating a summative simulation using an observation instrument. This type of evaluation is known as
   A. Peer evaluation—NO, this is people at the same level evaluating each other.
   B. **Interrater reliability evaluation—YES, this checks the evaluation with another expert.**
   C. Dual evaluation—NO, this is not what it is called.
   D. Rubric evaluation—NO, this is comparing procedures against a premade form.

6. Additional rigorous research and evidence-based practice appraisals are needed to ensure:
   A. Students are satisfied with simulation learning experiences.—NO, there are many studies about perceptions.
   B. Faculty are competent in providing simulation learning experiences.—NO, this is not something needed more study since there is established certification standards.
   C. Simulation is meeting the learners' outcomes.—NO, this is also a short-term evaluation that is done.
   D. **Simulation is impacting safe patient care.—YES, this is needed, additional long-term studies.**

7. High-quality simulation learning experiences should begin with:
   A. Resource management—NO, this does not ensure high-quality simulation.
   B. **Clear learning objectives—YES, this is the driver of the experience.**
   C. Participants in mind—NO, this is important, but not the first step
   D. Identification of appropriate technology—NO, this does not ensure high-quality simulation.

8. When choosing an evaluation tool for a simulation learning experience, it should reflect:

   A. The students involved—NO, this is not always necessary to have it specific to a certain discipline.
   B. The technology used—NO, this is not the important piece of evaluation.
   C. The faculty's expertise—NO, this is not the important piece of evaluation.
   D. The learning domain—YES, it should reflect knowledge, skills, or attitude.

9. Needed simulation research should be focused on which level of evaluation?

   A. Reaction—NO, this is perceptions of end users.
   B. Leaning—NO, this is meeting learning objectives.
   C. Behavior—NO, this is evaluating skills.
   D. Results—YES, this is translation into practice.

10. Which level of translational research is an evaluation of learning "carried over to patient care"?

    A. T-1—NO, this refers to learning in the simulation laboratory.
    B. T-2—YES, this is the carryover into patient care areas.
    C. T-3—NO, this is long-term improving patient care.
    D. T-4—NO, this is not a level.

CHAPTER 20 PRACTICE QUESTIONS

1. The novice healthcare simulation educator needs additional understanding of the governing principle of simulation education when she states:

   A. "Simulation is part of the routine learning for health professionals."—YES, it is not "routine."
   B. "Simulation assists society."—NO, it assists professionals to develop in their roles.
   C. "Simulation's goal is patient care outcomes."—NO, patient safety is the goal.
   D. "Using simulation assists in procedural practice."—NO, it does help professionals learn procedures.

2. Developing a social contract includes:

   A. Professionals understanding their roles—YES, professional development includes acquiring characteristics of a professional role.
   B. Society supporting the profession—NO, society does not just support the profession—it is reciprocal.
   C. Society trusting the works of the profession—NO, professionals have to gain trust.
   D. Being concerned with public values—NO, professional values are the concern.

3. Simulation standards of practice are developed by:

   A. Experts teaching simulation to novice educators—NO, it does not always need experts.
   B. Critical analysis of best practice—YES, it should use evidence to develop standards.

C. Solidifying practices—NO, things should remain flexible and be constantly updated.
D. Educators maintaining a specific set of skills—NO, skill sets change as professionals mature.

4. Continuous professional development (CPD) in simulation assists professionals to increase in:

    A. Career advancement—NO, this is not always the goal.
    B. Debriefing—NO, this is an aspect of good teaching.
    C. Communication—YES, it increases perception of different roles and points of view.
    D. Moulage—NO, this is an aspect of simulation development.

5. Continuous professional development (CPD) in simulation has been demonstrated to increase:

    A. Learner knowledge—YES, educating teachers promotes better achievement of student learning outcomes.
    B. Professional career attainment—NO, this is not always the outcome of CPD.
    C. Higher fidelity—NO, this is not always the outcome of CPD.
    D. Critical analysis—NO, this too is not always the end produce of CPD.

6. The graduate student needs a better understanding of continuous professional development (CPD) for healthcare simulation educators when he states that CPD:

    A. "Increases knowledge about systems, structures, and organizational cultures."—NO, this is true.
    B. "Is not needed to address basic knowledge skills, and attitudes."—YES, this is a piece of CPD.
    C. "Increases engagement in the learning processes."—NO, this should be given for educators.
    D. "Promotes learning outcomes for teachers and students."—NO, this is an outcome of CPD.

7. Considerations of organizations that healthcare simulation educators should embrace pertain to:

    A. Financial burden—YES, this must be considered when looking at the big picture.
    B. Their career trajectory—NO, this is an individual agenda.
    C. Future organizational structure and changes—NO, this is usually done by upper administration.
    D. Personal agendas of management—NO, this is an individual agenda.

8. Crucial conversations in professional healthcare situations many times include this subject:

    A. Promotion—NO, this is usually not crucial.
    B. Diversity—YES, this is a sensitive subject that needs to be discussed.
    C. Compensation—NO, this is usually not crucial.
    D. Leadership—NO, this is usually not crucial.

9. One of the attributes not included in developing self-efficacy in the simulation learning is:

    A. Relevancy—NO, this is included.
    B. Credibility—NO, this is included.
    C. Knowledge—NO, this is included.
    D. Critical thinking—YES, this is contained in knowledge and not separately included.

10. The third step of negotiating a professional role that can be fostered in a simulation scenario is:

    A. Feeling like an imposter—NO, this is the first step.
    B. Trial and error—NO, this is the second step.
    C. Taking the role seriously—YES, this is the third step.
    D. Transference—NO, this is the fourth step.

■ CHAPTER 21 PRACTICE QUESTIONS

1. Which of Kirkpatrick's levels of evaluation has been *least* heavily researched in simulation?

    A. Level 1, Reaction—NO, this has been researched.
    B. Level 2, Learning—NO, this has been researched.
    C. Level 3, Behavior—NO, this has been researched.
    D. Level 4, Results—YES, this needs long-term research.

2. Which is the best method to utilize to video record a team simulation?

    A. Show the entire video with no comments.—NO, it should be discussed.
    B. Bookmark while videotaping and show critical points both positive and negative.—YES, this homes in on the points of learning.
    C. Bookmark while videotaping and just show negative points.—NO, positive should be emphasized also.
    D. Send the video to students to watch on their own.—NO, this does not instruct.

3. What are the gaps in research? Select all that apply:

    A. Satisfaction—NO, there is research about satisfaction with simulation.
    B. Patient outcomes—YES, this is lacking.
    C. Confidence—NO, there is research about students' confidence with simulation.
    D. Valid measuring instruments—YES, reliable and valid instruments are needed.

4. How does one determine the validity of an instrument?

    A. Content experts review with high correlation of agreement—YES, this determines content validity.
    B. Piloted on 10 learners prior to use—NO, this pilots an instrument for item analysis.
    C. Colleague review—NO, they should be experts.
    D. The instrument measures the correct concepts.—NO, this is the opinion of one person.

5. A skilled simulation educator plans time in the simulation to include which of the following?

    A. A 10-minute debriefing—NO, it may take longer.
    B. Time to watch the entire video—NO, critical points need to be reviewed.
    C. A comprehensive orientation and prebriefing—YES, this is to decrease student anxiety.
    D. Ten minutes for students to write a reflection paper—NO, debriefing as a group may be more effective.

6. What is the gap in faculty simulation expertise identified in the national study of simulation programs? Check all that apply.

    A. Faculty development—YES, faculty needs a better understanding of simulation principles.
    B. Vendor education—NO, this is not necessarily going to impact students.
    C. Formal education—NO, this is not the most effective way to impact learning.
    D. Lack of Certified Healthcare Simulation Educators™—YES, this is excellent for faculty development.

7. Which component of Jeffries theoretical framework was changed?

    A. Facilitator—NO, this has remained the same.
    B. Student—YES, the student component has been expanded.
    C. Design characteristics—NO, this has remained the same.
    D. Outcomes—NO, this has remained the same.

8. Which organization offers certification in healthcare simulation education?

    A. International Nursing Association for Clinical Simulation & Learning (INACSL)—NO, this does not offer the certification.
    B. Society for Simulation in Healthcare (SSH)—YES, this organization is the leader in simulation certification.
    C. Association of Standardized Patient Educators (ASPE)—NO, this association does not offer the certification.
    D. American Nurses Credentialing Center (ANCC)—NO, this organization does not offer the certification.

9. From the national survey, what is the amount of simulation that can replace clinical experience?

    A. 20%—NO, this is incorrect.
    B. 25%—NO, this is incorrect.
    C. 50%—NO, this is incorrect.
    D. No evidence supports a particular percentage—YES.

10. Which of the following simulation modalities would best fit a mental health simulation?

    A. A virtual game—NO, this may not produce affective learning.
    B. A mannequin—NO, this may not produce affective learning.

C. A standardized patient\actor—YES, real people can best demonstrate emotions.

D. A video—NO, this may not produce affective learning.

CHAPTER 22 PRACTICE QUESTIONS

1. Which of the following leadership styles will most likely result in employee satisfaction?

   A. Transformational—YES, this places autonomy with the employees.
   B. Management by exception—NO, more engagement is needed.
   C. Laissez faire—NO, more engagement is needed.
   D. Transactional—NO, this hierarchical.

2. Which words most accurately describe retention? Retention_____.

   A. Is overrated; it is good for business to have a constant turnover of new enthusiastic personnel—NO, retention is important for maintenance of the simulation center.
   B. Is not something a manager needs to focus on—NO, retention is important for maintenance of the simulation center.
   C. Is an important part of the mission and strategic plan—NO, retention is important for maintenance of the simulation center.
   D. Is critical in maintaining quality and reducing expenses—YES, these are the elements that make retention important.

3. Which of the following is most important to increase realism and learner engagement in simulation?

   A. Inclusion of actor (standardized patient's) and confederates in the scenario—NO, this is not the most important element.
   B. Willingness of the learner to engage in the learning process—YES, this is the most important piece for a learning experience to be successful.
   C. Realistic smells, sounds, and images—NO, this is not the most important element.
   D. High-fidelity human patient simulators with voice modulators—NO, this is not the most important element.

4. Which statement most closely reflects the underlying attitude of a transformative leader?

   A. Failure is a way to grow.—YES, we learn from mistakes.
   B. Perfection is demanded.—NO, this is not transformative.
   C. Errors are largely caused by carelessness.—NO, this is not transformative.
   D. System policies and process rarely need updates.—NO, this is not transformative.

5. The individual who schedules events (the scheduler) in your simulation center cancels a high-priority user and, in his place, schedules a friend's group (a mid-priority user) in the center. You are the director of the center, and you just received an email complaint from your high-priority user. What initial action is the most appropriate in addressing this situation with the scheduler?

   A. Dismiss the scheduler.—NO, this increases turnover.
   B. Meet with the scheduler and clarify policy and expectations. Support the scheduler in rectifying the situation.—YES, help the scheduler to find a solution.
   C. Immediately place the scheduler on unpaid leave. Meet in a few days after you have straightened everything out.—NO, this is punitive.
   D. Stop by the scheduler's office and express your disappointment and frustration.—NO, this is punitive.

6. Which method is most likely to be successful for all users in keeping supplies organized in a larger center?

   A. Designate a place for each item and label everything.—YES, this organizes supplies.
   B. Keep secret stashes of hard-to-find items.—NO, this does not help organization.
   C. Lock supplies in cupboards.—NO, this does not help organization.
   D. Delegate one contact person as a gatekeeper for all supplies and equipment.—NO, this does not help accountability.

7. When managing supplies and equipment, it is important to _____.

   A. Track equipment repairs and warranty and service agreement information—NO, this is just one aspect.
   B. Track nondurable supplies and equipment for inventory and costs—NO, this is just one aspect.
   C. Determine what supplies and equipment and their costs are used in each scenario—NO, this is just one aspect.
   D. All of the above—YES, they are all important.

8. Which of the following need to be considered in scheduling an event?

   A. Personnel—NO, this is just one aspect.
   B. Mission, vision, and values—NO, this is just one aspect.
   C. Equipment and supplies—NO, this is just one aspect.
   D. All of the above—YES, they are all important.

9. Which one of the following can best help bring balance and effectiveness?

   A. Diligently learn and apply time-management skills.—NO, this is just one aspect, but it is really prioritizing.
   B. Consider what is essential and eliminate the nonessential.—YES, this is the ideal way to promote life balance.
   C. Apply the Six Sigma principles in your life.—NO, this is just one aspect, but it is rally prioritizing.
   D. Never open email first thing in the morning.—NO, this is just one aspect, but it is rally prioritizing.

10. You are setting up the room for a scenario and notice a piece of equipment is not working correctly. Select item with the best sequence for trouble shooting and correcting this problem.
    A. Call the sales representative/manufacturer, ensure the device is plugged in/charged, refer to the owner's manual for trouble-shooting, shut down the device and start it back up again.—NO, check all connections first.
    B. Ensure all cable connections are secure, repair or replace item, check to see whether the device is plugged in/charged, shut down the device and start it back up again.—NO, check all connections first then shut it down if needed.
    C. **Ensure all connections are secure, shut down the device and start it back up again, refer to owner's manual for trouble shooting, call representative/manufacturer.—YES, this would be the best sequence of events for troubleshooting.**
    D. Shut down the device and start it back up again, ensure the device is plugged in/charged, ensure all cable connections are secure, call the sales rep/manufacturer.—NO, check all connections first.

CHAPTER 23 PRACTICE QUESTIONS

1. A simulation educator is developing a self-study report for an accreditation process and is describing a simulation about the goals and responsibilities of a rapid-response team. This should be integrated in standard:
   A. Simulation℠ Participant Evaluation—NO, this references assessment of learning.
   B. **Simulation℠ Outcomes and Objectives—YES, this describes what the goals of the simulation scenario are.**
   C. Simulation℠ Facilitation—NO, this is about the simulation educator role.
   D. Simulation℠ Debriefing—NO, this is about the reflection and process improvement piece.

2. A simulation educator is developing a self-study report for accreditation and includes a section on personnel qualification; this information should be included in:
   A. Simulation℠ Debriefing—NO, this is about the reflection and process improvement piece.
   B. Simulation℠ Simulation Design—NO, this is about the instructional methods.
   C. Simulation℠ Professional Integrity—NO, this is about professionalism and ethics.
   D. **Simulation℠ Facilitation—YES, this is about the simulation educator.**

3. The U.S. Department of Education defines *accreditation* as
   A. The act or instance of choosing a candidate or organization for election or appointment or honor—NO, this is in reference to an individual.
   B. An activity that supports or provides active encouragement for the furtherance of cause, venture, or aim—NO, this is motivation.

C. The action or process of providing someone or something with an official document attesting to a status or level of achievement—NO, this is more of a certificate.

D. The status of public recognition that an accrediting agency grants to an educational institution or program that meets the agency's standards and requirements—YES, this states that a program meets and/or exceeds standards set forth.

4. Accreditation of your simulation center is a prestigious recognition that may lead to all of the following EXCEPT:

   A. Decreased student enrolment of the Simulation Lab's educational affiliates—YES, it should increase enrollment.
   B. Improved educational experience for students—NO, it should accomplish this.
   C. Forecasting benefits—NO, this, too, will be a product of accreditation.
   D. Improvements in business operations—NO, this will also be a benefit.

5. End-of-unit or chapter tests, end-of-term (midterm) exams and end-of-semester (final) exams are all examples of _____ assessments.

   A. High stakes—NO, these are standardized test that are usually given nationally.
   B. Summative—YES, these test produce a grade for an end unit or semester.
   C. Self—NO, these are facilitator or faculty made.
   D. Authentic—NO, this is not how tests are categorized.

6. When developing an accreditation self-study report, the simulation educator describes a student grievance incident and the due process that led to a resolution. This should be explained in which standard?

   A. Simulation^{SM} Simulation Design—NO, this is about the methodologies.
   B. Simulation^{SM} Outcomes and Objectives—NO, this is about goals.
   C. Simulation^{SM} Professional Integrity—YES, this is about ethical practice.
   D. Simulation^{SM} Security—NO, this is related to keeping elements safe.

7. A key ingredient for a successful accreditation process is to have a:

   A. Consultant—NO, this is not always needed.
   B. Simulation educator—YES, this is necessary to run a well-designed laboratory.
   C. Project manager—NO, this is not a necessity.
   D. Accreditations liaison—NO, this is not a necessity.

8. Simulation programs are accredited by:
   A. **International Nursing Association for Clinical Simulation and Learning (INACSL)—YES, this is the accreditation agency.**
   B. International Meeting on Simulation in Healthcare (IMSH)—NO, this is not the accreditation agency.
   C. Certified Healthcare Simulation Educator™ (CHSE™) Independent Accreditors—NO, this is not the accreditation agency.
   D. Society for Simulation in Healthcare (SSH)—NO, this is not the accreditation agency.

9. Best practice is a method that has been generally accepted as superior to any alternatives because it produces results that are supported by research. Which standard incorporates best practice from adult learning?
   A. **Simulation^{SM} Simulation Design—YES, this standard incorporates adult learning.**
   B. Simulation^{SM} Outcomes and Objectives—NO, this standard does not incorporate the principles of adult learning.
   C. Simulation^{SM} Facilitation—NO, this standard does not incorporate the principles of adult learning.
   D. Simulation^{SM} Debriefing—NO, this standard does not incorporate the principles of adult learning.

10. The use of standardized terminology has the goal of reducing negative consequences like confusion, misunderstanding, and poor learning outcomes. What are accepted sources for terminology in in situ simulation?
    A. Simulation^{SM} Simulation Protocols—NO, this is not the place to find terminology.
    B. Simulation^{SM} Participant Evaluation—NO, this is not the place to find terminology.
    C. Simulation^{SM} Professional Integrity—NO, this is not the place to find terminology.
    D. **Society for Simulation in Healthcare's *Healthcare Simulation Dictionary*—YES, this will have terminology.**

26 Answers and Rationales to Practice Test

1. Learners in a simulation laboratory who have a cognitive or physical disability receive:

    A. Special equipment—NO, this may be needed but it is not the overarching principle.
    B. More time—NO, this may be needed but it is not the overarching principle.
    C. Reasonable accommodations—YES, by law this is by law what is required.
    D. An individual educator—NO, this may not be reasonable.

2. The key concept of debriefing is to:

    A. Critique the event—NO, this is not an assessment strategy.
    B. Identify peer interaction—NO, this is about reflecting on one's own actions.
    C. Build consensus—NO, this is an individual or team process used for improvement.
    D. Develop improvement strategies—YES, this is the key concept.

3. The simulation educator understands that the best way to present a situation to a cohort of healthcare learners is to:

    A. Schedule specific time during each semester.—NO, this is effective but not the most effective method.
    B. Have students sign up on their own.—NO, this will cause scheduling problems.
    C. Use simulation as a remediation tool.—NO, simulation can be used as an effective learning tool also.
    D. Integrate simulation throughout the curriculum.—YES, it should be threaded throughout the curriculum.

4. For which of the following is videotaping most appropriate?

    A. Interviewing a patient (standardized patient [SP]) for professional development—YES, this activity demonstrates affective learning to the student.
    B. Megacode in Advanced Cardiac Life Support (ACLS)—NO, this concentrates on skills.
    C. Medication administration—NO, this concentrates on skills.
    D. Intraosseous vascular insertion—NO, this concentrates on skills.

5. According to Kern et al. (2009), the initial step in curriculum development to include in simulation is (Chapter 15):

   A. **Needs assessment—YES, the needs assessment will establish the reason for simulation.**
   B. Learner assessment—NO, this is important but comes second.
   C. Choosing the appropriate environment—NO, this is important but comes later than the needs assessment.
   D. Establishing learning objectives—NO, this is important but comes later than the needs assessment.

6. The novice simulation educator needs additional understanding when she states the following is a protection of students' ethical, legal, and regulatory rights in a simulation laboratory:

   A. Having codes of conduct—NO, this is needed to protect all students.
   B. Maintaining fair evaluation processes—NO, this is needed for equity.
   C. Having consent to record—NO, this is needed to protect information.
   D. **Implied consent for picture taking—YES, consent should be obtained.**

7. Which research method should be used to measure mastery learning?

   A. **Validated checklists—YES, this is an evaluative mechanism that records learning.**
   B. Multiple choice test—NO, this measures cognitive ability.
   C. Peer critique—NO, this is not expert evaluation.
   D. Focus group—NO, this elicits affective leaning.

8. The novice simulation educator needs further understanding when she states a mode of simulation includes

   A. Live scenarios—NO, this is interacting with real people or systems.
   B. Virtual learning—NO, this is interacting with simulated systems.
   C. Constructive theory—NO, this is interacting with simulated people and systems together.
   D. **Task trainers—YES, this is not an identified mode.**

9. What was Rossignol's (2017) conclusion when she compared oral debriefing to video-assisted debriefing (Chapter 21)?

   A. Video-assisted debriefing is better.—NO, one is not better than another.
   B. Oral debriefing is better.—NO, one is not better than another.
   C. **There is no significant difference between oral and video-assisted debriefing.—YES, both can be used effectively.**
   D. Repeated simulations increase psychological stress.—NO, this is not true.

10. In the medical education literature, simulation is a reliable tool for assessing which of these?

    A. Clinical outcomes—NO, this has not been developed completely to date.
    B. **Teamwork and communication—YES, there are reliable and valid tools to measure.**
    C. Patient outcomes—NO, this has not been developed completely to date.
    D. Knowledge—NO, this has not been developed completely to date.

11. Interprofessional education (IPE) is a form of:

    A. Experiential learning—YES, it encompasses active participation.
    B. Behavioralism—NO, this is a stimulus–response type of educational process.
    C. Deliberate practice—NO, this is a type of simulation learning.
    D. Self-directed learning—NO, this is usually module learning in which the students set the objectives.

12. When combined with simulation-based medical education, which teaching method improves skills acquisition?

    A. Deliberate practice—YES, this concentrates on improving skills.
    B. Didactic content—NO, this does not practice skills.
    C. Case studies—NO, this does not practice skills.
    D. Mock codes—NO, this does not practice skills over and over again.

13. Simulation educators understand that the purpose of formative evaluation is to provide:

    A. A grade for the activity—NO, this is a summative evaluation.
    B. Information for prebriefing—NO, this is preparatory information not evaluation.
    C. Constructive feedback—YES, so students can learn from the evaluation and improve.
    D. A pass/fail for the clinical skill—NO, this also would be summative.

14. The Certified Healthcare Simulation Educator™ observes the students missing an important assessment during a scenario and has the mannequin cough so the students listen to lung sounds. According to Meller (1997), this element of activity is a(n) (Chapter 14):

    A. Passive element—NO, this refers to the environment.
    B. Active element—NO, these are things preprogrammed into the scenario.
    C. Interactive element—YES, these are changes done by the certified healthcare educator.
    D. Transference—NO, this is applying knowledge.

15. Feedback is a process used in debriefing to:

    A. Provide a grade for the student.—NO, this is not an evaluation process.
    B. Identify remediation needs.—NO, this is not to identify remediation plans.
    C. Consider the student successful or unsuccessful.—NO, this is not an evaluation process.
    D. Promote desirable student development.—YES, this is the goal of feedback.

16. Professional conduct expected from a hired standardized patient (SP) includes:

    A. Articulation skills—NO, this is not listed as professional conduct.
    B. Knowledge of evaluation processes—NO, this is not listed as professional conduct.
    C. Emotional intelligence—YES, this is needed so SPs react appropriately to learners.
    D. Honesty—NO, this is not listed as professional conduct.

17. A new educator has developed a simulation scenario for his critical care course and after the scenario the educator should undertake the following activity first:

    A. Write another simulation scenario on a topic of interest.—NO, this is not the first step after a scenario.
    B. **Evaluate the students' feedback about the scenario.—YES, this can be done by allowing learners to provide their perceptions.**
    C. Determine the methods of evaluation to be used.—NO, this should already have been completed.
    D. Develop a schedule for the simulation activities.—NO, this should have been an initial step in planning.

18. An asset to using part-task trainers is:

    A. They are lightweight.—NO, some are actually cumbersome and heavy such as the entire torso.
    B. They are disposable.—NO, they are durable.
    C. They are small and store easily.—NO, some are large.
    D. **They are cost-effective.—YES, they are a less expensive mode of learning than high-fidelity mannequins.**

19. In planning the simulation event, the experienced simulation educator understands that:

    A. Student skills should all be at an acceptable level—NO, these may differ greatly.
    B. Scenarios that are difficult and challenging will produce better discussion in debriefing—No, this is not necessarily true.
    C. Topic areas should include common scenarios—NO, many times uncommon scenarios are needed.
    D. **Activities that will help meet student learning outcomes usually work the best—YES, simulation should be relevant to the course and assist learners in achieving the student learning outcomes.**

20. A nurse educator is developing goals for the simulation activities to be included in her course. A goal written in the affective domain is:

    A. "Learners will demonstrate the correct technique for inserting an intravenous catheter."—NO, this is the psychomotor domain.
    B. "Learners will demonstrate the correct technique for administering intramuscular medications."—NO, this is the psychomotor domain.
    C. **"Students will demonstrate empathy for the patient and family members."—YES, this is the affective domain.**
    D. "Learners will understand the steps of checking tube feeding residuals."—NO, this is the cognitive domain.

21. The following would be an example of a high-stakes simulation laboratory evaluation:

    A. **Performing an end-of-course objective structured clinical examination (OSCE)—YES, this is high stakes because it can result in failure in the course.**
    B. Completing one of four didactic tests given throughout the semester—NO, this is one of four so a poor grade may be able to be made up on the other three tests.

C. Deliberate practice of Foley catheter insertion in open laboratory hours—NO, this is practice.
D. A simulation scenario about a cardiac infarction that is recorded for review—NO, this is being reviewed so it is not high stakes if there is an opportunity for improvement.

22. The new simulation educator needs additional understanding of curriculum development when she states:
    A. "I need to identify every place where I can get resources."—NO, this needs to be done to implement a curriculum.
    B. "This curriculum needs to be evaluated in an ongoing fashion."—NO, this needs to be done to implement a curriculum.
    C. "I am positive that we have political support for this simulation curriculum."—NO, political support can change at any time.
    D. "We can address implementation barriers as they arise."—YES, barriers have to be anticipated to overcome right up front.

23. The healthcare simulation educator understands that the four main core competencies for interprofessional collaborative practice include:
    A. Leadership—NO, this is not a named core competency.
    B. Evidence-based practice—NO, this is not a named core competency.
    C. Reflection—NO, this is not a named core competency.
    D. Communication—YES, this is one of the four named core competencies.

24. In an advocacy-inquiry debriefing session the simulation educator correctly starts a process improvement when he states:
    A. "I am concerned because I noticed the team took four minutes to organize themselves."—YES, the educator starts with what was observed and of concern.
    B. "The team took too long to organize themselves."—NO, this is a direct observation on the learners.
    C. "Let's list what went well and what needs improvement."—NO, this is plus/delta technique.
    D. Can you all tell me as a group what took you so long?—NO, this is a "dirty question."

25. During a formative evaluation with a student after a simulation scenario about patient safety, the best response from the debriefer would be:
    A. "Not identifying the patient could result in you eventually losing your license."—NO, this is not a process improvement.
    B. "Your lack of safety in patient identification fails you."—NO, this would be summative.
    C. "Understanding patient safety is my priority."—NO, this focus is on the debriefer.
    D. "Can you think of how to increase patient safety in the next scenario."—YES, this is formative and requests reflection.

26. The most effective simulation method to teach intravenous (IV) insertion would be:
    A. Using a standardized patient—NO, this is an invasive procedure.
    B. **Using a part-task trainer with a standardized patient—YES, this has the ability to do the procedure without being invasive on a human and the standardized patient can provide emotion.**
    C. Using a high-fidelity mannequin—NO, this decreases realism.
    D. Using a peer who is role-playing—NO, this is an invasive procedure.

27. During a simulation scenario a student starts to have an anxiety attack and stands against the wall as if immobile. The best recourse for the simulation educator in this scenario is:
    A. **Stop the scenario and ask the student to come out then continue.—YES, the student needs to be cared for first.**
    B. Continue the scenario and provide feedback to the student individually immediately after.—NO, the condition warrants immediate intervention.
    C. Give the other students a "life saver" to focus their attention on the student having the anxiety attach.—NO, this will not meet the learning goals and the student with the anxiety attach needs attention.
    D. Stop the scenario and debrief the group.—NO, this is an individual problem and needs confidentiality.

28. One of the primary reasons to integrate simulation throughout a curriculum is to identify
    A. Skill attainment—NO, although this is a reason it is not the most salient reason.
    B. Missing procedures—NO, this is a curriculum stacking issue.
    C. **Knowledge gaps—YES, to assist students to fill in what they may not see or learn elsewhere.**
    D. At-risk students—NO, there are many methods to identify students at risk.

29. The Certified Healthcare Simulation Educator™ takes great care to make a patient wound on a part-task trainer look real. This will increase:
    A. **Physical fidelity—YES, this has to do with the human body realism.**
    B. Psychological fidelity—NO, this is preparing the students.
    C. Environmental fidelity—NO, this has to do with the surroundings.
    D. Equipment fidelity—NO, this has to do with the actual mannequins or prat-task trainers.

30. Standardized patients (SPs) should come out of character when:
    A. The student makes an error.—NO, the SP should stay in character and note or correct.
    B. The student requests further information.—NO, this SP should not have to teach.
    C. **The student is finished.—YES, when the scenario is over.**
    D. The student asks the SP to come out of character.—NO, this is not by student request.

31. The Certified Healthcare Simulation Educator™ prebriefs the students by allowing him or her to view and touch the mannequins. This will increase:

   A. Physical fidelity—NO, this has to do with the human body realism.
   B. Psychological fidelity—YES, this is preparing the students.
   C. Environmental fidelity—NO, this has to do with the surroundings.
   D. Equipment fidelity—NO, this has to do with the actual mannequins or prat-task trainers.

32. The novice Certified Healthcare Simulation Educator™ needs additional orientation when she states:

   A. "Increased realism will ensure the learning outcomes."—YES, realism does not ensure student learning outcomes alone.
   B. "Realism should be created within a safe environment."—NO, this may be true.
   C. "Realism increases the fidelity of the simulation scenario."—NO, this may be true.
   D. "Realism many assist the students to better understand the situation."—NO, this may be true.

33. The concept of deliberate practice builds on the understanding that

   A. People will keep trying to get things right.—NO, this is not necessarily true for all people.
   B. Deliberate practice will lead to perfection.—NO, the goal is not perfection.
   C. Repeated behaviors will become automatic habits.—YES, it trains the mind to repeat behaviors.
   D. Every attempt provides new understanding.—NO, it is just repeating behavior.

34. The Certified Healthcare Simulation Educator™ understands that one of the main core competencies for interprofessional collaborative is:

   A. Leadership—NO, this is not one of the core competencies.
   B. Responsibility—YES, this is one of the named four core competencies.
   C. Reflection—NO, this is not one of the core competencies.
   D. Demonstration—NO, this is not one of the core competencies.

35. The novice simulation educator needs a better understanding of the role of standardized/simulated patients when he states:

   A. "They can grade the student."—YES, they cannot; they are not educators.
   B. "They can provide feedback."—NO, they can and should do this.
   C. "They can be scripted."—NO, they are scripted.
   D. "They can display emotions."—NO, that is the asset of having them.

36. Microethical situations can be simulated and include all of the following except:

    A. Borderline medication administration practices—NO, this is a microethical concern that needs correction.
    B. Poor infection control practices—NO, this is a microethical concern that needs correction.
    C. Breeches in confidentiality—NO, this is a microethical concern that needs correction.
    D. Sexual misconduct—YES, this is a serious ethical issue.

37. The following is an example of a basic "sandwich" feedback approach:

    A. "You did a good patient assessment and need to improve on both heart sounds and lung sound stethoscope placement."—NO, this is positive, negative, negative.
    B. "The heart sound stethoscope placement was incorrect so let us review, but the lung sound stethoscope placement on the standardized patient was correct."—NO, this is negative then positive.
    C. "You did an overall thorough patient head-to-toe assessment but need practice in lung sound stethoscope placement, but your heart stethoscope placement was fine."—YES, this is positive, negative, positive.
    D. "Let us consider going over the placement of your stethoscope for the heart sounds one more time."—NO, this is negative.

38. In order to create a simulation scenario that appropriately uses the concept of "as if" it should:

    A. Have increased fidelity.—NO, this may not guarantee that fiction contract.
    B. Contain moulage.—NO, this may not guarantee that fiction contract.
    C. Contain believable information.—YES, it has to be feasible.
    D. Use a complex care case.—NO, this may not guarantee that fiction contract.

39. Simulation scenarios can evaluate students in all learning domains. One student states during a debriefing that he felt as if there was an ethical issue when the feeding tube was inserted in the patient. The domain that is reflected in this student's learning is:

    A. Cognitive—NO, this is knowledge.
    B. Psychomotor—NO, this is doing.
    C. Internalization—NO, this is taking on values.
    D. Affective—YES, this is attitudes.

40. The Certified Healthcare Simulation Educator™ writes a student learning outcome, "At the end of this scenario the students will demonstrate correct sterile technique." This student learning outcome is written in which domain?

    A. Cognitive—NO, this is knowledge.
    B. Psychomotor—YES, this is doing.
    C. Internalization—NO, this refers to taking on values.
    D. Affective—NO, this is attitude.

26 ANSWERS AND RATIONALES TO PRACTICE TEST ■ 405

41. Using a TeamSTEPPS approach, the simulation scenario should teach the CUS principles, which are:

    A. Concerned, Uncommunicated, Strategies—NO, this is not what the principle stands for.
    B. Cognitive, Uncomfortable, Safety—NO, this is not what the principle stands for.
    C. Cognitive, Uncommunicated, Scenario—NO, this is not what the principle stands for.
    D. Concerned, Uncomfortable, Safety—YES, this is what the principle stands for.

42. The Certified Healthcare Simulation Educator™ writes a student learning outcome, "At the end of this scenario the students will describe correct sterile technique." This student learning outcome is written in which domain?

    A. Cognition—YES, this is knowledge.
    B. Psychomotor— NO, this is doing.
    C. Internalization—NO, this is taking on values.
    D. Affective—NO, this is attitudes.

43. One of the most important professional development pieces about simulation for faculty is:

    A. Working the mannequins—NO, this is not the most important concept to grasp about simulation.
    B. Developing scenarios—NO, this is not the most important concept to grasp about simulation.
    C. Understanding debriefing—YES, debriefing is the most important aspect for learning to take place.
    D. Learning how to troubleshoot—NO, this is not the most important concept to grasp about simulation.

44. Common team problems identified during simulation include all of the following except:

    A. Lack of role understanding—NO, this is a common issue.
    B. No plan to correct mistakes—NO, this is a common issue.
    C. Lack of evaluation for the team effort—NO, this is a common issue.
    D. Lack of leadership—YES, teams do not have to have a leader to function within their roles appropriately.

45. The Certified Healthcare Simulation Educator™ understands that the four main core competencies for interprofessional collaborative practice include:

    A. Leadership—NO, this is not one of the core competencies.
    B. Delegation—NO, this is not one of the core competencies.
    C. Values—YES, this is one of the core competencies.
    D. Demonstration—NO, this is not one of the core competencies.

V DOMAIN IV: SIMULATION RESOURCES AND ENVIRONMENTS

46. A student gets upset during a team-based simulation scenario and raises her voice. The Certified Healthcare Simulation Educator™ debriefs her and discusses the behavior with her in order to promote which of Wong and Driscoll's (2008) affective learning domains (Chapter 14)?

    A. Receiving—NO, this is taking in knowledge.
    B. Valuing—NO, this is demonstrating a preference.
    C. Internalizing—YES, this is taking in the values of the profession.
    D. Organizing—NO, this is formulating knowledge.

47. In planning to use standardized patients for simulation, the experienced nurse educator knows that it is important to:

    A. Provide orientation and training for the people involved.—YES, depending on the role to be played, the standardized patients need guidance in what is required for the simulation to unfold as planned.
    B. Recruit only trained actors to serve as standardized patients.—NO, this is not always possible.
    C. Ensure that the actors are paid prior to the simulation day.—NO, they should preform the work first.
    D. Provide an exact script for the actors to follow.—NO, sometimes the actors can use their own history is appropriate.

48. To identify potential issues and problems that may occur with new simulation activities, the nurse educator should:

    A. Seek the input of students who will be participating.—NO, it should be already prepared for the students.
    B. Ask other faculty whether they can foresee any problems.—NO, this may not be the best way to identify potential difficulties.
    C. Conduct a run-through or field test of the new simulation.—YES, in addition to identifying potential problems, this is also an opportunity to ensure that necessary resources are available and the simulation is running seamlessly.
    D. Ask for suggestions from practice partners.—NO, this may also not be the best method to identify difficulties.

49. When prescreening standardized patient actors, the Certified Healthcare Simulation Educator™ should collect:

    A. A reference—NO, this is a great idea but not the main item needed.
    B. A curriculum vitae (CV)—YES, this will evaluate the experience.
    C. Application—NO, this is a great idea but not the main item needed.
    D. Video of acting skills—NO, this is a great idea but not the main item needed.

50. When observing a debriefing led by a novice educator, the experienced nurse educator would need to intervene when which statement is made?

    A. "Help me to understand why you did this."—NO, this is a question eliciting reflection.
    B. "How do you think the group did overall?"—NO, no this is having students reflect.

C. "You know this is the wrong way to do this."—YES, this sounds accusatory and will block further communication with the learners.
D. "Can you tell me what you were thinking at this time?"—NO, this is directly asking a student to reflect on their decision-making processes.

51. In planning to teach the students intravenous (IV) insertion, the nurse educator elects to use the computer-generated, three-dimensional (3-D) IV program to allow learners to practice the skill. This is an example of what type of simulation modality?

    A. High-fidelity—NO, it is VR.
    B. Virtual reality—YES, virtual reality includes 3-D imaging, interaction with the environment, and visual/auditory feedback.
    C. Task trainer—NO, it is VR.
    D. Standardized patient—NO, it is VR.

52. When discussing advantages of simulation, the nurse educator would not include which statement?

    A. "Simulation can substitute for some clinical hours in difficult to find specialty areas."—NO, this is true and very much an asset to simulation.
    B. "Simulation is useful in helping students to experience uncommon clinical situations."—NO, this is true.
    C. "Simulation can help students to develop confidence before entering the hospital setting."—NO, this is also true.
    D. "Simulation is something that can be done at the last minute if needed for makeup days."—YES, simulation should always be a planned activity to ensure the student learning outcomes will be met and the simulation is relevant and worthwhile.

53. A simulation educator is developing an interprofessional simulation experience involving physicians, registered nurses, emergency medical technicians (EMTs) and licensed practical nurses. Which standard's guidelines would the educator have to follow in order to reach learning outcomes shared by all specialties?

    A. Simulation[SM] Simulation Design—NO, this is not necessarily going to ensure interprofessional education objectives are met.
    B. Simulation[SM] Outcomes and Objectives—NO, this is not necessarily going to ensure interprofessional education objectives are met.
    C. Simulation[SM] Professional Integrity—NO, this is not necessarily going to ensure interprofessional education objectives are met.
    D. Simulation[SM] Simulation-Enhanced Interprofessional Education (Sim-IPE)—YES, this is the standard guideline.

54. The Simulation[SM] Debriefing standard contains the following learning goals except:

    A. Facilitate reflection on individual and team performance to achieve targeted performance improvement.—NO, this is included.
    B. Facilitate appropriate critical thinking, clinical judgment, reasoning, reflection, and reflective thinking.—NO, this is included.

C. Recognize unprofessional and unethical behavior during simulation and take steps to abate it.—YES, this happened in situ.
D. Allow facilitation to be modified based on assessed participant needs and the impact of the experience—NO, this is included.

55. Components of team training include leadership, and that role specifically includes which key component:
    A. A shared understanding—NO, this is associated with peer observation.
    B. Delegation—YES, leaders must appropriately delegate.
    C. Balance of work—NO, this is balance.
    D. Mutual trust—NO this is the concept of trust.

56. The Certified Healthcare Simulation Educator™ understand that the four main core competencies for interprofessional collaborative practice include
    A. Teamwork—YES, this is one of the four core competencies needed.
    B. Delegation—NO, this is not identified as a core competency.
    C. Prioritization—NO, this is not identified as a core competency.
    D. Demonstration—NO, this is not identified as a core competency.

57. Simulation can be a reliable method of evaluation when:
    A. There are effective evaluation tools—YES, that are reliable and valid.
    B. When simulation educators videotape students—NO, this may not ensure reliability if different evaluators are using different standards.
    C. Students understand the purpose of simulation—NO, this does not guarantee reliability in results.
    D. When students pass an objective test on the content learned in simulation—NO, this is a different evaluation mechanism.

58. When using simulation to understand students' perceptions, the experienced nurse educator would choose:
    A. Objective structured clinical exams (OSCEs)—NO, OSCEs are an objective assessment tool.
    B. Self-reporting surveys—YES, self-reporting is the students' perceptions.
    C. Skills checklists—NO, these are just completed or not.
    D. Direct questioning—NO, no this is yes or no.

59. What statement by the nurse educator would indicate that she has a poor understanding of designing simulation activities?
    A. "I will have students arrive at 0700 a.m., and we will see how long the simulation takes." YES, this is poor planning.
    B. "I will schedule small groups of learners for each simulation activity."—NO, simulation activities are more effective when learners are placed in smaller groups.
    C. "I will have the course faculty help develop objectives for the day."—NO, the objectives, outcomes, or goals should be done by the course instructor.
    D. "I will bring each group of students in for pre-briefing."—NO, it is good practice to orientate students.

60. When discussing plans for a simulation day with his mentor, the new nurse educator demonstrates lack of knowledge about simulation modalities by stating:

    A. "Intravenous (IV) arms are a great use of low-fidelity simulation."—NO, they are low-fidelity.
    B. "High-fidelity mannequins can be used effectively with new nursing students."—NO, they can be used effectively for even low-level skill attainment.
    C. "A task trainer can be effective in teaching new skills."—NO, task trainers are often used for procedural training and the practice of skills.
    D. **"Debriefing is an effective method for evaluating skill acquisition with task trainers."—YES, this is not the purpose of debriefing.**

61. The simulation educator gets the same results with six different groups of students using a newly made skills checkoff list for skill attainment of second year physical therapy students. The simulation educator understands this supports the interments:

    A. Credibility—NO, it is the reliability.
    B. Validity—NO, it is reliability.
    C. **Reliability—YES, it documents consistency multiple groups.**
    D. Content—NO, this is done in reference to validity not reliability.

62. The best description of a simulation educator who is a transformational leader is:

    A. **"She moves people towards the future by providing us with what simulation can do for learners."—YES, this futuristic view sets transformational leaders apart.**
    B. "She organizes the simulation laboratory so it is easy for students to learn."—NO, organization and management can be done by many types of leaders.
    C. "She supports faculty by developing scenarios that depict hard-to-get student clinical experiences."—NO, organization and management can be done by many types of leaders.
    D. "She is excellent at scheduling the simulation experiences needed for learners throughout the semester."—NO, organization and management can be done by many types of leaders.

63. A key concept of interprofessionality is:

    A. **Constant knowledge sharing—YES, this is the necessary element for interprofessional education and teamwork.**
    B. Leadership ability—NO, this is needed but not the "key" element.
    C. Delegation of tasks—NO, this is needed but not the "key" element.
    D. Prioritization of interventions—NO, this is needed but not the "key" element.

64. Debriefing should create a climate of:
    A. Mutual respect—NO, this is important but not the main climate-creating concept.
    B. Straightforwardness—NO, this is important but not the main climate-creating concept.
    C. Shared perspectives—NO, this process provides a time for the standardized patient or simulation educator to give the student her or his observations.
    D. Psychological safety—YES, this is necessary to open conversations and decrease vulnerability.

65. The best description of a simulation educator who is a transactional leader is:
    A. "She moves people toward the future by providing us with what simulation can do for learners."—NO, this is a transformational leader.
    B. "She organizes the simulation laboratory so it is easy for students to learn."—YES, this is a hierarchical leader who may sometimes micromanage.
    C. "She provides the resources needed so simulation educators can be creative."—NO, this is an attribute of a transformational leader.
    D. "She keeps the mission of the simulation laboratory learning environment in focus as meetings."—NO, this is an attribute of a transformational leader.

66. What level of proficiency is the Certified Healthcare Simulation Educator™ displaying when he uses a lifesaver who assists students to stay on track when the students demonstrate the first indication that they will deviate from the student learning outcomes?
    A. Advanced beginner—NO, at this level procedures are being followed.
    B. Competent—NO, at this level the person is organized, but still needs to plan.
    C. Proficient—NO, at this level the person is still learning from experiences.
    D. Expert—YES, this is an educator who can use intuition.

67. National studies have demonstrated that student learning outcomes in healthcare programs are:
    A. Negatively impacted by the overuse of simulation—NO, simulation positively impacts students to reach their SLOs.
    B. Positively impacted by the use of simulation—YES, simulation has been shown to positively impact the attainment of SLOs.
    C. Not significantly affected by simulation—NO, simulation positively impacts students to reach their SLOs.
    D. Obscured by simulation learning experiences—NO, simulation positively impacts students to reach their SLOs.

68. The reason that simulation laboratories are an appropriate place for diversity training is:
    A. Standardized patients (SPs) can pretend to be of any ethnicity or race.—NO, this is not the most important factor in diversity training.
    B. Mannequins can be altered with moulage to look like a minority patient.—NO, this is not the most important factor in diversity training.

26 ANSWERS AND RATIONALES TO PRACTICE TEST ■ 411

C. Learners do not bring their social determinants into the laboratory space with them.—NO, social determinants can never be negated in any place.

D. It is safe space where learning can take place for all under the guidance of experienced simulation educators.—YES, the environment facilitates an equal playing field (as much as humanly possible).

69. When healthcare students negotiate the role of a professional they begin by:

   A. Feeling like an imposter—YES, they have not connected with the role in the beginning.
   B. Using trial-and-error methods to learn—NO, this is after there is some small connection with the role.
   C. Start understanding the seriousness of the role—NO, this takes place later in the educational process.
   D. Gain confidence and socialize into role—NO, this is much later in the educational process of healthcare students.

70. When a healthcare learner enters a simulation scenario and stops for a moment to observe the surroundings and the placement of the patient in the room, this student demonstrates socialization in the form of:

   A. Understanding—NO, this is simple memory and usually does not include a reflective learning process.
   B. Expert—NO, this is someone who can use their intuition in a situation.
   C. Modulation frame—NO, this usually includes a reflective learning process.
   D. Primary frame—YES, this is being aware of surroundings.

71. When a healthcare learner enters a simulation scenario and reflects on a past simulation experience, the socialization is in the form of a(n):

   A. Understanding—NO, this is simply memory and usually does not include a reflective learning process.
   B. Expert—NO, this is someone who can use intuition in a situation.
   C. Modulation frame—YES, this usually includes a reflective learning process.
   D. Primary frame—NO, this is being aware of one's surroundings.

72. The novice simulation educator needs additional understanding when he states:

   A. "Minority students will do just as well in simulation because they are apt to join in like everyone else."—YES, this is not usually the case, minority students needs to feel welcomed and engaged.
   B. "Minority students can feel marginalized in the learning environment."—NO, this is true.
   C. "Minority students need to feel as if they belong in the scenario with everyone else."—NO, this is true.
   D. "Minority students may have more difficulty succeeding due to social determinants."—NO, this is true.

73. A student receives time and a half during classroom testing. During an evaluative scenario in the simulation laboratory, students have to read the patient's case history. The student who is accommodated in the classroom should:

    A. Be referred to the student services Americans With Disabilities Act (ADA) officer—YES, the educational organization's ADA officer has to supply an official letter describing accommodations.
    B. Be provided with time and half to read the case—NO, not without a letter from the ADA officer.
    C. Be held to the same clinical standards as all students—NO, if the accommodations are reasonable then they should be made by the ADA officer.
    D. Be provided a private testing time—NO, this is not the accommodation needed.

74. The goal of interprofessional education (IPE) is to:

    A. Have people understand each other's role.—NO, this may happen but it is not the ultimate goal.
    B. Make the working environment more congenial.—NO, this may happen but it is not the ultimate goal.
    C. Provide different perspectives about patient care.—NO, this may happen but it is not the ultimate goal.
    D. Provide safe patient care.—YES, patient safety is the goal.

75. When simulation educators discuss how students learn, store, and recall information, they are referring to:

    A. Worldviews—NO, this is just a description of how philosophies are formed.
    B. Philosophies—NO, these are grander concepts than theories.
    C. Teaching theories—NO, this is not a stand-alone theory.
    D. Learning theories—YES, these are the essence of a learning theory.

76. The simulation educator writes the following objective: "At the end of this simulation experience the learner will correctly demonstrate intravenous insertion." When reading this objective, it is understood that the simulation educator is using:

    A. Constructivism—NO, this is knowledge build by the student not preconceived by the simulation educator.
    B. Behaviorism—YES, this is a measurable outcome observable through behavior.
    C. Scaffolding—NO, this is constructing knowledge from simple to complex.
    D. Realism—NO, this is a view of the world that it can be empirically explained.

77. A simulation educator begins the presession by asking the students to recall information from the previous session a week ago in order to assist them to gain new related knowledge. The simulation educator is using which educational theory?

    A. Constructivism—YES, this is knowledge build by the student not preconceived by the simulation educator.
    B. Behaviorism—NO, this is measurable outcome observable through behavior.

    C. Scaffolding—NO, this is constructing knowledge from simple to complex.
    D. Realism—NO, this is a view of the world as one that can be empirically explained.

78. According to adult learning theory, which of the following learning preferences attributes is not associated with students in the simulation laboratory:

    A. Self-directedness in instruction—NO, this is an adult learning attribute.
    B. Motivation to learn—NO, this is an adult learning attribute.
    C. Independence in decision-making—NO, this is an adult learning attribute.
    D. **Seeking out theoretical knowledge—YES, this is not an adult learning attribute; adult learners are concerned with situation-specific learning events.**

79. The novice simulation educator needs a better understanding when he states:

    A. "Simulation can be used for pharmacology practice."—NO, this is true.
    B. **"Using simulation for basic science is difficult."—YES, it can be used fairly easily for basic science.**
    C. "Practicing skills is done well using part-task trainers."—NO, this is true.
    D. "Crisis management can be taught effectively with simulation."—NO, this is true.

80. A simulation educator is asking the standardized patients (SPs) for feedback about the learner's performance and skills. The simulation educator is using which educational philosophy?

    A. **Constructivism—YES, this is knowledge built by the student not preconceived by the simulation educator and it includes real-world feedback.**
    B. Behaviorism—NO, this is measurable outcome observable through behavior.
    C. Scaffolding—NO, this is constructing knowledge from simple to complex.
    D. Realism—NO, this is a view of the world as one that can be empirically explained.

81. A learner is trying over and over to gain skill placing a nasogastric tube on a part-task trainer. The student is displaying which concept in Kolb's experiential learning theory?

    A. Concrete experience—NO, this is basing learning in what is tangible.
    B. Abstract conceptualization—NO, this is thinking about situations and different perspectives.
    C. Reflective observation—NO, this is thinking about things before reacting.
    D. **Active experimentation—YES, this is hands-on learning.**

82. The novice simulation educator needs a better understanding of scenario learning objectives when he states:

    A. **"It is basically to get students to make up clinical hours."—YES, this is not the goal of simulation.**
    B. "It is to understand taking a health history on a patient."—NO, this is a goal of simulation.

C. "It is to understand patient teaching."—NO, this is a goal of simulation.
D. "It is to understand the proper physical assessment techniques."—NO, this is a goal of simulation.

83. A learner is watching the scenario of cardiac arrest on a patient and a resuscitation effort and chooses to be the "recorder" for the event. The student is displaying which concept in Kolb's experiential learning theory?

   A. Concrete experience—NO, this is basing learning in what is tangible.
   B. Abstract conceptualization—NO, this is thinking about situations and different perspectives.
   C. Reflective observation—YES, this is thinking about things before reacting.
   D. Active experimentation—NO, this is hands-on learning.

84. An example of closed-loop communication is:

   A. "Did you get a regular heart rhythm?"—NO, this is just asking a question; it does not verify information.
   B. "Please provide the patient with a shock."—NO, this is providing a command; it does not verify information.
   C. "Please let me know what you heard me say about the treatment plan."—YES, this verifies information.
   D. "Are you going to tell me what you would like first?"—NO, this is just asking a question; it does not verify information.

85. A learner approaches the simulation educator the day following a scenario that she participated in and tells the educator she has been thinking about her responses and thinks they could have been communicated better. The student is displaying which concept in Kolb's experiential learning theory?

   A. Concrete experience—NO, this is basing learning in what is tangible.
   B. Abstract conceptualization—YES, this is thinking about situations and different perspectives.
   C. Reflective observation—NO, this is thinking about things before reacting.
   D. Active experimentation—NO, this is hands-on learning.

86. During a simulation scenario, a student performs skills on the mannequin and reacts and changes directions appropriately when the cardiac monitor strip is different. The student is displaying which concept in Kolb's experiential learning theory?

   A. Concrete experience—YES, this is basing learning in what is tangible.
   B. Abstract conceptualization—NO, this is thinking about situations and different perspectives.
   C. Reflective observation—NO, this is thinking about things before reacting.
   D. Active experimentation—NO, this is hands-on learning.

87. A simulation educator is debriefing learners and provides them with Internet resources and poses questions that stretch their current knowledge base to

consider different approaches. The simulation educator is using which learning theory?

　A. Constructivism—NO, this is student-centered knowledge building from past experiences.
　B. Behaviorism—NO, this is stimulus–response learning.
　C. Scaffolding—YES, this is building knowledge through accessing resources and stretching students to the next level of understanding.
　D. Realism—NO, this is an empirical type of learning.

88. The novice simulation educator needs a better understanding of Kneebone's essential elements for successful simulation when he states simulation should:

　A. "Allow for deliberate practice."—NO, this is part of Kneebone's explanation of simulation.
　B. "Can include experiences as close to real life as possible."—NO, this is part of Kneebone's explanation of simulation.
　C. "Be learner centered."—NO, this is part of Kneebone's explanation of simulation.
　D. "Encourage students to learn skills using peer-tutoring."—YES, Kneebone calls for expert tutors to enhance learning.

89. A tool that shows validity between the simulation educator's responses and expectations is said to have:

　A. Content validity—NO, this refers to the appropriateness of each item and comprehensiveness of the measurement.
　B. Construct validity—NO, this refers to the process of establishing that an action accurately represents the concept being evaluated.
　C. Face validity—NO, this asks whether the evaluation tool appears to be measuring the concept it is supposed to measure?
　D. Predictive validity—YES, this asks whether there is a correlation between the responses and an expectation.

90. Reflective debriefing techniques encourage the standardized patients (SPs) to understand the student's:

　A. Frame of reference—YES, this helps to understand why students make assumptions.
　B. Social determinants—NO, this is not part of the considerations but it does play into all the students do.
　C. Prior learning—NO, this is not part of the considerations but it does play into all the students do.
　D. Role and responsibilities—NO, this is not part of the considerations.

91. The effective application of the Simulation^{SM} Simulation Operations standard will guarantee the following:

　A. Reduced engagement of the simulation team—NO, this is not a component.
　B. Variability in student performance in the simulation lab—NO, this is not a component.

C. Successful advancement of the simulation program director—NO, this is not a component.
D. **Improve interprofessional collaboration—YES, it will help the team effort.**

92. An effective method of studying for the Certified Nurse Educator (CNE) examination is:

    A. Reviewing the Society for Simulation in Healthcare (SSH) website—NO, this is helpful but will not suffice for studying.
    B. Reading the handbook—NO, this is helpful but will not suffice for studying.
    C. **Establishing a peer study group—YES, evidence shows this as an effective study mechanism.**
    D. Asking others about test specifics—NO, this is not appropriate ethically.

93. During a scenario using a part-task trainer haptic body part and a computer to insert a central line, students ask why they need the leg and torso when they can see them on the computer. The simulation educator's best answer is:

    A. "It is to get you to visualize the anatomy in three dimensions (3-D)."—NO, this is not the main purpose for using a haptic body part.
    B. "So students understand where to place the line."—NO, this is not the main purpose for using a haptic body part.
    C. **"To get the real feel of the puncture site."—YES, it familiarizes the students with how it may feel to touch patients.**
    D. "To further demonstrate the technique."—NO, this is not the main purpose for using a haptic body part.

94. Standardized patient instructions should include:

    A. Being flexible and telling the student what they feel—NO, this is usually not the intention.
    B. Sharing personal experiences—NO, this does not meet the objectives.
    C. **Answers to questions that may be asked—YES, it is important to anticipate answers that keep the student learning outcomes on track.**
    D. Going off script at will—NO, this does not meet the objectives.

95. Using moulage is appropriate for:

    A. Promoting simulation as a learning experiences—NO, it is not necessarily needed as a marketing tool.
    B. Meeting objectives—NO, but if it assists in helping students meet the learning objectives it should be used.
    C. **Increasing realism—YES, it should increase realism.**
    D. Decreasing student anxiety—NO, it is not specific to anxiety.

96. Closed-loop communication includes:

    A. Eye contact—NO, although this is encouraged when able.
    B. Team members of different disciplines—NO, same-discipline professionals can engage in closed-loop communication.
    C. Technology—NO, technology may not be necessary.
    D. **Repeating what was said—YES, making sure the message received was intended.**

97. The "B" in situation, background, assessment, and recommendation (SBAR) communication reminds one to remember:

    A. The assessment findings—NO, this is the "A."
    B. The patient's medications—NO, this is part of the background usually.
    C. The blood test results—NO, this is usually part of the background.
    D. The patient's healthcare history—YES, this is all inclusive of what is needed from the past health history of the patient.

98. During standardized patient case development by a novice simulation educator, the mentor realizes more understanding is needed when the educator prioritizes the:

    A. Setting—NO, this is important.
    B. Standardized patient role—NO, this is important.
    C. Student role—YES, this is not usually predicted beforehand if the scenario is built for the students' learning.
    D. Timing—NO, this is important.

99. When simulation evaluation checklists are subjective, it is helpful to use:

    A. Two evaluators—NO, this is not necessary if the tool has validity.
    B. Descriptions—YES, this is helpful if it is subjective.
    C. The student's input—NO, this is part of a self-evaluation.
    D. The standardized patient's input—NO, this may or may not be used.

100. The "S" in situation, background, assessment, and recommendation (SBAR) communication should be succinctly used for:

    A. Introduction—NO, this should be done initially so the receiver knows who is speaking.
    B. Healthcare history—YES, this is why there is communication.
    C. Prescription recommendation—NO, this is part of it but is not the whole situation.
    D. Symptoms—NO, this is part of it but is not the whole situation.

Index

abstract conceptualization (AC), 168
AC. *See* abstract conceptualization
accommodative learners, 39
accreditation, 323–325. *See also* standards of simulation programs
    Society for Simulation in Healthcare (SSH) accredits simulation programs, 325
ACLS. *See* Advanced Cardiac Life Support
active elements, 172
active experimentation (AE), 168
adult learners, 84, 152, 170–171, 238
adult learning, 84–85
Advanced Cardiac Life Support (ACLS), 283
advanced certification, 5
advocacy–inquiry debriefing, 231
advocating for simulation, 31–32
AE. *See* active experimentation
affective learning, 283
Agency for Healthcare Research and Quality (AHRQ), 68, 81, 259–260
AHRQ. *See* Agency for Healthcare Research and Quality
American Heart Association Basic Life Support (BLS), 283
analytical learners, 39
andragogy, 170–171
annual report, 305
application processing, 4
Approaches and Study Skills Inventory for Students (ASSIST), 182
ARCS model, 183
as-if concept, 173
ASPE. *See* Association of Standardized Patient Educators
assertive educator, 42
assimilation, 228
ASSIST. *See* Approaches and Study Skills Inventory for Students
Association of Standardized Patient Educators (ASPE), 4, 287
aural or auditory (a) learners, 37
avatar, 148–149, 150, 154–157

baby boomer generation, 40
Basic Principles of Curriculum and Instruction, 167

behaviorism, 167
belongingness, 48
block scheduling, 300–301
Bloom's taxonomy, 185–186
BLS. *See* American Heart Association Basic Life Support
box-type simulation trainers, 141
Brophy model, 183
budget, 306–308
business plan, 306

caffeine, 18
California Critical Thinking Disposition Inventory, 179
capital equipment, 307, 308
cardiopulmonary resuscitation, 10
case study analysis debriefing, 230
CE. *See* concrete experience
certification
    advanced, 5
    initial, 4
    recertification/renewal, 5
    simulation, use of, 3
Certified Healthcare Simulation Educators™ (CHSEs™), 105, 267–270, 280, 324
checklists, 15
Choo's positive characteristics for educators, 44
CHSEs™. *See* Certified Healthcare Simulation Educators™
cleansing wipes, 101
cleanup and resetting, 100–101
Clinical Simulation Evaluation Tool (CSET), 282
closed-loop communication, 83
CLSST. *See* Cooperative Learning with Simulation-based Skills Training
code of conduct and confidential guidelines, 68–69
cognitive development process, 152
cognitive scaffolding, 169
collaboration educator, 43
collaborative agenda, 246
communities of interest, 313
computer-based simulations, 129–130
computer-based testing, 17
computer-based testing sites, 4

concrete experience (CE), 168
confederates, 121, 128
Confidential Structured Report of Performance (CSRP) online, 4
constructed reality, 126
constructive feedback, 242
constructive simulation, 127
constructivism, 167
Cooperative Learning with Simulation-based Skills Training (CLSST), 259
Core Competencies for Interprofessional Collaborative Practice, 56
counseling of an employee/learner, 317
crisis resource management (CRM), 82
critical reflection, 70, 80
critical thinking, 177–179
CRM. *See* crisis resource management
crucial conversations, 270
CSET. *See* Clinical Simulation Evaluation Tool
CSRP online. *See* Confidential Structured Report of Performance online
cultural humility, 45
culturally diverse learners, 45–46

DASH©. *See* Debriefing Assessment for Simulation in Healthcare©
debriefing, 133, 184, 284–285, 327
  advocacy–inquiry, 231
  as an assessment process, 229
  background, 224
  case study analysis, 230
  defining attributes of, 226–228
  difficulties, 233
  environment, 232–233
  facilitator role in, 229
  foundations, 238
  learning process and, 225
  for meaningful learning, 231
  method of, 231
  models, 243–246
  oral (Socratic) questioning, 228
  Plus-Delta, 232
  process, 84, 224–225
  research, 285–286
  selection of SPs for, 240–242
  simulation educator, 3–5, 8–9, 27–32, 45, 84, 126, 130, 134, 143, 166, 225, 227–228, 231–233, 281, 288, 289, 324, 325, 327, 329
  SPs competencies, 238–240
  starting, 246
  steps to ensure quality, 248
  structured, 230
  techniques, 232
  3-D model of, 231

Debriefing Assessment for Simulation in Healthcare© (DASH©), 261
Debriefing with Good Judgment, 231, 284
decision/interpretation, 186
deep learning, 181
delegator, 42
deliberate practice (DP), 80, 171, 174, 201
demonstrator, 42
DeYoung's motivational tips, 183
diversity
  attributes, 36
  culturally diverse learners, 45–46
  effect on simulation scenarios, 46–47
  in learning styles, 36–40
  in teaching styles of healthcare educators, 41–45
dossier, 273
DP. *See* deliberate practice

EBSP. *See* evidence-based simulation practice
educational philosophies and theories, 166–167. *See also* interprofessional education (IPE)
Educational Practices in Simulation Scale (EPSS), 261
educational principles, 9
educational strategy, 281
EES. *See* Employee Education System
effective simulation, 198
eligibility for certification
  advanced, 5
  initial, 4
ELT. *See* experimental learning theory
emergency medical technicians (EMTs), 309
emotions, 227
empirical knowledge, 181
Employee Education System (EES), 287
EMTs. *See* emergency medical technicians
English as a second language (ESL) learner, 46
environment management, 188–189. *See also* physical space
environmental fidelity, 173
EPSS. *See* Educational Practices in Simulation Scale
equipment fidelity, 173
equipment/technology, understanding, 16–17
escape plan, 30
ESL learner. *See* English as a second language learner
esthetic knowledge, 181
ethical knowledge, 181
ethical standards and principles in, healthcare simulation education
  history, 68
  professional development through simulation, 70–71
  safe learning environment, 68–70

evaluation of simulation activities, 251–261, 282–283
  behavior measures, 283
  formative evaluation, 69, 257–258
  individual learner, 253–255
  instruments for, 260
  Kirkpatrick's levels of evaluation, 256, 257, 282–283
  Miller's pyramid model, 256–257
  peer evaluation, 259
  self-evaluation, 258–259
  in simulation-based team training (SBTT), 251–252, 259–260
  in simulation-based training (SBT), 252–253, 259–260
  simulation-based training (SBT) learner evaluation, 256
  summative evaluation, 69, 258
  Translational Science Research (TSR) phases, 256
events, scheduling of, 298
evidence, use of in healthcare simulation, 269–270
evidence-based healthcare simulation, 269–270
evidence-based simulation practice (EBSP), 180, 241, 269–270
examination
  preparing for success in, 14–16
  qualification requirements, 14
  strategies for answering questions, 18–21
  test areas covered in, 13–22
  test plan for, 7
experiential learning, 83–84, 199, 223
experimental learning theory (ELT), 168–169
expert, 42, 270–271
extrapolation, 186
extrinsic needs, 182

facilitative educator, 43
facilitator, 42
faculty development, resources for, 30–31
faculty mentorship, 29–30
faculty training, 28
FAME, 180
feasibility, 204
fees for certification, 4
fiction contract, 173, 280
fidelity, 140, 173
first come, first served scheduling, 301
fishbowl method, 233
food for improving brain power and energy, 15
formal authority, 42
formative evaluation, 69, 257–258. *See also* evaluation of simulation activities

frames, 48, 180–181
functional fidelity, 86

Gagne's condition of learning, 187
generalization, 186
Generation X, 40
Generation Y, 40
generational learners, 40
global learners, 38
Goffman's theory of frame analysis, 180–181
Grasha's teaching styles, 42

haptic technology, 141
HCAT. *See* Health Assessment Communication Assessment Tool
Health Assessment Communication Assessment Tool (HCAT), 284
Health Insurance Portability and Accountability Act of 1996 (HIPAA), 68
healthcare faculty, 199
healthcare professionals, 15, 20, 55, 56, 63, 79–81, 84, 105, 149, 166, 173, 181, 186, 188, 251, 269, 271, 280
healthcare simulation, 85, 87
Hertzberg's motivation-hygiene theory, 316
Hicks and Burkus attributes of "master teachers," 44
high-fidelity simulation, 85–87
high-fidelity simulators, 134
HIPAA. *See* Health Insurance Portability and Accountability Act of 1996
hospital-based simulation, 284
House, Chassie, and Spohn's teaching behaviors, 43
HPS. *See* human patient simulator
human factors, 204–205
human patient simulator (HPS), 16, 121
hybrid simulation methodology, 17
  foundations, 126–127
  issues of, 133–134
  scenario development, 131
  stakeholder education, 130–131
  standardized participant training, 131–133
  typology and modes, 127–130

INACSL. *See* International Nursing Association for Clinical Simulation & Learning
INACSL Standards of Best Practice: Simulation^{SM}, 253
integrated practice model, 58
integration, 227
interactive elements, 172
interactivity, 185

internal review board (IRB) training, 316
internalizing, 175
International Nursing Association for Clinical Simulation & Learning (INACSL), 4, 69, 253, 280, 284, 287, 323, 326–328
interprofessional collaborative practice, 56
    core competencies, 58
interprofessional education (IPE), 204, 314
    background, 54–57
    general competencies, 57–62
    history of, 54
    IC (interprofessional communication) competencies, 60–61
    pearls and pitfalls implementing, 61
    RR (Roles and Responsibilities) competencies, 59–60
    TT (teams and teamwork) competencies, 61–62
    VE (values/ethics) competencies, 59
Interprofessional Education Collaborative (IPEC), 56–58, 188
interprofessionality, 57–58
intrinsic motivation, 182
intuitive learners, 38
IPE. See interprofessional education
IPEC. See Interprofessional Education Collaborative
ISBAR Communication, 83

Jung's theory of psychological types, 44
just-in-time education, 140

Kelly's teaching effectiveness, 43
kinesthetic (k) or active learners, 37
Kirkpatrick's levels of evaluation, 256, 257, 282–283
knowing, theories of, 181
Kolb's learning styles, 39

Laucken's theory of conceptualizing reality, 174
leadership styles and retention, 316
learner and learning disabilities, 47
learner evaluations, 69, 253
learner socialization, 184–185
learner-centered education, 204
learners' locus of control, 182
learning. See also virtual learning (VL)
    defined, 166
    domains, 175–176
    experiences, 282
learning continuum, 58
learning process, 84
learning style, 36–40
learning theories
    experimental learning theory (ELT), 168–169
    scaffolding learning theory, 169
    social learning theory, 170

lifesaver from outside the scenario, 318
lifesavers, 46, 47, 318
live simulation, 127
logbooks, 308
low-fidelity simulators, 134

makeup, 97–98
    remover, 101
mannequin-based simulations, 129
mannequin-patient simulation specialist, 130
mannequin-patient technician, 130
mastery experiences, 170
MBTI. See Myers-Briggs Type Indicator
medium fidelity, 134
mentorship programs, 270
metacognition, 179
Millennials, 40
Miller's pyramid model, 256–257
mindfulness, 179
mission statement, 306
mixed simulation, 17
mnemonics, 15
modulation frames, 48
modulations, 181
motivation factors, 316
motivational theories, 182–183
moulage, 93, 309
    basic moulage kit, 95–96
    basic supplies, 95
    cleanup and resetting, 100–101
    educational basis for use of, 94–95
    for HPS, 98–99
    makeup, 97–98
    preparing substances, 96
    special effect basics, 99–100
    for SPs, 96–97
mSTREET (modular Synthetic Training, Research, Evaluation and Extrapolation Tool), 157
MTV generation, 40
multimodal/mixture (m) learners, 37–38
Myers-Briggs Type Indicator (MBTI), 44

National Center for Interprofessional Education and Practice, 56
natural primary frames, 180
nexters, 40

Office of Nursing Services (ONS), 289
Office of Patient Care Services (PCS), 287, 289
ONS. See Office of Nursing Services
operations management, 298
    business plan, 306
    personnel and nonpersonnel issues, 315–319
    physical space, 308–310

policies, 310
   preparing for event, 301–303
   scheduling, 298–301
   tracking center activities, 303–308
organizing, 175
"outside" the scenario or simulation, 47

participants, 281
participants, standardized. *See* standardized participants; standardized (simulated) patients (SPs)
part-task trainers (PTTs), 128, 139–140
   advantages of, 142–143
   box-type simulation trainers, 141
   complex, 141
   curriculum development using, 141–142
   definition, 140–141
passive elements, 172
patient safety, 165, 205
patient-controlled anesthesia (PCA) pump, 310
PBL. *See* problem-based learning
PCS. *See* Office of Patient Care Services
PEARLS. *See* Promoting Excellence and Reflective Learning in Simulation
pedagogy, 170–171
peer evaluation, 259
perfect practice, 85
personal knowledge, 181
Peter Winter Institute for Simulation, 309
phenomenal mode of thinking, 176–177
physical fidelity, 86–87, 134, 173
physical mode of thinking, 176
physical space, 308–310
   modifying the physical environment, 309–310
   organizing, 308
physiological states, 170
planning simulation activities
   designing, 216
   evaluation methods, 215
   evaluation tools, 216
   evaluation, types of, 215
   goal definition, 214
   learning objectives, 214–215
   needs assessment, 210
   preparations, 218–219
   resource identification, 217
   selecting modality, 216–217
   simulation team, 217–218
Plus-Delta debriefing, 232
policies and procedure manuals, 308
portfolio, 273
positive change process, 270
positive feedback, 242
prebriefing, 280–281
prescenario checklist, 304–305

primary frames, 48, 180
problem-based learning (PBL), 188
professional development
   expertise, 270–271
   mentoring, 271–273
   staying current, 268–269
   through simulation, 70–71, 268
professional portfolio/dossier, 273
professional role, 272
professional values and capabilities (test area), 8–9
Promoting Excellence and Reflective Learning in Simulation (PEARLS), 231
psychological fidelity, 87, 134, 173
psychological safety, 245
psychometrician, 130
psychomotor domain, 283

Quirk's teaching styles, 42–43

randomized control trials, 284
reactions to simulation, 282
reading (R) or writing learners, 37
realism, 35, 173–175, 204
reality shock, 184
reception, 227
recertification standards, 21
recertification/renewal of certification, 5
reference materials, 308
reflection, 188, 226–227
reflective learners, 39
reflective observation (RO), 168
reliability, 204, 260
research
   debriefing, 284–285
   frameworks, 286
   prebriefing, 280–281
   resources, 287–289
   simulation, 281–284
resource identification, 217
resources for faculty development, 30–31
responding stage in learning development, 175
RO. *See* reflective observation
role-play options, 243

safe learning environment, 68–70
SBAR communication, 83
SBAR mnemonic, 15
SBE. *See* simulation-based education
SBL. *See* simulation-based learning
SBLES. *See* Simulation-Based Learning Evaluation Scale
SBTT. *See* simulation-based team training
scaffolding learning theory, 169
scenario development, 131

scenario lifesavers, 318
scheduler, 300
scheduling, 298–301
    block, 300–301
    calendar, 299
    first come, first served, 301
    methods to track, 298–299
scoring, 186
SDL. *See* self-directed learning
SDS. *See* Simulation Design Scale
Second Life, 31
self-directed learning (SDL), 188
self-efficacy, 170, 270–271
self-evaluation, 258–259
semantical mode of thinking, 176
serious games, 149–150
serious gaming, 184–185
SimLEARN, 287
simulation, 8–9, 197
    advocating for, 31–32
    debriefing, 327
    facilitation methods, 327
    faculty mentorship, 29–30
    faculty training, 28
    high-fidelity, 85–87
    knowledge acquisition, 28
    learning as a social practice, 48
    methodology, 83–85
    outcomes and objectives, 327
    participant evaluation, 327–328
    practicing in a, benefits, 13–14
    professional integrity, 328
    realism in, 35, 173–175, 204
    research, 281–284
    resources for faculty development, 30–31
    Sim-IPE, 328
    simulation design, 326–327
    simulation glossary, 328
    simulation operations, 328
    socialization during, 48–49
simulation activities. *See also* moulage; planning simulation activities
    designing, 216
    evaluation of, 251–261
simulation centers
    human resource policies and procedures, 311
    managers and administrators, 314–315
    organizational documents for, 310–311
    personnel and human capital, 312–313
    personnel and nonpersonnel issues, 315–319
    physical security, 312
    physical space, 308–310
    policies, procedure, and practices, 310–314
    stakeholders and communities of interest, 313–314
    tracking center activities, 303–308
    users of, 314–315
    using in situ simulation, 312
Simulation Design Scale (SDS), 260
simulation education, ethical standards and principles in, healthcare, 3
simulation educator, 3, 5, 9, 27–31, 45, 69–71, 80, 84, 85, 126, 130, 134, 143, 166, 182, 190, 225, 227–228, 231–233, 289, 324, 325, 329
simulation environments
    interprofessional learning, 188–189
    self-directed learning (SDL), 188
simulation event
    delivery of a, 301–303
    timeline, 303
simulation learning frameworks
    Doerr and Murray, 172
    Kirkpatrick, 172
    Kneebone, 171
    Meller, 172
simulation organizations for healthcare educators, 288
simulation scenarios, 308
simulation team, 217–218
simulation-based education (SBE), 280, 328
simulation-based evaluation, 186. *See also* evaluation of simulation activities
simulation-based experience, 69, 253
simulation-based healthcare education and evaluation
    curriculum development, 198–201
    deliberate practice (DP), 201
    integrating simulation, 202–203
    learning domains, 201–202
    simulation concepts, 203–205
simulation-based learning (SBL), 80
Simulation-Based Learning Evaluation Scale (SBLES), 187
simulation-based team training (SBTT), 251–252, 259–260
simulation-based training (SBT), 251–252, 259–260
simulation-based training (SBT) learner evaluation, 253
simulation-enhanced interprofessional education, 287
simulator, 140
simulator briefing, 184
situational awareness, 85
skill equipment checklists, 308
SLOs. *See* student learning outcomes
social aspects, 184
social cognitive theory (SCT) of behavior, 270
social practice, 184
social primary frames, 180
socialization during simulation, 48–49

Society for Simulation in Healthcare (SSH), 3, 287, 325
SP Program Information Sheet, 241
special effect basics, 99–100
SPs. *See* standardized (simulated) patients
SSH. *See* Society for Simulation in Healthcare
stakeholder education, 130–131
stakeholders, 313–314
standardized participants, 128–129. *See also* standardized (simulated) patients (SPs)
   debriefing and feedback activities
      preparing for, 242–243
      selection for, 240–242
   debriefing competencies, 238–240
   information meeting, 241–242
   training, 131–133
standardized (simulated) patients (SPs), 16, 17, 70, 96–97, 105, 128, 173
   case development, 106
   case template, 116–119
   as confederates, 121
   core competencies, 238–240
   debriefing competencies, 238
   door sign, 109
   educator, 130
   evaluation checklist, 110
   feedback, 116–119
   flexibility, 106
   focus and objectives, 108–109
   identifying the setting, 107
   orientation, education, and training of, 119–120
   position and attire, 107–108
   questions and answers, 109
   role in learner evaluation and feedback, 120–121
   role of, 107
   sample cases, 111–116
   selecting, 240
   simulation cases, 111–116
   student checklist, 115–116
   student evaluation criteria and passing score, 111
   student participant, 108
   timing of simulation scenario, 106–107
   training, 131–133
standards of simulation programs, 325–326. *See also* accreditation; ethical standards and principles in, healthcare simulation education
   debriefing process, 327
   facilitation methods, 327
   outcomes and objectives, 327
   participant evaluation, 327–328
   professional integrity of participant, 328
   Sim-IPE, 328
   simulation design, 326–327

   simulation facilitation, 327
   simulation glossary, 328
   simulation operations, 328
   terminology, 328
Story and Butt's teaching delivery, 44
strategic learning, 181–182
strategic plan, 306
structured debriefing, 230
student learning outcomes (SLOs), 8, 168
suggestive educator, 42
summative evaluations, 69, 258. *See also* evaluation of simulation activities
surface learning, 182. *See also* learning
suspending disbelief, 173–174

tactile learners, 38
task fidelity, 86
task trainers, 16
Taxonomy of Educational Objectives, 185
teaching simulation, 185
Teaching Style Inventory (TSI), 44
Team Performance Observation Tool (TPOT), 187, 260
Team Strategies and Tools to Enhance Performance and Patient Safety, 81
team training, 80–82
Team-Based Competencies: Building a Shared Foundation for Education and Clinical Practice, 56
team-based learning, 174–175
team-learning principals, 81
TeamSTEPPS, 81, 259
teamwork, 204
termination of an employee, 317
test anxiety, strategies to ease, 17–18
test areas covered in examination
   educating and assessing learners, 8–9
   knowledge of simulation principles, 9
   professional values and capabilities, 8–9
   simulation resources, 9
test plan for examination, 7
thinking, modes of, 176–177
3-D computer-based simulated healthcare environment, 148–151
3-D model of debriefing, 231
TPOT. *See* Team Performance Observation Tool
track scheduling, 298–299. *See also* scheduling
tracking center activities, 303–308
transactional leadership, 8
transformational leadership, 8
Translational Science Research (TSR) phases, 256
troubleshooting, 319

unexpected events, 318
unknowing, 181
user manuals, 308

validity, 204, 260
values statement, 306
valuing, 175
VARK learning style, 36–37
VEM. *See* Vroom's expectancy model
verbal (linguistic) learners, 38
verbal persuasion, 170
Veterans Health Administration (VHA), 287, 289
VHA. *See* Veterans Health Administration
vicarious experiences, 170
virtual learning (VL), 148–149. *See also* learning
  advantages and disadvantages, 152–154
  websites, 156–157
virtual patients (VPs), 149
virtual reality (VR)
  theoretical frameworks, 151–152
  virtual learning, 148–151
virtual reality simulation (VRS), 16, 148
  entering and designing, 154–155
virtual simulation, 127

virtual worlds (VWs), 147–150
vision statement, 306
visual (v) or spatial learners, 36–37
VL. *See* virtual learning
VL platforms, 150–151
Voki platform, 151
VPs. *See* virtual patients
VR. *See* virtual reality
Vroom's expectancy model (VEM), 183
VRS. *See* virtual reality simulation
VWs. *See* virtual worlds
Vygotsky's activity theory, 152

Watson–Glaser Critical Thinking Appraisal (WGCTA), 179
WGCTA. *See* Watson–Glaser Critical Thinking Appraisal
what ifs, 30
"within" the scenario or simulation, 47